D1566823

PHARMACEUTICAL AND CLINICAL CALCULATIONS

HOW TO ORDER THIS BOOK

BY PHONE: 800-233-9936 or 717-291-5609, 8AM–5PM Eastern Time

BY FAX: 717-295-4538

BY MAIL: Order Department
Technomic Publishing Company, Inc.
851 New Holland Avenue, Box 3535
Lancaster, PA 17604, U.S.A.

BY CREDIT CARD: American Express, VISA, MasterCard

BY WWW SITE: http://www.techpub.com

PERMISSION TO PHOTOCOPY—POLICY STATEMENT

PHARMACEUTICAL AND CLINICAL CALCULATIONS

2nd EDITION

Mansoor A. Khan, Ph.D.
Indra K. Reddy, Ph.D.

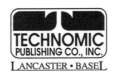

TECHNOMIC
PUBLISHING CO., INC.
LANCASTER • BASEL

Pharmaceutical and Clinical Calculations
aTECHNOMIC®publication

Technomic Publishing Company, Inc.
851 New Holland Avenue, Box 3535
Lancaster, Pennsylvania 17604 U.S.A.

Printed in the United States of America
10   9   8   7   6   5   4   3   2   1

Main entry under title:
  Pharmaceutical and Clinical Calculations, Second Edition

A Technomic Publishing Company book
Bibliography: p.
Includes index p. 393

Library of Congress Catalog Card No. 99-69344
ISBN No. 1-56676-812-8

Pharmacists for the 21st Century must be patient-focused clinical practitioners. While the pharmacist's primary duty has always been to ensure that
his/her patients receive accurately prepared, highest quality therapeutic agents,
today's pharmacist must also be knowledgeable and skilled at calculating
individualized doses of the various medications by considering the unique
clinical characteristics of his/her patients. The goal is to ensure that all patients
receive the highest quality pharmaceutical care possible by minimizing potential medication related problems. When all the elements of patient care are
considered, our patients will receive optimal outcomes from their drug therapy.
This is the critical duty of today's pharmacist.

A basic premise of delivering quality pharmaceutical care is ensuring that
the pharmaceutical products that the pharmacist prepares and dispenses to his/
her patients contain the correct dose of the medication. Thus, the first steps
toward patient-centered pharmaceutical care are learning how to accurately
interpret a prescription or medication order, calculate the appropriate amounts
of ingredients and precisely weigh and measure ingredients. Following closely
is learning how to accurately calculate and measure the appropriate dose of
medication that meets the patient's unique clinical needs.

In *Pharmaceutical and Clinical Calculations,* second edition, Drs. Mansoor
Khan and Indra Reddy have provided a contemporary resource that can help
pharmacy students learn the basic principles of how to accurately interpret
prescriptions and medication orders, measure, calculate and compound quality
dosage forms. In the latter chapters, the student can learn multiple methods
to accurately and safely dose patients. The computational methods to accom-
plish these ends are clearly presented, and the examples used to demonstrate
the concepts are relevant to contemporary practice. Pharmacy students will

be presented with these very same problems in live patients during clinical rotations. This book can also be a reference source for practitioners who need to "refresh" basic concepts in measurements and calculations to ensure safe and effective drug therapy for their patients. The concepts and methods presented serve as foundational knowledge and skills for all patient-centered pharmacists as they seek to serve their patients with the highest level of care.

ARTHUR A. NELSON, JR., R.PH., PH.D.
Dean and Professor
School of Pharmacy
Texas Tech University Health Sciences Center
Amarillo, Texas

Pharmaceutical and clinical calculations are critical to the delivery of safe, effective, and competent patient care and professional practice. The current shift in pharmacy education from product-oriented practices to patient-oriented practices makes the calculations even more challenging. Many students in pharmacy and health science programs and beginning practitioners in the related areas struggle to master these essential skills. Although many books are available on theoretical and applied concepts of calculations involving medication dosages, only a few reflect the emphasis on pharmaceutical care and the contemporary pharmacy practice.

The present text is designed for Pharm. D. or undergraduate students in baccalaureate curriculum in pharmacy, contemporary pharmacy practice professionals, and other health care professionals. It provides calculations involving various dosage forms in a well-organized and easy to comprehend manner.

The book contains fifteen chapters. Chapter 1 presents a review of prerequisite mathematics, which includes Roman numerals, fractions and decimals, ratios and proportions, dilution and concentration expressions, and density and specific gravity. Chapter 2 deals with systems of measurement. The metric system is emphasized since it is federally mandated. Though the apothecary system of measurement is fast declining, a few prescriptions still appear with these units in professional practice. An explanation of various systems of measurement and the interconversions are provided in this chapter. Chapter 3, ''Prescription and Medication Orders,'' not only provides a thorough explanation of types and components of prescriptions, but also lists abbreviations, most commonly prescribed drugs with their brand and generic names, directions for use, and errors and omissions in prescriptions. In Chapter 4, principles of weighing and measuring including the *aliquot* method for solids, as well as liquids, are discussed.

Chapters 5 through 7 deal with essential calculations involving different dosage forms including oral liquid, solid, and semisolid dosage forms. Chapter 5 embodies calculations pertaining to syrups, elixirs, and suspensions. The calculations involving percentage strength, dilution and concentration, and milliequivalents and milliosmoles are included in this chapter. Extemporaneous filling of powders in capsules and calculations involving trituration, levigation, and geometric mixing are provided in Chapter 6. Calculations involving semisolid dosage forms including *alligation alternate* and *alligation medial* are presented in Chapter 7.

A variety of dosage forms are applied topically to the eye, nose, and ear. Chapter 8 provides calculations involving isotonicity, pH, and buffering of topical dosage forms. Chapter 9 deals with calculations involving suppositories. Chapter 10 features calculations associated with parenteral medications, which include rate of flow of intravenous fluids, insulin and heparin administration, and reconstitution of powdered medications. Calculations involving calories, nitrogen, protein-calorie percentage, parenteral hyperalimentation, and resting energy expenditure assessments are presented in Chapter 11.

The clinical calculations are included in the book to provide necessary background for the clinical pharmacy practice. Knowledge of clinical pharmacokinetics is essential in providing an optimum drug concentration at the receptor site to obtain the desired therapeutic response and to minimize the drug's adverse or toxic effects. For an optimal therapeutic response, the clinical pharmacist must select a suitable drug and determine an appropriate dose with the available strengths and a convenient dosing interval. To perform this task, serum or plasma drug concentrations have to be analyzed, the pharmacokinetic parameters have to be evaluated, the drug dose has to be adjusted, and the dosing interval needs to be determined. Chapter 12 deals with the determination of pharmacokinetic parameters, loading and maintenance doses, and tailoring of doses for patients with renal damage. Chapter 13 presents calculations involving doses and dose adjustments that are required in pediatric and geriatric patients. Emphasis is placed on the calculations involving the use of aminoglycosides and critical care. Calculations involving strengths of vaccines and toxoids are presented in Chapter 14. Chapter 15 deals with calculations involving radiopharmaceuticals including mean life, half-life, radioactive decay, and percentage activity. Key concepts are highlighted throughout the text for emphasis and easy retrieval. The examples presented throughout the text reflect the practice environment in community, hospital, and nuclear pharmacy settings. Answers to all the practice and review problems are provided at the end of the book. Although every effort was made to maintain the accuracy of doses and other product related information, the readers should not use this book as the only source of information for professional practice.

The authors would like to acknowledge Drs. Michael DeGennaro, Amir Shojaei, and Abdel-Azim Zaghloul for their helpful comments and suggestions on various chapters of the book, Dr. Steven Strauss and Ms. Susan Farmer of Technomic Publishing Company, Inc. for their excellent cooperation and coordination, and Mr. Fred Mills, R.Ph., for providing specific case studies and information on errors and omissions. The authors would like to acknowledge with thanks the faculty at several pharmacy schools for their active participation in the survey prior to undertaking the task of writing this book. The participation and input by these faculty not only made us realize the immediate need for this book, but also helped us organize it. Finally, the authors would like to thank their wives, Ms. Rehana Khan and Ms. Neelima Reddy for their inspiration, encouragement, and forbearance throughout this endeavor, which made work a pleasure.

Mansoor A. Khan
Indra K. Reddy

CHAPTER 1

Prerequisite Mathematics Review

NUMBERS AND NUMERALS

A number is a total quantity or amount, whereas a numeral is a word, sign, or group of words and signs representing a number.

ARABIC AND ROMAN NUMERALS

Arabic Numerals

Arabic numerals, such a 1, 2, 3, etc., are used universally to indicate quantities. These numerals, which are represented by a zero and nine digits, are easy to read and less likely to be confused.

Roman Numerals

Roman numerals are used with the apothecary's system of measurement to designate quantities on prescription. In the Roman system of counting, letters of the alphabet (both uppercase and lowercase) such as I or i, V or v, and X or x are used to designate numbers. A few commonly used Roman numerals and their Arabic equivalents are given in Table 1.1.

In the usage of Roman numerals, the following set of rules apply:

(1) When a Roman numeral is repeated, it doubles its value; when a Roman numeral is repeated three times, it triples its value.

1

TABLE 1.1.   Roman Numerals and
Their Arabic Equivalents.

Roman Numeral	Arabic Numeral
I (or i)	1
II (or ii)	2
III or (iii)	3
IV (or iv)	4
V (or v)	5
VI (or vi)	6
VII (or vii)	7
VIII (or viii)	8
IX (or ix)	9
X (or x)	10
XX (or xx)	20
XXX (or xxx)	30
L (or l)	50
C (or c)	100
D (or d)	500
M (or m)	1000

Examples:

I = 1, II = 2, III = 3

X = 10, XX = 20, XXX = 30

(2) When Roman numeral(s) of lesser value follows one of a greater value, they are added.

Examples:

VII = 5 + 1 + 1 = 7

XVI = 10 + 5 + 1 = 16

(3) When Roman numeral(s) of lesser value precedes one of a greater value, they are subtracted from the greater value numeral.

Examples:

IV = 5 − 1 = 4

IX = 10 − 1 = 9

(4) When Roman numeral of a lesser value is placed between two greater values, it is first subtracted from the greater numeral placed after it, and then that value is added to the other numeral(s) (i.e., subtraction rule applies first, then the addition rule).

Examples:

XXIX = 10 + 10 + (10 − 1) = 29

XIV = 10 + (5 − 1) = 14

(5) Roman numerals may not be repeated more than three times in succession.

Example: 4 is written as IV but not as IIII

(6) When possible, largest value numerals should be used.

Example: 15 is written as XV but not as VVV

Roman numerals are sometimes combined with the abbreviation for one half, ss. The abbreviation should always be at the end of a Roman numeral. Generally, Roman numerals are written in lowercase when used with ss, such as iss to indicate 1½.

FRACTIONS

A *fraction* is a portion of a whole number. Fractions contain two numbers: the bottom number (referred to as *denominator*) and the top number (referred to as *numerator*). The denominator in the fraction is the total number of parts into which the whole number is divided. The numerator in the fraction is the number of parts we have.

A *proper fraction* should always be less than 1, i.e., the numerator is smaller than the denominator.

Examples:

5/8, 7/8, 3/8

A proper fraction such as 3/8 may be read as "3 of 8 parts" or as "3 divided by 8."

An *improper fraction* has a numerator that is equal to or greater than the denominator. It is therefore equal to or greater than one.

Examples:

2/2 = 1, 5/4, 6/5

To reduce the improper fraction, divide the numerator by the denominator.

Examples:

8/8 = 8 ÷ 8 = 1

6/4 = 6 ÷ 4 = $1\frac{2}{4}$

9/4 = 9 ÷ 4 = $2\frac{1}{4}$

To reduce the fraction to its *lowest terms* (which may be referred to as "simplifying the fraction"), find the largest number (referred to as *greatest common divisor*) that will divide evenly into each term.

Examples:

15/20 = 15 ÷ 5/20 ÷ 5 = 3/4

12/18 = 12 ÷ 6/18 ÷ 6 = 2/3

7/21 = 7 ÷ 7/21 ÷ 7 = 1/3

Addition of Fractions

To add fractions, the following steps may be used:

(1) Find a *least common denominator* or the smallest number that divides all the denominators evenly.
(2) Change each fraction so that it has that denominator but retains its original value.
(3) Add the numerators.
(4) Reduce the resulting fraction to its lowest terms.

Example:

4/6 + 2.4/4 + 2/5

By changing each fraction such that it has the same denominator without changing the value of the fraction, we get:

40/60 + 36/60 + 24/60

= 100/60

= $1\frac{40}{60}$ or $1\frac{2}{3}$

Some numbers are expressed as *mixed numbers* (a whole number and a fraction). To change mixed numbers to improper fractions, multiply the whole number by the denominator of the fraction and then add the numerator.

Examples:

$10\frac{5}{8}$ = 85/8

$3\frac{5}{6}$ = 23/6

Subtraction of Fractions

To subtract fractions, the following steps may be used:

(1) Find a *least common denominator* or the smallest number that is divided by all the denominators evenly.
(2) Change each fraction so that it has that denominator but retains its original value.
(3) Subtract the numerators.
(4) Reduce the resulting fraction to its lowest terms.

Example:

5/6 − 4/5

= 25/30 − 24/30

= 1/30

If one of the numbers is a mixed number, change it to an improper fraction and then subtract.

Example:

$4\frac{1}{4} - 4/5$

$= 17/4 - 4/5$

$= 85/20 - 16/20$

$= 69/20$ or $3\frac{9}{20}$

Multiplication of Fractions

To multiply fractions, following steps may be used:

(1) Fractions are multiplied by multiplying the two numerators to obtain the numerator of the answer and then multiplying the two denominators to obtain the denominator of the answer.

Example:

$3/5 \times 1/2 = 3/10$

(2) Reduce your answer to lowest terms, when possible.
(3) When possible, divide the numerator of any of the fractions and the denominator of any of the fractions by the same number. Then multiply the denominators and reduce the fraction to its lowest terms.

Example:

$2/3 \times 7/8$

$= 1/3 \times 7/4$

$= 7/12$

(4) To multiply a fraction with a whole number, assume the denominator of the whole number to be 1. Then multiply the numerator and denominator in the same way as explained above in step 1.

Example:

$4 \times 5/6$

$= 20/6 = 10/3$ or $3\frac{1}{3}$

(5) When there are mixed numbers in the problem, change them to improper fractions and then multiply.

Example:

$2\frac{1}{3} \times 3\frac{1}{4}$

$= 7/3 \times 13/4$

$= 91/12$

$= 7\frac{7}{12}$

In the division of fractions, the following terms are used:

Dividend = The number to be divided
Divisor = The number by which the dividend is divided
Quotient = The number obtained by dividing the dividend with the divisor, i.e., *dividend ÷ divisor = quotient;* this expression may be read as "dividend is divided by divisor to obtain the quotient"

Division of Fractions

To divide a whole number or a fraction by a proper or improper fraction, invert the divisor and multiply.

Example:

$4/5 \div 2/3$

$= 4/5 \times 3/2$

$= 6/5$ or $1\frac{1}{5}$

Note: Whole numbers are assumed to have a denominator of 1.
When there is a mixed number in the problem, first change it to an improper function, then invert the divisor, and multiply.

Example:

$4\frac{6}{9} \div 6/8$

$= 42/9 \div 6/8$

$= 42/9 \times 8/6$

$= 7/9 \times 8/1$

$= 56/9$ or $6\frac{2}{9}$

DECIMALS

Decimals are another means of expressing a fractional amount. A decimal is a fraction whose denominator is 10 or a multiple of 10.

Example:

$0.8 = 8/10$

$0.08 = 8/100$

$0.008 = 8/1000$

A *decimal mixed number* is a whole number and a decimal fraction.

Example:

$4.3 = 4\frac{3}{10}$

Each position to the left of the decimal is ten times the previous place and each position to the right is one-tenth the previous place. The position to the left or right of the decimal point is referred to as *place value*, which determines the size of the denominator. Figure 1.1 indicates the *place value* of the numerals to the left and right of the decimal point.

Adding zeros to a decimal without changing the place value of the numerals does not affect the value of the number. However, adding or subtracting zeros between the decimal point and the numeral does change the value of the number.

Example:

0.4, 0.40, or 0.400; all these represent four-tenths

But, 0.4 = four-tenths

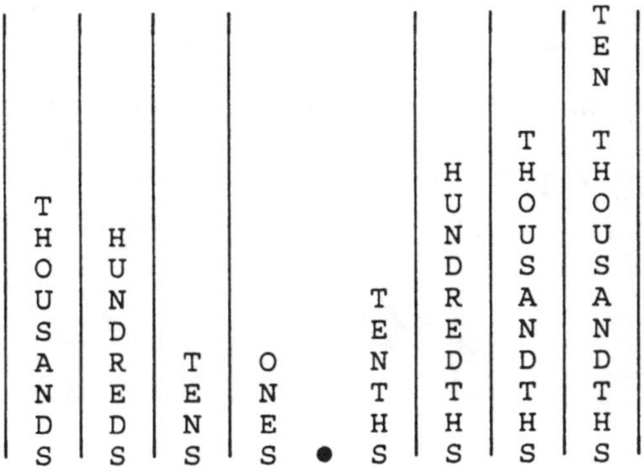

```
                                            T
                                            E
                                            N
                              T     T
                        H     H     H
    T                   U     O     O
    H     H             N     U     U
    O     U             D     S     S
    U     N       T     R     A     A
    S     D       E     E     N     N
    A     R   T   N     D     D     D
    N     E   E   T     T     T     T
    D     D   N   H     H     H     H
    S     S   S   S  •  S     S     S
```

FIGURE 1.1. Place values of numerals.

0.04 = four-hundredths

0.004 = four-thousandths

Addition and Subtraction

To add or subtract decimals, line up the numbers so that all numbers with the same place value are in the same column, and then add or subtract.

Examples:

Addition:
```
 16.24
  8.12
 12.62
 36.98
```

Subtraction:
```
 43.78
− 8.43
 35.35
```

Multiplication

To multiply decimals, multiply the numerals as usual and move the decimal point in the answer to the left as many places as there are in the sum of the decimal places in the two numbers being multiplied.

Example:

8.23 × 6.76 (sum of the decimal places in the two numbers is 4)

823 × 676 = 556348

55.6348

Division

To divide decimals, following steps may be used:

(1) Change the divisor to a whole number by moving the decimal point to the right.
(2) Move the decimal point in the dividend to the right the same number of places.
(3) Divide.
(4) Place the decimal point in the quotient above the decimal in the dividend.

Example:

Divide 26 by 2.006

Change the divisor and dividend to whole numbers by moving the decimal point to the right:

Dividend = 26000
Divisor = 2006
Divide

```
                 12.961
2006. ) 26000.000
           2006
           5940
           4012
           1928 0
           1805 4
            122 60
            120 36
              2 240
              2 006
                234
```

Practice Problems

(1) Write the following in Roman numerals:

   a. 28
   b. 15
   c. 17
   d. 23

(2) Convert the following Roman numerals to Arabic numerals:

   a. xlvi
   b. lxxiv
   c. xlvii
   d. xxxix

(3) Perform the following operations and indicate your answer in Arabic numbers:

   a. XII + VII
   b. XXVI − XII
   c. XXIV ÷ VI
   d. XIX × IX

(4) Perform the following operations and indicate your answer in Roman numbers:

   a. 18 + 13
   b. 48 ÷ 6
   c. 625 ÷ 25
   d. 17 + 15 + 23 − 6

(5) Interpret the *quantity* in each of the following:

   a. Caps. no. lxiv
   b. Tabs no. xlvii
   c. Pil. no. xlv
   d. Caps. no. xvi

(6) A bottle of Children's Tylenol® contains 30 teaspoonfuls of liquid. If each dose is ½ teaspoonful, how many doses are available in this bottle?

(7) A prescription contains 3/5 gr of ingredient A, 2/4 gr of ingredient B, 6/20 gr of ingredient C, and 4/15 gr of ingredient D. Calculate the total weight of the four ingredients in the prescription?

(8) A patient needs to take ½ tablet of Medication A and 1½ tablets of Medication B, both three times a day for 7 days. How many tablets does the patient receive over seven days for each of the medication?

(9) A pharmacist had 10 g of codeine sulfate. If he used it in preparing 5 capsules each containing 0.025 g, 10 capsules each containing 0.010 g, and 12 capsules each containing 0.015 g, how many g of codeine sulfate were left after he prepared all the capsules?

(10) A tablet contains 1/20 gr of ingredient A, 1/4 gr of ingredient B, 1/12 gr of ingredient C, and enough of ingredient D to make a total of 20 gr. How many grains of ingredient D are in the tablet?

RATIO AND PROPORTION

Ratio

A ratio indicates a relation or comparison of two like quantities. It can be expressed as a quotient, a fraction, a percentage, or a decimal.

Examples:

Quotient
   $1 \div 2 = 1{:}2$ or 1 is to 2

Fraction
   $1/4 = 1{:}4$ or 1 is to 4

Percentage
   20% or 20:100 or 20 is to 100

Decimal
   $0.15 = 15/100 = 15{:}100$ or 15 is to 100

If the two terms of a ratio are multiplied or divided by the same number, the value of the ratio will not change. For example, the ratio of 30:6 (or 30/6) has a value of 5. If both terms are multiplied by 3, the ratio becomes 90:18 (or 90/18) and still has the same value of 5.

Ratios having the same values are equivalent. Cross products of two equivalent ratios are equal, i.e., the product of the numerator of one and the denominator of the other always equals the product of the denominator of one and the numerator of the other.

Example:

$4/5 = 12/15$

Cross products of the above equivalent ratios are equal, i.e., $4 \times 15 = 5 \times 12 = 60$

Proportion

Two equal fractions can be written as a proportion. Thus, a proportion is a statement of equality between two fractions or ratios. The following forms may be used to express the proportions:

$$a:b = c:d$$

$$a:b::c:d$$

$$a/b = c/d$$

Examples of equal fractions written as proportions:

$$12/15 = 4/5$$

$$3/6 = 21/42$$

$$8/16 = 22/44$$

A proportion when written as $1/2 = 5/10$ can be read as "one is to two as five is to ten," and $8/16 = 22/44$ may be read as "8 is to 16 as 22 is to 44."

When a proportion is written as $1:2 = 5:10$, the outside numbers (1 and 10) may be referred to as "extremes" and the inside numbers (2 and 5) as "means." When two fractions are equal, their cross products are also equal. Stated in another way, the product of the extremes equals the product of the means. Therefore, $1/2 = 5/10$ can be written as $1 \times 10 = 2 \times 5$.

If one of the terms in a proportion is unknown, it can be designated as X. The value of "X" can be calculated by setting up a proportion and solving for the unknown, X, as follows:

(1) Find the product of means and extremes, i.e., cross multiply the terms.
(2) Solve for X by dividing each side of the equation by the number that X was multiplied by.

Example:

$1/2 = X/4$; find the value of X

$1:2 = X:4$; $1 \times 4 = 2 \times X$ or $4 = 2X$

$$4/2 = 2X/2$$

$$X = 2$$

Use of proportion is very common in dosage calculations, especially in finding out the drug concentration per teaspoonful or in the preparation of bulk or stock solutions of certain medications. In a given proportion, when any three terms are known, the missing term can be determined. Thus, for example, if $a/b = c/d$, then:

$$a = bc/d$$

$$b = ad/c$$

$$c = ad/b$$

$$d = bc/a$$

For example, to find out how many milligrams of the drug demerol is present in 5 mL when there are 15 mg of demerol in 1 mL, a proportion can be set as:

$$\text{drug:volume} = \text{drug:volume}$$

$$15 \text{ mg:1 mL} = X \text{ mg:5 mL}$$

$$X = 15 \times 5 = 75 \text{ mg}$$

PERCENTAGE

The word *percent* means hundredths of a whole and is represented by the symbol %. Therefore, 1% is the same as the fraction 1/100 or the decimal fraction 0.01.

Examples:

5% = 5/100 or 1/20

To express a percent as a decimal, note that percent means division by 100; with decimals, division by 100 is accomplished by moving the decimal point two places to the left.

Examples:

50% = 0.50

5% = 0.05

To change a fraction to a percent, first change the fraction to a decimal and then multiply it by 100. If the number is already presented as a decimal, directly multiply by 100.

Examples:

1/25 = 0.04 = 4%

1/20 = 0.05 = 5%

The word *percentage* indicates "rate per hundred" and indicates *parts per 100 parts*. A percentage may also be expressed as a ratio, given as a fraction or decimal fraction. For example, 15% indicates 15 parts of 100 parts and may also be expressed as 15/100 or 0.15.

To convert the percentage of a number to equivalent decimal fraction, first drop the percent sign and then divide the numerator by 100.

Examples:

15% of 100 is same as 15/100, or 0.15

0.15% = 0.15/100 = 0.0015

PERCENT CONCENTRATION EXPRESSIONS

The concentration of a solution may be expressed in terms of the quantity of solute in a definite volume of solution or as the quantity of solute in a definite weight of solution. The quantity (or amount) is an absolute value (e.g., 10 mL, 5 g, 5 mg, etc.), whereas concentration is the quantity of a substance in relation to a definite volume or weight of other substance (e.g., 2 g/5 g, 4 mL/5 mL, 5 mg/1 mL, etc.).

(1) *Percent weight-in-volume, % w/v:* number of grams of a constituent (solute) in 100 mL of liquid preparation (solution)

(2) *Percent weight-in-weight (percent by weight), % w/w:* number of grams of a constituent (solute) in 100 g of preparation (solution)

(3) *Percent volume-in-volume (percent by volume), % v/v:* number of milliliters of a constituent (solute) in 100 mL of preparation (solution)

(4) *Milligram percent, mg%:* number of milligrams of a constituent (solute) in 100 mL of preparation (solution)

Example 1:

If 4 g of sucrose are dissolved in enough water to make 250 mL of solution, what is the concentration in terms of % w/v of the solution?

By the method of proportion:

$$\frac{4g}{250 \text{ mL}} = \frac{X \text{ g}}{100 \text{ mL}}$$

Solving for X, we get:

$$X = (100 \times 4) \div 250 = 1.6 \text{ g}$$

answer: 1.6 g in 100 mL is 1.6% w/v

Example 2:

An injection contains 40 mg pentobarbital sodium in each milliliter of solution. What is the concentration in terms of % w/v of the solution?
By the method of proportion:

$$\frac{40 \text{ mg}}{1 \text{ mL}} = \frac{X \text{ mg}}{100 \text{ mL}}$$

Solving for X, we get:

$$X = (100 \times 40) = 4000 \text{ mg or 4 g}$$

answer: 4 g in 100 mL is 4% w/v

Example 3:

How many grams of zinc chloride should be used in preparing 5 L of the mouth wash containing 1/10% w/v of zinc chloride?

$$1/10\% = 0.1\% = 0.1 \text{ g in 100 mL}$$

By the method of proportion:

$$\frac{0.1 \text{ g}}{100 \text{ mL}} = \frac{X \text{ g}}{5000 \text{ mL}}$$

$$X = (0.1 \times 5000)/100$$

answer: $= 5.0$ g

Practice Problems

(1) A pharmacist dispenses 180 prescriptions a day. How many more prescriptions does he need to dispense each day to bring a 15% increase?

(2) If an ophthalmic solution contains 10 mg of pilocarpine in each milliliter of solution, how many milliliters of solution would be needed to deliver 0.5 mg of pilocarpine?

(3) A pharmacist prepared a solution containing 10 million units of potassium penicillin per 20 mL. How many units of potassium penicillin will a 0.50-mL solution contain?

(4) A cough syrup contains 5 mg of brompheniramine maleate in each 5-mL dose. How many milligrams of brompheniramine maleate would be contained in a 120-mL container of the syrup?

(5) What is the percentage strength, expressed as % w/w, of a solution prepared by dissolving 60 g of potassium chloride in 150 mL of water?

(6) How many grams of antipyrine should be used in preparing 5% of a 60-mL solution of antipyrine?

(7) How many milligrams of a drug should be used in preparing 5 L of a 0.01% drug solution?

(8) How many liters of 2% w/v iodine tincture can be made from 108 g of iodine?

(9) How many milliliters of 0.9% w/v sodium chloride solution can be made from 325 g of sodium chloride?

(10) If a physician orders 25 mg of a drug for a patient, how many milliliters of a 2.5% w/v solution of the drug should be used?

DILUTION AND CONCENTRATION

When ratio strengths are provided, convert them to percentage strengths and then set up a proportion. When proportional parts are used in a dosage calculation, reduce them to lowest terms.

When a solution of a given strength is diluted, its strength will be reduced. For example, a 100 mL of a solution containing 10 g of a substance has a strength of 1:10 or 10% w/v. If this solution is diluted to 200 mL, i.e., the volume of the solution is doubled by adding 100 mL of solvent, the original strength will be reduced by one-half to 1:20 or 5% w/v.

To calculate the strength of a solution prepared by diluting a solution of known quantity and strength, a proportion may be set up as follows:

$$Q_1 \times C_1 = Q_2 \times C_2$$

where

Q_1 = known quantity
C_1 = known concentration
Q_2 = final quantity after dilution
C_2 = final concentration after dilution

From this expression, strength or final concentration of the solution can be determined. To calculate the volume of solution of desired strength that can be made by diluting a known quantity of a solution, similar expression is used.

Example 1:

If 5 mL of a 20% w/v aqueous solution of furosemide is diluted to 10 mL, what will be the final strength of furosemide?

$$5 \text{ (mL)} \times 20 \text{ (\% w/v)} = 10 \text{ (mL)} \times X \text{ (\% w/v)}$$

$$X = 5 \times 20/10 = 10\% \text{ w/v}$$

Example 2:

If phenobarbital elixir containing 4% w/v phenobarbital is evaporated to 90% of its volume, what is the strength of phenobarbital in the remaining product?

$$100 \text{ (mL)} \times 4 \text{ (\% w/v)} = 90 \text{ (mL)} \times X \text{ (\% w/v)}$$

$$X = 400/90 = 4.44\% \text{ w/v}$$

Example 3:

How many milliliters of a 0.01:20 v/v solution of methyl salicylate in alcohol can be made from 100 mL of 2% v/v solution?

$$0.01:20 = 0.01/20 = 0.0005 = 0.05\%$$

$$100 \text{ (mL)} \times 2 \ (\% \text{ v/v}) = X \text{ (mL)} \times 0.05 \ (\% \text{ v/v})$$

$$X = 200/0.05 = 4000 \text{ mL}$$

For very dilute solutions, concentration may be expressed in parts per million (ppm). For example, 5 ppm corresponds to 0.0005%.

Practice Problems

(1) How many milliliters of a 1:50 w/v solution of ferrous sulfate should be used to prepare 1 L of a 1:400 w/v solution?

(2) If 150 mL of a 20% w/v chlorobutanol are diluted to 5 gallons, what will be the percentage strength of the dilution?

(3) If 200 mL of a 10% w/v solution are diluted to 2 L, what will be the percentage strength?

(4) How many milliliters of water should be added to 200 mL of a 1:125 w/v solution to make a solution such that 50 mL diluted to 100 mL will provide a 1:4000 dilution?

(5) How many milliliters of water should be added to 100 mL of a 1:10 w/v solution to make a solution such that 20 mL diluted to 100 mL will provide a 1:2000 dilution?

(6) What is the strength of a potassium chloride solution obtained by evaporating 600 mL of a 10% w/v solution to 250 mL?

(7) How many liters of water for injection must be added to 2 L of a 50% w/v dextrose injection to reduce the concentration to 5% w/v?

(8) How many milliliters of a 0.1% w/v benzalkonium chloride solution should be used to prepare 1 L of a 1:4000 solution?

(9) How many milliliters of water should be added to a liter of 1:2000 w/v solution to make a 1:5000 w/v solution?

(10) How much water should be added to 1500 mL of 75% v/v ethyl alcohol to prepare a 50% v/v solution?

DENSITY AND SPECIFIC GRAVITY

The pharmacist often uses measurable quantities such as density and specific gravity when interconverting between weight (mass) and volume.

Density

Density is a derived quantity combining mass and volume. It is defined as mass per unit volume of a substance at a fixed temperature and pressure. It is usually expressed in CGS system, i.e., as grams per cubic centimeter (g/cm³) or simply as grams per milliliter (g/mL). In SI units, it may be expressed as kilograms per cubic meter. It may also be expressed as number of grains per fluidounce, or the number of pounds per gallon.

Density may be calculated by dividing the mass of a substance by its volume. For example, if 100 mL of Lugol's solution weighs 120 g, its density is:

$$\frac{120 \text{ (g)}}{100 \text{ (mL)}} = 1.2 \text{ g/mL}$$

Specific Gravity

Specific gravity is the ratio of the density of a substance to the density of water, the values for both substances being determined at the same temperature or at another specified temperature. For practical purposes, it may be defined as the ratio of the mass of a substance to the mass of an equal volume of water at the similar temperature. The official pharmaceutical compendia uses 25°C to express specific gravity.

Specific gravity may be calculated by dividing the mass of a given substance by the weight of an equal volume of water. For example, if 100 mL of simple syrup, NF weighs 131.3, and 100 mL of water, at the same temperature, weighs 100 g, the specific gravity of the simple syrup is:

$$\frac{\text{Weight of 100 mL of simple syrup}}{\text{Weight of 100 mL of water}}$$

$$\frac{131.3}{100} = 1.313$$

Note: The values of density and specific gravity, in metric system, are numerically equal, i.e., when expressed in g/cc, the values of density and specific gravity are the same. For example, a density of 1.2 g/cc equals specific gravity of 1.2.

Specific Volume

Specific volume is the ratio of volume of a substance to the volume of an equal weight of another substance taken as a standard, the volumes for both substances being determined at the same temperature.

Specific volume may be calculated by dividing the volume of a given mass of the substance by the volume of an equal mass of water. For example, if

100 g of a syrup measures 85 mL, and 100 g of water, at the same temperature, measures 100 mL, the specific volume of that syrup is:

$$\frac{\text{Volume of 100 g of syrup}}{\text{Volume of 100 g of water}}$$

$$\frac{85 \; (\text{mL})}{100 \; (\text{mL})} = 0.85$$

Note: The specific gravity and specific volume are reciprocals of each other, i.e., the product of their multiplication is 1.

If the specific gravity of the solution is known, interconversions between % w/v and % w/v are possible using the following expression:

$$\frac{\text{Percent weight-in-weight}}{\text{(\% w/w) of the solution}} = \frac{\begin{array}{c}\text{Percent weight-in-volume} \\ \text{(\% w/v) of the solution}\end{array}}{\begin{array}{c}\text{Specific gravity of} \\ \text{the solution}\end{array}}$$

Example 1:

How many milliliters of 90% (w/w) sulfuric acid having a specific gravity of 1.788 should be used in preparing a liter of 8% (w/v) acid?

$$90\% \; \text{w/w} \times 1.788 = 160.92\% \; \text{w/v}$$

$$1000 \; \text{mL} \times 8\% \; \text{w/v} = 160.92\% \; \text{w/v} \times X \; \text{mL}$$

$$\text{answer: } X = 49.7 \; \text{or} \; 50 \; \text{mL}$$

Example 2:

A pharmacist mixes 100 mL of 35% (w/w) hydrochloric acid with enough purified water to make 400 mL. If the specific gravity of hydrochloric acid is 1.20, calculate the percentage strength (w/v) of the final solution.

$$100 \; \text{mL} \times 35\% \; (\text{w/w}) = 400 \; \text{mL} \times X \; (\text{w/w})$$

$$X = \frac{100 \times 35}{400} = 8.75\% \; \text{w/w}$$

$$\text{answer: } 8.75 \times 1.20 = 10.5\% \; \text{w/v}$$

Example 3:

How many milliliters of a 64% (w/w) sorbitol solution having a specific gravity 1.26, should be used in preparing a liter of a 10% (w/v) solution?

$$64\% \text{ w/w} \times 1.26 = 80.64\% \text{ w/v}$$

$$1000 \text{ mL} \times 10\% \text{ w/v} = X \text{ mL} \times 80.64\% \text{ w/v}$$

$$X = \frac{1000 \times 10}{80.64} = 124 \text{ mL}$$

answer: 124 mL

Practice Problems

(1) If a liter of mannitol solution weighs 1285 g, what is its specific gravity?

(2) If 50 mL of glycerin weighs 135 g, what is its specific gravity?

(3) The specific gravity of ethyl alcohol is 0.820. What is its specific volume?

(4) If 68 g of a sulfuric acid solution measures 55.5 mL, what is its specific volume?

(5) What is the weight of 15 mL of propylene glycol having a specific gravity of 1.24?

(6) What is the weight, in grams, of 250 mL of iodine solution having a specific gravity of 1.28?

(7) What is the volume of 50 g of potassium chloride solution with a specific gravity of 1.30?

(8) What is the weight, in kilograms, of 1 gallon of dextrose solution having a specific gravity of 1.25?

(9) The strength of syrup USP solution is 65% w/w and its specific gravity is 1.313. What is its concentration in % w/v?

(10) How many milliliters of 36.5% w/w hydrochloric acid are needed to prepare one gallon of 25% w/v acid? The specific gravity of hydrochloric acid is 1.20.

CHAPTER 2

Systems of Measurement

The knowledge and application of pharmaceutical and clinical calculations are essential for the practice of pharmacy and related health professions. Many calculations have been simplified by the shift from apothecary to metric system of measurements. However, a significant proportion of calculation errors occur because of simple mistakes in arithmetic. Further, the dosage forms prepared by pharmaceutical companies undergo several inspections and quality control tests. Such a luxury is almost impossible to find in a pharmacy or hospital setting. Therefore it is imperative that the health care professionals be extremely careful in performing pharmaceutical and clinical calculations. In the present chapter, a brief introduction is provided for the three systems of measurement and their interconversions:

- metric system
- apothecary and avoirdupois systems
- household system
- interconversions

THE METRIC SYSTEM

The metric system, which is federally mandated and appears in the official listing of drugs in the *United States Pharmacopoeia* (USP), is a logically organized system of measurement. It was first developed by the French. The basic units multiplied or divided by 10 comprise the metric system. Therefore, a knowledge of decimals, reviewed in Chapter 1, is useful for this system.

In the metric system, the three primary or fundamental units are: the meter for length, the liter for volume, and the gram for weight. In addition to these basic units, the metric system includes multiples of basic units with a prefix to indicate its relationship with the basic unit. For example, a milliliter represents 1/1000 or 0.001 part of a liter. A milligram represents 0.001 g and a kilogram represents 1000 times the gram. A pharmacist rarely uses the secondary or the derived units of the metric system. Therefore, secondary units such as Joules or Newton are not included in this book. The table of measurements in Table 2.1 is very important for the pharmacists.

The pharmacist should be able to perform interconversions from a microgram to a centigram or from a nanogram to a microgram. The following general guidelines may be helpful:

(1) To prevent the mistake of overlooking a decimal point, precede the decimal point with a zero if the value is less than one, i.e., writing 0.8 g is better than .8 g. As a practical example, if a prescription is written for Dexamethasone Oral Solution .5 mg/.5 mL, one possible mistake could be dispensing 0.5 mg/5 mL solution. This under-medication to the patient would most likely be avoided if 0.5 mg/0.5 mL is written.

(2) To convert milligram (large unit) to microgram (small unit), multiply by 1000 or move the decimal point three places to the right.

(3) To convert microgram (small unit) to centigram (large unit), divide by 10,000 or simply move the decimal point four places to the left.

(4) To add, subtract, multiply or divide different metric units, first convert all the units to the same denomination. For example, to subtract 54 mg from 0.28 g, solve as 280 mg − 54 mg = 226 mg.
    Note:
    • Gram is represented by g or G whereas a grain is represented by gr.
    • Milliliters are sometimes represented by cc, which is a cubic centimeter (cm³). This is very useful, especially when a conversion from a volume unit to a length unit or vice versa is needed.
    • μg can also be represented by mcg. As an example, Cytotec®, which contains the drug misoprostol, is available in strengths of 100 mcg and 200 mcg.

TABLE 2.1.   Metric Weights.

0.001 kilogram (kg)	=	1 gram (g)
0.01 hectogram (hg)	=	1 gram (g)
0.1 dekagram (dkg)	=	1 gram (g)
10 decigram (dg)	=	1 gram (g)
100 centigram (cg)	=	1 gram (g)
1000 milligram (mg)	=	1 gram (g)
1,000,000 microgram (μg)	=	1 gram (g)
1,000,000,000 nanogram (ng)	=	1 gram (g)

TABLE 2.2.   Metric Volume.

0.001 kiloliter (kL)	=	1 liter (L)
0.01 hectoliter (hL)	=	1 liter (L)
0.1 dekaliter (dkL)	=	1 liter (L)
10 deciliter (dL)	=	1 liter (L)
100 centiliter (cL)	=	1 liter (L)
1000 milliliter (mL)	=	1 liter (L)
1,000,000 microliter (μL)	=	1 liter (L)
1,000,000,000 nanoliter (nL)	=	1 liter (L)

(5) One should be careful with decimal points on prescriptions. When recording a prescription by telephone, decimal points should not be used unless needed. For example, *Norpramine® 10.0 mg* could be mistaken for *Norpramine® 100 mg*. The excess drug may cause adverse reactions such as blurred vision, confusion, flushing, fainting, etc., in the patients.

The above rules can be similarly applied to the conversions of volume and length measurements. While the weight and volume measurements are the most commonly used, the measure of length is used in measurements such as the patient's height and body surface area. The liquid and length measures are provided in Tables 2.2 and 2.3.

Example 1:

If a chlorpheniramine maleate tablet weighs 0.26 gram, one-fourth of the same tablet weighs how many milligrams?
Since the answer is required in milligrams, convert the weight of the tablet into milligrams first.

$$0.26 \text{ g} = 0.26 \times 1000 = 260 \text{ mg}$$

$$1/4 \times 260 \text{ mg} = 65 \text{ mg}$$

answer: 65 mg

TABLE 2.3.   Metric Length.

0.001 kilometer (km)	=	1 meter (m)
0.01 hectometer (hm)	=	1 meter (m)
0.1 dekameter (dkm)	=	1 meter (m)
10 decimeter (dm)	=	1 meter (m)
100 centimeter (cm)	=	1 meter (m)
1000 millimeter (mm)	=	1 meter (m)
1,000,000 micrometer (μm)	=	1 meter (m)
1,000,000,000 nanometer (nm)	=	1 meter (m)

Example 2:

If a vial of gentamycin contains 80 mg of drug in 2 mL, how many micrograms of the drug are present in 0.025 mL?

$$80 \text{ mg} = 80,000 \text{ } \mu g$$

By the method of proportion, if 80,000 μg are contained in 2 mL, how many micrograms are contained in 0.025 mL?

$$2 \text{ mL}/80,000 = 0.025 \text{ mL}/X$$

$$\text{answer: } X = 1000 \text{ } \mu g$$

Example 3:

Add 1.25 g, 35 mg, and 80 μg, and express the result in milligrams. Convert all the units to the same denomination and then perform the computation.

$$1.25 \text{ g} = 1250 \text{ mg, and } 80 \text{ } \mu g = 0.08 \text{ mg}$$

$$\text{Therefore, } 1250 + 35 + 0.08 = 1285.08 \text{ mg}$$

$$\text{answer: } 1285.08 \text{ mg}$$

Practice Problems

(1) 30 g of Bactroban® ointment contains 2% mupirocin. If one gram of the ointment is applied to an affected area, how many milligrams of mupirocin is used?

(2) Pediaprofen® pediatric suspension contains 80 mg of ibuprofen in 5 mL of the suspension. While taking 2.5 mL of this medication, the patient spilled 0.5 mL of the suspension. How many grams of ibuprofen did the patient receive?

(3) Diprosone® lotion contains 0.05% betamethasone diproprionate. How many microliters of the lotion will contain 2.5 μg of the drug?

(4) Fer-In-Sol® drops contain 75 mg of ferrous sulfate in 0.6 mL of the solution. If a pharmacist dispensed 90 mL of the solution, how many grams of ferrous sulfate was dispensed?

(5) Feldene® tablets contain 20 mg of piroxicam per tablet. If 20 dekagrams of piroxicam is provided, how many tablets can be prepared with this amount?

(6) When an intravenous solution containing 0.2 g of a sulfa drug in 1 L of the solution is administered to a patient at the rate of 100 mL per hour, how many micrograms of the drug will the patient receive in a two-minute period?

(7) When dividing 0.32 g of a drug into 800 equal doses, how many μg of the drug will be present in each dose?

(8) The four ingredients of a chewable tablet weigh 0.3 g, 115 mg, 5000 μg, and 0.003 kg. How many milligrams will the tablet weigh?

(9) If 200 μL, 0.4 mL, 0.006 cL, and 0.0008 dL of a preservative solution are removed from a container, how many milliliters of the solution have been removed?

(10) The following amounts of alcohol have been removed from a stock bottle containing 1.5 L: 0.00005 kL, 50 mL, 0.05 dkL, and 5 dL. How much alcohol will be left in the original stock bottle?

APOTHECARIES' SYSTEM

Unlike the metric system which has units for weight, volume, and length, the apothecaries' system has units for weight and volume only. This is an old system and its use is rapidly declining. However, some physicians still prescribe using this system. A few drug labels that were originally produced under the apothecaries' system, still state the apothecaries' equivalent on the label. As a few examples, phenobarbital, aspirin, codeine, sodium bicarbonate, and potassium iodide labels appear in the metric as well as apothecary units. Moreover, a few questions have also appeared in the apothecaries' units in pharmacist licensing examinations. Therefore, pharmacists are still required to learn this system.

The basic unit for weight is grain (gr) and that of volume is minim (m). Unlike the metric units, the amount is expressed in Roman numerals after the apothecaries' symbol. For example, ½ grain is expressed as gr ss but not ½ gr. Twenty minims is expressed as m xx. Sometimes physicians also use Arabic numerals in the apothecary system. For example 12 ounces can be written as ʒ XII or 4 ounces as 4 ʒ. Tables 2.4 and 2.5 show the relationships

TABLE 2.4. *Apothecaries' Liquid Measures.*

60 minims (m)	=	1 fluid dram (fʒ)
8 fluid drams (fʒ)	=	1 fluid ounce (fʒ)
16 fluid ounces (fʒ)	=	1 pint (pt or O)
2 pints (O)	=	1 quart (qt)
4 quarts (qt)	=	1 gallon (gal or C)

TABLE 2.5.   *Apothecaries' Weight Measures.*

20 grains	=	1 scruple (ᴈ)
3 scruples	=	1 dram (ʒ)
8 drams (ʒ)	=	1 ounce (ʒ)
12 ounces (ʒ)	=	1 pound (lb)
1 pound (lb)	=	5760 grains (gr)

between measures of liquid volume and solid weight in the apothecaries' system.

Example 1:

If a prescription calls for gr ii thyroid desiccated tablets and the pharmacist has gr ss tablets in stock, how many tablets of gr ss should be provided?

$$gr\ ii = 2\ grains$$

$$gr\ ss = \tfrac{1}{2}\ grain$$

$$2 \div \tfrac{1}{2} = 4\ tablets\ of\ gr\ ss$$

answer: 4 tablets of gr ss

Example 2:

How many doses of ʒ iv are present in O iiss of Maalox®?

$$O\ iiss = 2\tfrac{1}{2}\ pints$$

$$= 2.5 \times 16\ ounces = 40\ ounces$$

$$= 40 \times 8 = 320\ fluidrams$$

$$= 320/4 = 80\ doses$$

answer: 80 doses

Example 3:

A doctor ordered morphine sulfate gr 2/5 and the pharmacist has a stock solution of gr 1/8 per milliliter of morphine sulfate. How many milliliters of the stock solution is required to fill the prescription?

gr 2/5 = 0.4 grains needed

gr 1/8 = 0.125 grains per mL

0.125/mL = 0.4/X

X = 0.4/0.125 = 3.2

answer: 3.2 mL of the stock solution

Practice Problems

(1) If two quarts of acetaminophen elixir are present in the inventory, how many fℨ iv prescriptions can be filled?

(2) If you fill approximately twelve prescriptions of fℨ-vi Ventolin® syrup per day, how many gallons of the syrup would be used in fifteen days?

(3) How many minims of a topical keratolytic solution are contained in a 4 fluidram bottle?

(4) If thirty-six APAP suppositories of 2 gr each are dispensed, how many scruples of drug are dispensed?

(5) How many apothecary ounces are present in lbs iiiss?

(6) How many fluidrams remain after 4 fluidrams, 60 minims, and ½ fluid-ounce of guaifenesin are removed from a one pint container?

(7) How many ounces are present in gr CXX?

(8) A prescription requires gr 1/200 of a drug. If a pharmacist has gr 1/100 scored-tablets, how many tablets should be dispensed?

(9) If a generic syrup costs $14 for ½ oz (apoth) and the brand syrup costs $32 for the same amount of syrup, what is the dollar difference for one gallon of the drug?

(10) The container for Seconal® sodium capsules shows a strength of 100 mg (1½ gr) of the drug secobarbital sodium. If an ounce of drug is available, how many capsules can be prepared?

THE AVOIRDUPOIS SYSTEM

The avoirdupois system is also an old system used by the pharmacist, in the past, for ordering bulk chemicals. Since this system is no longer used, practice problems on this topic will not be provided. However, for reference considerations, the following conversions of avoirdupois weights are provided:

$$1 \text{ ounce (oz)} = 437.5 \text{ grains}$$

$$1 \text{ pound (lb)} = 7000 \text{ grains}$$

THE HOUSEHOLD SYSTEM

Though inaccurate, the use of the household system of measurements is on the rise because of an increased home health care delivery. In this system, the patients use household measuring devices such as the teaspoon, dessertspoon, tablespoon, wine-glass, coffee cup, etc. In the past, a drop has been used as an equivalent of a minim. But such a measure should be discouraged because of many factors affecting the drop size which include the density of the medication, temperature, surface tension, diameter and opening of the dropper, and the angle of the dropper. The official medicinal dropper (USP-NF) has an external diameter of 3 mm, and delivers 20 drops per mL of water at 25°C. Some manufacturers provide specially calibrated droppers with their products. A few examples of medications containing droppers include Tylenol® pediatric drops, Advil® pediatric drops, and Neosynephrine® nasal drops. Several ear, nose, and eye medications are now available in calibrated containers which provide drops by gently pressing the containers. Sometimes, the health care professonal has to calibrate the dropper for measuring small quantities such as 0.1 mL or 0.15 mL, when the calibrated dropper is not supplied by the manufacturer. The calibration procedure is outlined in the following section.

Calibration of the Medicinal Dropper

A dropper is calibrated by counting the number of drops required to transfer 2 mL of the intended liquid from its original container to a 5-mL measuring cylinder. For example, if it takes 40 drops to measure 2 mL of a liquid, then the number of drops to measure 0.15 mL of the liquid is obtained by the method of proportion as follows:

$$40 \text{ drops}/2 \text{ mL} = X \text{ drops}/0.15$$

$$X = 3 \text{ drops}$$

answer: 3 drops

The household measures are shown in Table 2.6.

It is important to remember that the household system of measurement should not be used for calculations in compounding or conversions from one system to the other. Household system of measures is designed for the

TABLE 2.6.   Household Measures.

1 teaspoonful* (tsp)	=	5 mL
1 dessertspoonful (dssp)	=	8 mL
1 tablespoonful (tbsp)	=	15 mL
1 ounce	=	2 tbsp or 30 mL
1 wine-glass	=	1 ounce
1 coffee cup	=	6 fluidounces
1 glass	=	8 fluidounces
1 quart (qt)	=	1 liter

* Some physicians denote this by ℨ. If this symbol appears in the directions for patient, it is equivalent to 5 mL. If the symbol appears in the compounding or the enlargement/reduction of formulae, it is equivalent to 3.69 mL by the apothecary measure.

convenience to the patient. Therefore this system is used for the directions on labels for the patients.

Example 1:

Suprax® suspension contains 100 mg/5 mL of the drug cefixime. If the patient takes one teaspoonful of the suspension twice daily for ten days, how many grams of the drug does the patient consume?

$$5 \text{ mL} \times 2 = 10 \text{ mL daily}$$

$$10 \times 10 = 100 \text{ mL, total dose}$$

$$0.1 \text{ g/5 mL} = X \text{ g/100}$$

$$X = 2 \text{ g}$$

answer: 2 g

Example 2:

In calibrating a medicinal dropper, 2 mL of a pediatric solution resulted in 48 drops. If it is desired to administer 0.08 mL of the medication to a baby, approximately how many drops should be given?
  By the method of proportion:

$$48 \text{ drops/2 mL} = X \text{ drops/0.08 mL}$$

$$X = 1.922 \text{ or 2 drops}$$

answer: 2 drops

Example 3:

If a teaspoonful of Tussi-Organidin® syrup is to be given three times daily for five days, how many fluidounces of the medication should be dispensed?

$$5 \times 3 = 15 \text{ mL daily}$$

$$15 \times 5 = 75 \text{ mL or } 2\frac{1}{2} \text{ fluidounces}$$

answer: $2\frac{1}{2}$ fluidounces

Practice Problems

(1) A pharmacist dispensed 4 fluidounces of an antacid suspension with instructions that the patient take two tablespoonfuls of the medication four times a day. How long will the medication last?

(2) Children's Advil® is available in a suspension form containing ibuprofen in a strength of 100 mg/5 mL of the suspension. If the patient receives one teaspoonful of the medication three times daily, how many grams of the drug will be consumed by the patient in two days?

(3) It is required to administer 0.3 mL of an otic solution using a new medicinal dropper. How many drops of the solution is to be administered when it is determined that 45 drops measure 2 mL of the otic solution?

(4) For a patient suffering from diarrhea, a doctor advised the patient to take one glassful of an electrolyte solution three times a day. The patient took one coffee-cupful of medication three times for one day. How much extra medication was the patient supposed to take?

(5) If a patient needs one teaspoonful of Alupent® oral liquid three times a day for ten days, how many fluidounces of medication should the pharmacist dispense?

(6) A patient received 8 fluidounces of Kaopectate® with the instructions of taking two teaspoonfuls of medication after each bowel movement. If the patient took Kaopectate® after ten such bowel movements, how many milliliters of the medication should be left in the container?

(7) A child received 5 f℥ of amoxicillin suspension containing 125 mg/5 mL. If one teaspoonful was taken three times a day, how many grams of amoxicillin did the child take in one week?

(8) How many teaspoonfuls equal the volume of a coffee cup?

(9) Is it true that one-half tablespoon equals one teaspoon?

(10) If a prescription is required for Phenergan VC with Codeine, two teaspoonfuls at bedtime for fifteen days, how many fluidounces of the syrup would the pharmacist dispense?

TABLE 2.7. Conversion Equivalents of the
Measurement Systems.

Apothecary	Metric	Household
1 minim (m)	0.06 mL	—
16.23 m	1 mL	—
1 fluidram (f℥)	3.69 mL	1 teaspoonful or 5 mL
1/2 fluidounce (f℥)	15 mL	1 tablespoonful
1 f℥	29.57 mL	2 tablespoonfuls
1 pint (O)	473 mL	500 mL
1 quart (qt)	946 mL	1 liter

INTERCONVERSIONS

In a pharmaceutical or clinical setting, health care professionals encounter more than one system of measurement. Therefore, it becomes necessary to convert all quantities to the same system of measurement. Depending upon the circumstances and the degree of accuracy required, a particular system would be preferred over the others. Some commonly used equivalents in pharmacy practice are shown in Tables 2.7 and 2.8.

A pharmacy or health care institution may use a particular set of equivalents as their established standards for interconversion. The health care professionals working in that environment must use those standards. If such standards are

TABLE 2.8. Approximate Equivalents Used by
Health Professionals.

Apothecary	Metric	Commonly Used Equivalent
1 grain (gr)	64.8 mg	65 mg*
1 ounce (℥)	31.1 g	30 g
1 pound	373.2 g	454 g**
1 minim	0.062 mL	0.06 mL
1 fluidounce	29.57 mL	30 mL
128 f℥	3785 mL	1 gallon (C)
—	1 kg	2.2 lb

* It should be remembered that this conversion is only approximate. Several other approximations have been used on the labels of certain tablets. For example. Saccharin tablets from Eli Lilly Company shows ½ gr (32 mg) on its label whereas the phenobarbital tablets from the same company have 30 mg (½ gr) on its label. Similarly sodium bicarbonate tablets from Eli Lilly have 5 grs (325 mg) on its label and potassium iodide from the same company has 300 mg (5 grs) on its container label. In the present book, it is advised to use one grain equivalent as 65 mg.
** This amount represents the equivalent of 1 avoirdupois pound. Since the pound is a bulk quantity, use of the avoirdupois system of measurements unit is more common.

not established, generally, the equivalents shown in the right column of Table 2.8 may be used.

Example 1:

Accupril® tablets are available in strengths of 5 mg and 40 mg of the drug quinapril HCl. Express these strengths in grains.

$$65 \text{ mg/1 grain} = 5/X$$

$$X = 0.076 \text{ or } 1/13 \text{ grains}$$

$$65 \text{ mg/1 grain} = 40/X$$

$$X = 0.62 = 1/1.6 = 5/8 \text{ grains}$$

answer: The range of available Accupril® tablets in grains is 1/13 to 5/8.

Example 2:

Daypro®, a nonsteroidal antiinflammatory agent, has a maximum daily dose requirement of 26 mg/kg/day. What is the maximum number of Daypro® 600 mg tablets that can be given to a 127-lb patient?

$$26 \text{ mg/2.2 lbs} = X \text{ mg/127 lb}$$

$$X = 1501 \text{ mg}$$

$$600 \text{ mg/1 tab} = 1501 \text{ mg}/X$$

$$X = 2.5 \text{ tablets}$$

answer: 2.5 tablets

Example 3:

Tylenol with codeine® elixir contains 12 mg of codeine per 5 mL of the elixir. If a pharmacist dispenses 4 fluidounces of the elixir to a patient, how many grains of codeine does the patient receive?

$$12 \text{ mg/5 mL} = X/120 \text{ mL}$$

$$X = 288 \text{ mg}$$

$$65 \text{ mg/1 gr} = 288 \text{ mg}/X$$

$$X = 4.43 \text{ grains}$$

answer: 4.43 grains

Practice Problems

(1) A Halcion® tablet contains 0.25 mg of triazolam. How many grains of the drug triazolam would be present in 100 tablets of Halcion®?

(2) If a quart of suspension contains 2 g of a drug, how many grains would be present in a gallon of the suspension?

(3) A Carafate® tablet contains 1 g of sucralfate. How many ounces of sucralfate would be present in ten Carafate® tablets?

(4) How many Hismanal® tablets (5 mg) would contain an ounce of astemizole?

(5) A prescription requires gr ii of phenolphthalein in f℥ iv of an emulsion. If the patient takes 2 tbsp of the emulsion at bedtime, how many milligrams of phenolphthalein does this dose represent?

(6) If a prescription requires ℥ii of camphor for ℥ii of an ointment, how many grams of camphor are needed to prepare a pound of the ointment?

(7) Zovirax® tablets, containing the antiviral drug acyclovir, are usually given in a dose of 80 mg/kg/day for five days for treating chickenpox. If the patient weighs 165 lb, how many ounce(s) of acyclovir would the patient consume if he has to take the full dose prescribed?

(8) If a physician prescribes 1½ grains of phenobarbital sodium from the Eli Lilly Company, how many grams of drug would it contain?

(9) Mr. John Doe has been suffering from diarrhea and Dr. Brown wants him to take 30 mL of Kaopectate®. How many tablespoonfuls of Kaopectate® should Mr. Doe take?

(10) Mrs. Straker has been advised by her physician to take at least 1.2 L of an electrolyte solution per day. How many glassfuls of the electrolyte solution should she take per day?

CHAPTER 3

Prescription and Medication Orders

The interpretation of prescription medication orders is one of the most important requirements of professional pharmacy practice. According to the National Association of Boards of Pharmacy's (NABP's) Model State Pharmacy Act,

The "Practice of Pharmacy" shall mean the interpretation and evaluation of prescription orders; the compounding, dispensing, labelling of drugs and devices (except labeling by a manufacturer, packer, or distributor of Non-Prescription Drugs and commercially packaged legend drugs and devices); the participation in drug selection and drug utilization reviews; the proper and safe storage of drugs and devices and the maintenance of proper records, therefore; the responsibility of advising where necessary or where regulated, of therapeutic values, content, hazards and use of drugs and devices; and the offering or performing of those acts, services, operations or transactions necessary in the conduct, operation, management and control of pharmacy.

The Model State Pharmacy Act of the NABP also defines drugs which are to be dispensed with or without prescription.

"Prescription Drug or Legend Drug" shall mean a drug which, under Federal Law is required, prior to being dispensed or delivered, to be labeled with either of the following statements: (1) "Caution: Federal law prohibits dispensing without prescription" (2) "Caution: Federal law restricts this drug to use by or on the order of a licensed veterinarian"; or a drug which is required by any applicable Federal or State Law or regulation to be dispensed on prescription only or is restricted to use by practitioners only.

Non-prescription drugs are defined as "Non-narcotic medicines or drugs which may be sold without a prescription and which are prepackaged for use by the consumer and labelled in accordance with the requirements of the statutes and regulation of this State and the Federal Government.''

The definitions provided above underscore the importance of understanding and interpreting prescriptions. A prescription is defined as an order for medication from a doctor, dentist, veterinarian, or any other licensed health care professional authorized to prescribe in that state. It shows the relationship between the prescriber, patient, and the pharmacist, in which the latter provides the medication to the patient.

TYPES OF PRESCRIPTIONS

Pharmacists receive prescriptions by telephone, fax, as written prescriptions from individual prescribers, practicing in a group, or hospitals and other institutions. Telephone orders are reduced to a written prescription (hard copy) by pharmacists. Generally, prescriptions include printed forms called "prescription blanks" which include the name, address, and telephone number of the prescriber; a provision to write the name, address, age or date of birth of the patient; and the ℞ symbol. "Medication orders" are prescription equivalents which are written by practitioners (prescribers) in a hospital or a similar institution. Components of medication orders with appropriate examples are presented in the subsequent section.

COMPONENTS OF PRESCRIPTIONS

Generally, a prescription consists of the following parts (see the sample prescription in Figure 3.1):

(1) Prescriber's name, degree, address and telephone number. In the case of prescriptions coming from a hospital or a multicenter clinic, the hospital or clinic's name, address and telephone numbers appear at the top. In such a case, the physician's name and degree would appear near his/her signature.

(2) Patient's name, address, age, and the date of prescription.

(3) The *Superscription,* which is represented by the Latin sign. ℞. This sign represents "take thou" or "you take" or "recipe." Sometimes, this sign is also used to denote the pharmacy itself.

(4) The *Inscription* is the general content of the prescription. It states the name and strength of the medication, either as its brand (proprietary) or generic (nonproprietary) name. In the case of compounded prescriptions, the *inscription* states the name and strength of active ingredients.

```
┌─────────────────────────────────────────────────┐
│        ┌───────────────────────────────┐         │
│        │      Henry Huxtable, M.D.      │         │
│        │     61-40 Flushing Avenue      │         │
│        │       Monroe, LA 71208         │         │
│        │      Phone No. 555-1234        │         │
│        └───────────────────────────────┘         │
│                                                   │
│   Name : Lisa Taylor           Age: 70           │
│   Address: 96 Havana Blvd., FL 31207  Date: 2/28/96│
│                                                   │
│   ℞                                               │
│                                                   │
│          Cafergot Suppositories                   │
│                   #12                             │
│                                                   │
│                                                   │
│          Sig: In. rect, i HS, prn pain.           │
│                                                   │
│                                                   │
│                                                   │
│   REFILL  None                                    │
│                                                   │
│   DAW  ✓                                          │
│                           HHuxtable               │
│                     DEA # AD 7973142              │
│                                                   │
└─────────────────────────────────────────────────┘
```

FIGURE 3.1. Sample prescription.

(5) The *Subscription* represents the directions to the dispenser and indicates the type of dosage form or the number of dosage units. For compounded prescriptions, the subscription is written using English or Latin abbreviations. A few examples are provided as follows:

- M. et ft. sol. Disp ℥ vi (Mix and make solution. Dispense six fluidounces)
- Ft. ung. Disp ℥ ii (Make ointment and dispense two ounces)
- Ft. cap. DTD xii (Make capsules and let twelve such doses be given)

(6) The *Signa,* also known as *transcription* represents the directions to the patient. These directions are written in English or Latin or a combination of both. Latin directions in prescriptions are declining, but since they are still used, it is important to learn them. A few examples are provided below:

- ii caps bid, 7 days (Take two capsules twice daily for seven days)
- gtt. iii a.u. hs (Instill three drops in both the ears at bedtime)
- In rect. prn pain (Insert rectally as needed for pain)

(7) The prescriber's signature.

(8) The refill directions, in which the information about how many times, if authorized, a prescription can be refilled is provided.

(9) Other information, such as "Dispense as Written."

(10) Drug Enforcement Administration (DEA) registration number and/or the state registration number of the prescribing authority.

LABEL ON THE CONTAINER

It is a legal requirement to affix a prescription label on the immediate container of prescription medications. The pharmacist is responsible for the accuracy of the label. It should bear the name, address, and the telephone number of the pharmacy, the date of dispensing, the prescription number, the prescriber's name, the name and address of the patient, and the directions for use of the medication. Some states require additional information. The name and strength of the medication, and the refill directions are also written frequently. The label for a sample prescription is in Figure 3.2.

MEDICATION ORDER

While prescriptions are written in an outpatient setting, medication orders

---

NORTHEAST PHARMACY
169 Hillside Avenue
Monroe, LA 71206   555-0342

R # 123456   Date: 2/28/96
Taylor, Lisa
96 Havana Blvd.
Insert one suppository rectally at
bed time, as needed for pain.
Cafergot suppositories # 12
                H. Huxtable, M.D.

FIGURE 3.2. Sample label.

HILL HEALTH CARE HOSPITAL LITTLE ROCK, ARKANSA				
PHYSICIAN'S ORDER SHEET Please Use Ball Point Pen and Press Firmly. You are making more than one copy		Rodman, Brown 41-22 Passedena Little Rock, AK ID# 87654	Admit 2/26/96 DOB 7/7/42 Dr. L. Burley Room 107	

ORDERED		PHYSICIAN'S ORDERS	NURSE NOTED	
DATE	TIME	START A NEW SECTION WITH EACH SET OF ORDERS	HOUR	NAME
2/26	0900	Dynapen 250 mg. PO q6h		
2/26	0900	Darvon Compound 65 PO q4h prn pain		
2/26	0900	Vibramycin 0.2 g po stat	0940	L. Ito
		L. Burley, M.D.		

FIGURE 3.3. Sample medication order.

(Figure 3.3) are written in an institutional setting. A medication order is also known as a drug order or a physician's order. These orders generally contain the name, age or date of birth, hospital ID number, room number, the date of admission to hospital, and any patient allergies. Sometimes the patient's diagnosis is included. Besides patient information, the following information about the medication is included:

- date and time of the medication order
- name of the drug (brand or generic)
- dosage form
- route of administration, e.g., oral, sublingual, intramuscular, intravenous, rectal, etc.
- administration schedule, e.g., times per day, milliliters per hour, at bedtime, etc.
- other information such as some restrictions or specifications
- prescriber's signature
- provision for the pharmacist's or nurse's notes

COMMON LATIN TERMS AND ABBREVIATIONS

Terms Related to Quantities

Abbreviation	Term/Phrase	Meaning
aa	Ana	Of each
q.s.	Quantum sufficiat	Sufficient quantity
ad lib.	Ad libitum	Freely, at pleasure
℥	Ounce	One ounce
f℥	Fluidounce	One fluidounce
O or pt	Pint	One pint
qt	Quart	One quart
gal	Gallon	One gallon
m	Minim	One minim
ʒ	Dram or drachm	One drachm
fʒ	Fluid drachm	One fluid drachm
gr	Grain	One grain
э	Scruple	One scruple

Terms Related to Administration Times

Abbreviation	Term/Phrase	Meaning
qd	Quaque die	Once daily
bid	Bis in die	Twice daily
tid	Ter in die	Three times daily
qid	Quarter in die	Four times daily
am or AM	Ante meridium	In the morning
pm or PM	Post meridium	In the evening
h.s.	Hora somni	At bedtime
a.c.	Ante cibos	Before meals
p.c.	Post cibos	After meals
i.c.	Inter cibos	Between meals
om	Omne mane	Every morning
on	Omne nocte	Every night
p.r.n.	Pro re nata	When required
q.h.	Quaque hora	Every hour
q2h	Quaque secunda hora	Every two hours
q3h	Quaque tertia hora	Every three hours
q4h	Quaque quarta hora	Every four hours
q6h	Quaque sex hora	Every six hours
q8h	Quaque octo hora	Every eight hours

Terms Related to Preparations or Remedies

Abbreviation	Term/Phrase	Meaning
amp	Ampul	Ampul
aq	Aqua	Water
aur or oto	Auristillae	Ear drops
cap	Capsula	A capsule
comp	Compositus	Compounded
cm or crem	Cremor	A cream
garg	gargarisma	Gargle
gtt	Guttae	Drops
inj.	Injectio	An injection
liq.	Liquor	A solution
mist.	Mistura	A mixture
Neb.	Nebula	A nebulizer
pil.	Pilula	A pill
pulv.	Pulvis	A powder
suppos.	Suppositorium	A suppository
troch.	Trochiscus	A lozenge

Instructions for Preparations

Abbreviation	Term/Phrase	Meaning
div.	Divide	Divide
ft	Fiat	Let it be made
m. ft.	Misce fiat	Mix to make
d.t.d.	dentur tales doses	Such doses be given
e.m.p.	ex modo prescriptio	In the manner prescribed
s	sine	Without

Method of Application

Abbreviation	Term/Phrase	Meaning
o.d. or OD	Oculus dexter	Right eye
o.l. or OL	Oculus Laevus	Left eye
o.u. or O_2	Oculo utro	Each eye or both eyes
o.s. or OS	Oculo sinister	Left eye
a.d. or AD	Aurio dextra	Right ear
a.l. or AL	Aurio Laeva	Left ear
e.m.p.	Ex. modo-prescriptio	As directed
u.d.	Ut. dictum	As directed
c	Cum	With
dext	Dexter	Right

Names for Ingredients and Products

Common Names	Meaning
Acidi tannici	Tannic acid
Ac. Sal.	Salicylic acid
Ac. Sal. Ac.	Aspirin
Aq. hamamelis	Witch hazel
Burrow's solution	Aluminum acetate solution
Camphorated oil	Camphor liniment
Camphorated Tr of opium	Paregoric
Cocoa butter	Theobroma oil
Epsom salt	Magnesium sulfate
Hydrous wool fat	Lanolin
L.C.D.	Liquid coal tar solution
Liq. calcis	Lime water
Lugol's solution	Strong iodine solution
Methylrosaniline Cl	Gentian violet
Olei lini	Linseed oil
Oleum ricini	Castor oil
Oleum morrhuae	Cod liver oil
Pulv. amyli	Starch
S.V.R.	Alcohol USP
Sweet oil	Olive oil
Whitfield's ont.	Benzoic and salicylic acids ointment

Miscellaneous

Abbreviation	Meaning
AA	Apply to affected area
AUD	Apply as directed
ASA	Acetyl salicylic acid
APAP	Acetaminophen
BCP	Birth control pills
BIW	Twice a week
BM	Bowel movement
BP	Blood pressure
BS	Blood sugar
BSA	Body surface area
ċ	With
CHF	Congestive heart failure
DSS	Doccusate

EES	Erythromycin ethyl succinate
et	and
fl	Fluid
FA	Folic acid
HA	Headache
HC	Hydrocortisone
HCTZ	Hydrochlorothiazide
HT	Hypertension
ID	Intradermal
IM	Intramuscular
INH	Isoniazid
IOP	Intraocular pressure
IV	Intravenous
IVP	Intravenous push
IVPB	Intravenous piggy bag
MVI	Multivitamin infusion
MOM	Milk of magnesia
N & V	Nausea and vomiting
NR	Nonrepeatable or no refill
NTG	Nitroglycerin
PBZ	Pyribenzamine
PPA	Phenylpropanolamine
SOB	Shortness of breath
SC	Subcutaneous
SL	Sublingual
tal. dos	Such doses
TIW	Thrice a week
TPN	Total parenteral nutrition
URI	Upper respiratory infection
UTI	Urinary tract infection

Vehicles

Abbreviation	Meaning
aq. bull	Boiling water
DW/or aq. dist	Distilled water
D5W	Dextrose 5% in water
NS or NSS	Normal saline (10.9% sodium chloride)
½NS	Half strength of normal saline
RL	Ringer's lactate

MEDICATIONS AND THEIR DIRECTIONS FOR USE

The following medications represent the most frequently prescribed dosage forms and their commonly prescribed *signa*. While the dosage forms may be available in several strengths, only one strength is listed here. The generic names of drugs are provided in parentheses. When the most frequently prescribed drug is generic, the brand name is provided in parentheses.

- Accupril® 5 mg (quinapril HCl): One tab qd
- Aciphex® 20 mg (rabeprazole sodium): One tab qd
- Actos® 7.5-45 mg (pioglitazone HCL): One tab qd
- Adalat® CC 60 mg (nifedipine): One tab Qd, ac
- Advil® (ibuprofen) Children's Suspension: tsp-iid
- Aldactone® 50 mg (spironolactone): One tab Qd
- Aldoril® 25 (methyldopa + HCTZ): One tab bid
- Allegra® 60 mg (Fexoferadine HCl): One cap bid
- Allopurinol 100 mg (Zyloprim®): One tab tid. pc.
- Alupent® Inhaler (metaproterenol sulfate): 2–3 puffs q 3–4 h
- Alupent® Syrup (metaproterenol sulfate): tsp-ii tid. ac
- Ambien® 5 mg (zolpidem tartrate): 2 tabs qd. hs
- Amoxil® 125 mg 5 mL (amoxicillin): tsp tid 7 days
- Anaprox DS® (naproxen sodium): One tab, bid. pc
- Antivert® 25 mg (meclizine HCl): One tab Qd, one hour prior to travel
- Aspirin 325 mg: 2 tabs qid. prn pain
- Atarax® 50 mg (hydroxyeine HCl): i tab, qid
- Ativan® 1 mg (lorazepam): tid. 1–2 tabs
- Atrovent® Inhaler tipratoprium bromide: 1–2 tabs inhalations qid. ud
- Augmentin® 125 mg/5 mL (amoxicillin ÷ clauvinate): One tsp tid. 7 days
- Avalide® 150-300 mg (irbesartan/12.5 mg HCTZ): One tab qd
- Avandia® 4-8 mg (rosiglitazone maleate): One tab qd (8 mg) or bid (4 mg)
- Axid® 300 mg (nizatidine): iqhs
- Azmacort® Inhaler (triamcinolone acetonide): 1–2 inhalations tid.-qid
- Bactrim® DS sulfamethoxazole ÷ trimethoprim): One tab bid. 10 days
- Bactroban® (mupirocin): Apply tid. (or Atid)
- BCP (estrogen + progestin): One tab qd. ud
- Beclovent® (beclomethasone dipropionate): One puffs-ii. qid. ud
- Beconase® (beclomethasone dipropionate): 2 inhalations in each nostril, bid
- Bentyl® 20 mg (dicyclomine HCl): One tab bid. ac
- Betoptic® (betaxolol HCl): gtt-ii ou bid. ud

- Biaxin® 250 mg (clarithromycin): One tab q12h. 7–14 days
- Blocadren® 10 mg (timolol maleate): One tab qd. prn migraine
- Brethaire® (terbutaline sulfate): puffs-ii q 4–6 h
- Bumex® 1 mg (bumetanide): One tab qd
- Buspar® 5 mg (buspirone HCl): One tab tid.
- Calan SR® 240 mg (verapamil HCl): One tab qd
- Capoten® 50 mg (captopril): tab-ss bid star, i tid. ld
- Carafate® Suspension (sucralfate): tsp-ii qid. 4 weeks
- Cardene® 30 mg (nicardipine HCl): One cap tid. ic
- Cardizem® 30 mg (diltiazem HCl): One tab qid
- Cardura® 4 mg (doxazocin mesylate): One tab qd
- Cartia-XT® 120-300 mg (diltiazem HCl): One tab qd
- Cartrol® 5 mg (carteolol HCl): One tab qd star. ii-qd
- Cataflam® 50 mg (diclofenac potassium): I tablet, tid.
- Catapress TTS®-2 Patch (clonidine HCl: Apply to upper arm or chest. q7d. ud
- Ceclor® 250 mg (cefaclor): One cap q8h. finish all
- Ceftin® 250 mg (cefuroxime axetil): One tab bid. finish all.pc
- Cefzil® Suspension 125 mg/5 mL (cefprozil): tsp-i bid. 10 days
- Celebrex® 100-200 mg (celecoxib): One cap bid (100 mg)/one cap qd (200 mg)
- Celexa® 20-40 mg (citalopram hydrobromide): One tab qd
- Chlordiazepoxide 10 mg (Librium®): One tab tid. pc
- Cipro® 500 mg (ciprofloxacin HCl): One tab q12h. 14 days.ac
- Claritin® 10 mg (loratadine): One tab qd. ac
- Cleocin-T® Topical Solution (clindamycin HCl): AA tid. UD
- Clinoril® 200 mg (sulindac): One tab bid. pc. 10 days
- Clonidine® 0.2 mg (Catapress®): One tab, bid
- Clozaril® 25 mg (clozapine): 2 tabs, bid
- Cogentin® 1 mg (benztropine mesylate): 2 tabs qd
- Compazine® Suppositories 25 mg (prochlorperazine): In rect bid
- Corgard® 80 mg (nadolol): 2 qd
- Cortisporin Otic® Solution (neomycin, polymyxin and hydrocortisone): gtt-iv au qid, UD
- Coumadin® 5 mg (warfarin sodium): i qd
- Cozaar® 25 mg (losartan potassium): 1–2 tabs qd
- Cytotec® 100 mcg (misoprostol): One tab qid. pc
- Dalmane® 15 mg (flurazepam HCl): caps-ii qhs
- Darvocet-N 100 (apap/Propoxyphene napsylate): One tab q4h. prn pain
- Daypro® (oxaprozin): ii-qd. pc
- Deconamine Syrup® (cpm and pseudoephedrine): tsp-i. ud
- Deltasone® 50 mg (prednisone): One tab qd. Then reduce the dose gradually as directed.

- Demadex® 10 mg (torsemide): i qd
- Demerol® 50 mg (meperidine HCl): 2 tab, q3h. prn
- Demulen® 35 mcg/1mg (ethinyl estradiol and ethyrodiol diacetate): One tab qd, UD
- Depakene® (valproic acid): 1 tab qd. pc
- Depakote® 125 mg (divalproex Na): 1–2 caps tid.
- Desogen® 0.15 mg/30 mcg (desogestrel and ethinyl estradiol): One tab qd, UD
- Desyrel® 150 mg (trazodone HCl): i qd
- Dexamethasone Oral 2 mg (Decadron®): I qd. om
- Diabeta® 2.5 mg (glyburide): i qd. om
- Diflucan® 100 mg (fluconazole): ii stat, i qd
- Dilacor® XR 180 mg (diltiazem HCl): i qd
- Dilantin® 50 mg Infatabs (phenytoin): ss tab, tid.
- Diphenhydramine HCl Syrup (Benadryl®): tsp-i tid., and ii hs
- Ditropan® (oxybutynin cl): One tab, ac. prn pain
- Dolobid® 250 mg (diflunisal): ii tid. pc
- Donnatal® Extentab (PB + hyoscyamine + atropine + scopolamine): i tid.
- Doral® 15 mg (quazepam): 1/2 tab, qhs
- Doxepin® 75 mg (Sinequan®, Adapin®): One tab qd
- Doxycycline 100 mg (Vibramycin®): One cap bid. 10 days
- Duricef® 1g (cefadroxil monohydrate): i qd. 10 days
- Dyazide® (triamterene + HCTZ): 1 cap qd
- Dynacirc® 5 mg (isradipine): i qd
- E-Mycin® 333 mg (erythromycin): i q8h. p.c., 7 days
- EES® (erythromycin): i q6h. 7 days
- Effexor® 25 mg (verilafaxine HCl): One tab tid.
- Elavil® 50 mg (amitriptyline): One tab qhs
- Eldepryl® (selegiline): i bid
- Elocon® cm (mometasone furoate): AA qd
- Entex® LA (phenylpropanolamine – guaifenesin): i bid
- Equagesic® (meprobamate + aspirin): 2 tabs. qid. prn
- Eryc® (erythromycin): i q6h. 14 days
- Erythromycin 500 mg (PCE®, E-Mycin®. Ilisone®): i q12h, 10 days
- Estrace® 2 mg (estradiol): i qd. cycles of three weeks followed by a week off
- Estraderm® 0.1 mg (estradiol): AUD. BIW
- Eulexin® (flutamide): 2 caps. q8h
- Felbatol® (felbamate): i qid
- Feldene® 20 mg caps (piroxicam): i qd. pc
- Fioricet® (apap. butalbital, caffeine): 2 caps, q4h prn. pain
- Fiorinal® (aspirin, butalbital. caffeine): 2 caps. q4h prn. pain
- Fiorinal® with codeine: 2 caps. q4h. prn pain

- Flagyl® 500 mg (metronidazole): One tab tid. for 5–10 days
- Flexeril® (cyclobenzaprine HCl): i tid.
- Flonase™ 50 mcg per actuation (fluticasone propionate): 2 sprays in each nostril qd
- Floxin® 300 mg tabs (ofloxacin): i q12h. 14 days
- Fosamax® 5 mg (alendronate Na): One tab qd
- Glucophage® 500 mg (metformin HCl): One tab bid, ic
- Glucotrol® 5 mg (glipizide): One tab qd
- Glynase™ PresTab™ 1.5 mg (glyburide): i qd. c breakfast
- Glyset® 25-100 mg (miglitol): One tab tid with the first bite of each meal
- Habitrol® 14 mg (nicotine TDDS): i patch qd. 8 wks
- Halcion® 0.125 mg tabs (triazolam): 1–2 qhs
- Haldol® 0.5 mg (haloperidol): One tab bid
- HCTZ 25 mg tabs (Esidrix®. Hydrodiuril®): ii qd
- HC 10 mg tabs (Cortef®): ii bid
- Hismanal® tabs (astemizole): i qd
- Hydralazine HCl 50 mg tabs (Apresoline®): i qid
- Hydroxyzine 50 mg tabs (Atarax®, Vistaril®): i qid
- Hytrin® 5 mg (terazocin): One tab qd
- Ibuprofen 400 mg tabs (Motrin®): i qid. pc
- Imdur® 30 mg (isosorbide mononitrate): One tab qd
- Imipramine 25 mg (Tofranil®): 2 tabs, qhs
- Imitrex™ 25 mg tab and 6 mg vial (sumatriptan succinate): One tab prn migraine
- Imodium® 2 mg (loperimide HCl): ii stat, i after each BM
- Inderal® 40 mg tab (propranolol HCl): i tid.
- Indocin® 50 mg tabs (indomethacin): i tid. pc
- Insulin NPH (Novolin® Ilentin®, Humulin®): icc, qd sc
- Intal® Inhaler (cromolyn sodium): inhalations-ii. qid. UD
- Ionamin® 15 mg (phentermine resin): One cap ac
- Isoptin® 80 mg (verapamil HCl): i tid.
- Isosorbide Dinitrate 20 mg (Isordil®, Sorbitrate®): One tab, q6h
- K-Dur® 20 meq tabs (potassium chloride): ii qd
- K-Lor® oral solution (potassium bicarbonate/citrate): M in glassful of OJ and drink
- K-Tab® (potassium supplement): ii bid
- Keflet® 250 mg cap (cephalexin): 1–2 tabs qid, 7 days
- Keflex® 500 mg caps (cephalexin): i qid. 7 days
- Kerlone® 10 mg tabs (betaxolol HCl): ii qd
- Klonopin® 1 mg tab (clonazepam): ss tid.
- Lamisil® 250 mg (terbinafine HCl): One qd for six weeks
- Lanoxin® 0.25 mg tabs (digoxin): ss qd
- Lasix® 40 mg (furosemide): One tab qd

- Lescol® 20 mg cap (fluvastatin Na): One tab, qd, hs
- Levaquin® 250-500 mg (levofloxacin): One tab qd
- Levoxyl® 0.125-0.200 mg (levothyroxine): One tab qd
- Lidex® Ont 0.05% (fluocinomide): AA qd
- Lipitor® 10 mg (atorvastatin Ca): One tab qd
- Lithionate® and Lithotabs
- Lithium Carbonate 300 mg tab (Eskalith®. Lithobid®): ii tid.
- Lodine® 300 mg (Etodolac®): One tab tid. pc
- Loestrin FE® 1 mg/20 mcg/75 mg (norethindrone, ethinyl estradiol, ferrous fumarate): 1 qd
- Lomotil® (diphenoxylate HCl + atropine sulfate): tsp-tid. prn diarrhea
- Lopid® 600 mg (gemfibrozil): One tab bid. ac
- Lopressor® 50 mg (metoprolol tartrate): 2 tab qd
- Lorabid® (loracarbet): One tab bid. ac. 7 days
- Lorcet® Plus & Lorcet 10/650
- Lorelco® 250 mg (probucol): 2 tab qd
- Lortab® 5/500 (apap + hydrocodone bitartrate): q4-6h, prn pain
- Lotensin® 10 mg tabs (benazepril HCl): i qd
- Lotrimin® cm 1% (clotrimazole): AA bid. UD
- Lotrisone® (clotrimazole + betamethasone dipropionate): AA tid.
- Lozol® 1.25 mg tab (indapamide): ii qd
- Macrodantin® 50 mg tabs (Nitrofurantoin macrocrystals): i qid. 7 days
- Maxair® Autohaler (pirbuterol acetate): puffs-ii q4-6h. UD
- Maxalt® 5-10 mg (rizatriptan benzoate): One tab qd (max 30 mg/24 hr)
- Maxaquin® tabs (lomefloxacin HCl): i qid. 14 days
- Maxzide® 25-mg (triamterene/HCTZ): 2 caps qd
- Mecliziné HCl 50 mg tabs (Antivert®): One tab prior to travel
- Meclomen® 50 mg tabs (meclofenamate): i qid. pc
- Medrol® 4 mg tab (methylprednisolone): ii qd
- Mellaril® 50 mg tab (thioridazine HCl): i tid.
- Meridia® 5-15 mg (sibutramine HCl): One tab qd (10 mg)
- Methyldópa 250 mg tab (Aldomet®): ii bid
- Metronidazole 250 mg tab (Flagyl®): i tid. 7 days
- Mevacor® 20 mg tab (lovastatin): i qd, pm
- Micro-K Extencaps® 8 meq (potassium chloride): ii qd
- Micronase® 2.5 mg tab (glyburide): i qd
- Minipress® 2 mg tab (prazocin HCl): i qd, hs
- Minocin® 50 mg tab (minocycline HCl): i qid, finish all
- Monopril® 10 mg tabs (fosinopril sodium): i bid, ac
- Motrin® 600 mg tabs (ibuprofen): i tid., pc
- Mycelex® vaginal cm (clotrimazole): Ins one applicatorful hs, 7 days
- Naldecon® Syrup (cpm + ppa + phenylephrine + phenyltoloxamine): tsp-q3-4h, prn allergy

- Nalfon® 300 mg tab (fenoprofen): 1–2 tid., pc
- Naprosyn® 500 mg tab (naproxen sodium): i bid, pc
- Nasacort® (triamcinolone acetonide): Two sprays in each nostril, qd
- Nasalcrom® (cromolyn sodium): One spray in each nostril, qid
- Nasalide® (flunisolide): Two sprays in each nostril, bid
- Neurontin® 300 mg (gabapentin): One tid
- Nicoderm® 14 mg (nicotine TDDS): One patch q24h, ud
- Nitro-Dur® 0.3 mg/hr (NTG TDDS): One pacth qd. ud
- Nitroglycerin 2.5 mg tab (Nitro-Bid®): i tid.
- NTG Oint: Apply ½″ q8h over 2 1/4 and 3 ½″ area
- NTG SL 0.3 mg tab (Nitrostat®): One SL, prn
- Nitrostat® 0.3 mg (NTG): One SL, prn
- Nizoral® tab (ketoconazole): 1–2 qd
- Nolvadex® tab (tamoxifen citrate): i AM & i PM
- Normodyne® 200 mg (labetolol HCl): One tab bid. ic
- Noroxin® (norfloxacin): One tab q12h, 14 days
- Norpramin® 50 mg (desipramine HCl): One tab bid
- Norvasc® 5 mg (amiodipine besylate): One tab qd
- Nystatin tab 500,000 units (mycostatin): One troche 5 X daily, 14 days
- Ogen® 1.25 mg (estropipate): 1–2 tab qd. ic
- Omnicef® 300 mg (celdinir): One cap bid
- Omnipen® 250 mg (ampicillin): One qid, 7–10 days
- Organidin® liquid elixir (iodinated glycerol): i-tsp, qid
- Ornade® spansule (cpm + ppa): i q12h
- Ortho-Cept® 0.15 mg/30 mcg (desogestrel and ethinyl estradiol): One qd, UD
- Ortho-Cyclen® 0.25 mg/35 mcg (norgestimae and ethinyl estradiol): One qd, UD
- Ortho-Novum® 1 mg/35 mcg (norethindrone and ethinyl estradiol): One qd UD
- Orudis® 50 mg (ketoprofen): i cap q6h, prn pain. pc
- Ovral® 0.5 mg/50 mcg (norgestrel and ethinyl estradiol): One qd, UD
- Pamelor® 25 mg (nortriptyline HCl): i cap. tid.
- Parlodel® 2.5 mg (bromocriptine mesylate): One tab qd
- Paxil® 20 mg (paroxetine HCl): One tab, qAM
- PCE® 333 mg (erythromycin): One tab q8h, finish all
- Pediazole® susp (erythromycin es + sulfisoxazole acetyl): tsp-i q6h. 10 days
- Penicillin VK 250 mg (Pen-Vee K®): One tab qid, 10 days
- Pepcid® 20 mg (famotidine): ii qd. hs
- Percocet® (apap/oxycodone): One tab, q6h, prn pain
- Percodan® (aspirin + oxycodone HCl + oxycodone terephthalate): One tab. q6h. prn pain

- Peridex® (chlorhexidine gluconate): 15 mL bid, swish for 30 sec and spit it out
- Persantin® 50 mg (dipyridamole): 2 tab qid, 30 min ac
- Phenergan® 25 mg (promethazine HCl): 1–2 tab, q4–6h. prn
- Phenergan® with codeine Liq: tsp-i q4–6h, prn
- Phenobarbital® 15 mg (phenobarbital): One tab bid
- PB 30 mg tab (Barbital®): One tab tid, prn sedation
- Pilocarpine (Pilocar®): 1–2 gtt ou, q4h, ud
- Plendil® 5 mg (felodipine): One tab, qd
- Poly-Vi-Flor® 0.25 liq dps (vit + fluoride): One dropperful po. qd
- Ponstel® Kapseals (mefenamic acid): i q6h, prn pain
- Potassium chloride 10 meq (K-Dur®, Slow-K®, Ten-K®, Micro-K, Klor-Con®): 2 tabs bid
- Pravachol® 10 mg (pravastatin sodium): 1–2 qd, hs
- Pred Forte® (prednisolone acetate): gtt-i ou qid, ud
- Prednisone 5 mg (Deltasone®, Orasone®): 2 tabs tid, ud
- Prelone® 15 mg per 5 mL syrup (prednisolone): one tsp qd. Then reduce the dose gradually as directed.
- Premarin® 0.9 mg (conjugated estrogens): One tab qd, ud
- Premarin® vag cm: In vag ii applicatorful. Cycles of 3 wks on and 1 wk off.
- Prempro® 0.625 mg/2.5 mg (conjugated estrogens and medroxyprogesterone acetate): I qd
- Prevacid® 15 mg (lansoprasole): One cap, ac for 4 wks
- Prilosec® (omeprazole): One tab qd, 6 wks
- Prinivil® 10 mg (lisinopril): One tab. qd, ac
- Procainamide 500 mg (Procan SR®): One tab. q3h
- Procardia® XL 30 mg (nifedipine): One tab. qd
- Prochlorperazine 10 mg (Compazine®): One tab qd. prn nausea
- Propine® (dipivefrin HCl) gtt-i ou, q12h. UD
- Propulsid® (Cisapride): One tab tid, ac & i hs
- Proscar® (finasteride): One tab, qd, ud
- Prosom® 1 mg (estazolam): One tab. qhs
- Prostep® 22 mg/day (nicotine TDDS): i patch/day 4–8 wks, ud
- Proventil® Inhaler (albuterol): puffs i–ii q4–6h, ud
- Proventil® 4 mg tab: i tid
- Provera® 5 mg (medroxyprogesterone acetate): 1–2 tab qd, ud
- Prozac® 20 mg (fluoxetine HCl): One tab bid
- Pyridium® 200 mg (phenazopyridine HCl): One tab tid, pc, 2 days
- Questran® powder (cholestyramine): One packet mix c a glassful of water and drink daily
- Quinidine gluconate (Quinaglute Dura-Tabs®): One tab q8-12h
- Quinidine sulfate 300 mg (Quinidex Extentabs®): One tab, tid

- Reglan® 5 mg (metoclopramide HCl): One tab bid, ac and i hs
- Relafen® 500 mg (nabumetone): 2 tab qd. pc
- Restoril® 15 mg (temazepam): One tab, qhs
- Retin-A® cm 0.1% (tretinoin): AA qhs
- Retrovir® (zidovudine, AZT): i q4h. ATC
- Rhincort® 50 mcg per actuation (budesonide): Puffs-ii au bid
- Risperdal® 1 mg (risperidone): One tab bid
- Ritalin® 10 mg (methylphenidate): One tab tid, ac
- Robaxin® 500 mg (methocarbomol): One tab qid
- Rogaine® (minoxidil): 1cc AA bid
- Rythmol® 150 mg (propafenone HCl): One tab, q8H
- Seldane® (terfenadine): One tab, bid
- Septra® DS (sulfamethoxazole/tmp): One tab, bid, 10 days
- Serax® 15 mg (oxazepam): One tab, tid
- Serevent® 25 mcg per actuation (salmeterol xinafoate): Puffs-ii q12h, UD
- Serzone® 50 mg (nefazodone HCl): Tabs-ii bid
- Sinemet® 25–100 (carbidopa + levodopa): One tab, tid
- Sinequan® 25 mg (doxepin HCl): One tab bid
- Slo-Bid® 100 mg (theophylline): 2 caps, bid, UD
- Slo-Phyllin® 200 mg (theophylline): One tab, bid
- Slow-K® (potassium chloride): One tab, qd
- Soma® (carisoprodol): One tab tid, & hs
- Sonata® 5-10 mg (zaleplon): One tab qhs
- Sporanox® (itraconazole): 2 tab qd
- Sumycin® 250 mg (tetracycline HCl): One cap qid, 7 days
- Suprax® 200 mg (cefixime): i bid, finish all
- Synthroid® 100 mcg (levothyroxine sodium): One tab qd, ac
- Tagamet® 400 mg (cimetidine): One tab, bid, 8 wks
- Talwin NX® (pentazocine ÷ naloxone): One tab q3-4h. prn pain
- Tegretol® 100 mg (carbamazepine): One tab, bid
- Tenex® 1 mg (guanfacine HCl): One tab, qhs
- Tenoretic® 50 mg (atenolol + chlorthalidone): One tab, qd
- Tenormin® 50 mg (atenolol): One tab, qd
- Terazol® 7 cm (terconazole): i applicatorful in vag, qhs, 7 days
- Terazol® 3 suppository: One sup in v qhs, 3 days
- Tetracycline HCl 250 mg (Achromycin®. Sumycin®): One cap, qid, ac
- Theo-Dur® 300 mg (theophylline): One tab, q12h
- Theo-24® 200 mg (theophylline): 2 caps qd, ac
- Theo-Dur Sprinkle® 75 mg (theophylline): caps-ii, bid, UD
- Thyroid 60 mg tabs: i qd
- Ticlid® (ticlopidine HCl): One tab, bid, ic
- Tilade® (nedocromil sodium): 2 puffs, qid, UD

- Timoptic® (timolol maleate): gtt-i ou bid
- Tobradex® ophthalmic oint (tobramycin and dexamethasone): Apply ½ ou tid
- Tobrex® op oint (tobramycin): a ou, qid, UD
- Tofranil® 50 mg (imipramine HCl): One tab qd
- Tolazamide 250 mg (Tolinase®): i tab, qd
- Tolectin DS® (tolmetin sodium): One tab, tid, pc
- Toprol-XL™ 50 mg (metoprolol succinate): One qd
- Toradol® tab (ketorolac tromethamine): i q4–6h, prn, UD
- Trandate® 200 mg (laberolol HCl): ss tab, bid, ic
- Transderm-Nitro® 0.2 mg/hr (NTG TDDS): i patch qd. UD
- Transderm-Scop® (scopolamine): i patch. biw. UD
- Tranxene® 15 mg (clorazepate dipotassium): One tab, bid, pc
- Trental® (pentoxifylline): One tab, bid, 8 wks
- Triamcinolone 4 mg (Aristocort®, Kenacort®): One tab, qd
- Triavil® 4–10 (amitriptyline HCl + perphenazine): One tab, tid
- Tri-Levlen® 0.05 mg/30 mcg (levonorgesterol and ethinyl estradiol): One qd, UD
- Triphasil® (levonorgesterol and ethinyl estradiol): One qd, UD
- Trusopt® ophthalmic solution (dorzolamide HCl): gtt-ii ou tid
- Tuss-Ornade® (caramiphen edisylate/ppa): One cap, q12h
- Tussi-Organidin® (iodinated glycerol): 1–2 isp, q4h
- Tussionex® Suspension (chlorpheniramine and hydrocodone): tsp i q12h
- Tylenol® #3 (apap + codeine phosphate): 1–2 tab, q4h, prn
- Tylox® (apap + oxycodone): One cap, q6h, prn
- Ultram® 50 mg (tramadol HCl): One tab q4–6h
- Valium® 5 mg (diazepam): One tab bid, prn
- Vancenase AQ® (beclomethasone dipropionate): i inh in each nostril, tid, UD
- Vanceril® Inh (beclomethasone dipropionate): puffs-ii tid-qid, UD
- Vantin® 100 mg (cefpodoxime proxetil): One tab bid, 14 days
- Vascor® 300 mg (bepridil HCl): One tab qd
- Vaseretic® 10–25 (enalapril maleate + HCTZ): 1–2 tab qd
- Vasotec® 5 mg (enalapril maleate): One tab, qd
- Veetids® 250 mg (penicillin V potassium): One qid, 7 days
- Velosef® 250 mg (cephradine): One cap q6h, finish all
- Ventolin® Inh (albuterol): puffs-ii q4–6h
- Ventolin® tabs 2 mg (albuterol sulfate): i tid
- Verapamil 80 mg tab (Calan®, Isoptin®): i tid, UD
- Verelan® 180 mg (verapamil HCl SR): i cap. bid
- Viagra® 25-100 mg (sildenafil citrate): One tab qd, one hour before sexual activity
- Vibramycin® 100 mg (doxycycline hyclate): One cap bid, 7 days

- Vicodin ES® (apap + hydrocodone bitartrate): 1–2 tabs q4–6h. prn pain
- Vioxx® 12.5-25 mg (rofecoxib): One tab qd
- Visken® 5 mg (pindolol): One tab, bid
- Vistaril® 25 mg (hydroxyzine pamoate): 1–2 caps qid. for N & V
- Voltaren® 50 mg (diclofenac sodium): One tab bid, pc
- Wellbutrin® 100 mg (bupropion HCl): One tab bid
- Xalaton® Ophthalmic solution (latanoprost): gtt-i ou qd
- Xanax® 1 mg (alprazolam): One tab bid
- Zantac® 150 mg (Ranitidine HCl): One tab bid
- Zebeta® 5-10 mg (bisoprolol fumarate): one tab qd
- Zestril® 10 mg (Lisinopril): One tab qd
- Ziac® 2.5 mg (bisoprolol fumarate and hydrochlorothiazide): One tab qd
- Zithromax® 250 mg (Azithromycin): ii stat. 1 qd, 5 days
- Zocor® 10 mg (Simvastatin): One tab qhs
- Zofran® 4 mg (Odantsetron HCl): 2 tab tid
- Zoloft® 50 mg (Sertraline HCl): One tab qd
- Zovirax® 200 mg (Acyclovir): One cap q4h. 10 days
- Zyloprim® 100 mg (allopurinol): One tab bid
- Zyrtec® 5 mg (cetirizine HCl): One tab qd

PRESCRIPTION PROBLEMS

A pharmacist or a nurse has to perform some simple mathematical computations related to the dosage form strength, the quantity of medication, dates for the refills, and the medication costs, etc. As a few examples, very often, the prescribing authority writes the dosage regimen for a particular strength of a medication but doesn't write the total units of the medication. The pharmacist or the nurse then calculate the number of dosage units and dispenses them. Sometime the medication available in the pharmacy is of a different strength than the one prescribed. The number of dosage units and the directions for administration have to be modified by a few calculations. The following are a few examples of the prescription problems.

Example 1:
℞

Amoxicillin 125 mg/5 mL

Sig: ii tsp tid, 7 days

How many f℥ of amoxicillin suspension would the patient receive?

$$2 \times 5 \text{ mL} = 10 \text{ mL, each dose}$$

$$10 \times 3 = 30 \text{ mL per day}$$

$$30 \times 7 = 210 \text{ mL or f℥ vii for seven days}$$

answer: 7 fluidounces

Example 2:

℞
   HCTZ   50 mg
            #XC

   Sig: i tab q AM for HPB

Re: 1

If this prescription was filled on April 15, when would the refill be due? Ninety tablets were dispensed with instructions to take one tablet every morning for high blood pressure. The medication would last for 90 days.

answer: the refill would be due on July 15

Example 3:

℞

   Keflex caps   500 mg

   Sig: i cap bid. 10 days

If the pharmacist has only 250 mg capsules in the inventory, how many capsules should be given to the patient?
20 capsules of 500 mg can be substituted with 40 capsules of 250 mg.

answer: 40 capsules

Practice Problems

(1) ℞

      Insulin 100 units/cc
                #10 cc

      Sig: 10 units bid, sc
      How many days would the medication last?

(2) ℞

>   Dr. Zogg's otic drops
>   15 cc
>
>   Sig: 0.1 cc au tid, prn pain

If a calibrated dropper delivers 40 drops per 2 mL, how many drops should the patient instill in each each every time?

(3) ℞

>   Aspirin   gr v
>   Caffeine   gr i
>   Lactose qs
>
>   Ft. cap. DTD #xx

How many grams of aspirin are needed for the above prescription?

Refer to the sample medication order (Figure 3.3) to answer questions 4 and 5.

(4) Assume that the patient has taken the medication at 6 P.M. but continues to suffer from pain. At what time should the next dose be taken?

(5) If doxycycline is authorized, how many 100 mg tablets would the patient need? When should the medication be administered?

(6) ℞

>   Chloral hydrate elixir
>
>   Sig: i dose of 250 mg, po hs

How many teaspoonfuls of chloral hydrate with a strength of gr viiss/5 mL should be administered to the patient and at what time of day?

(7) ℞

>   Erythromycin liquid (125 mg/tsp)
>
>   Sig: 250 mg qid po 10 days

If the medication was dispensed from a bottle containing one pint, how many milliliters of medication would be left in the original container?

(8) ℞

Atropine Sulfate 0.3 mg

Sig: Administer intramuscularly

If the available atropine vial label reads gr 1/150 per mL, how many milliliters of the injection should be administered?

(9) A 44-lb patient is to receive amoxicillin dosed at 100 mg per kg of body weight daily for 10 days. How many mL of an amoxicillin suspension (250 mg/tsp) should be dispensed?

(10) ℞

ppt sulfur
benzoic acid, aa 5% w/w
salicylic acid 10% w/w
hydrophilic ointment qs

Disp: 60 g

How many grams of sulfur are required for the prescription?

ERRORS AND OMISSIONS

Prescription errors are unintentional mistakes in the prescription, transcription, dispensing, and administration of medications. The patient either receives the medication incorrectly or fails to receive it altogether. Some prescription errors include wrong patient, incorrect medication, inappropriate dose, wrong time, wrong route of administration, and wrong rate of administration. For example, the profile of a patient shows that he is allergic to codeine, and yet he receives Tylenol® #3 by an error.

To prevent prescription or medication errors, it is a good practice to follow the "five rights principle" as a check: the right medication—in the right dose—to the right patients—at the right time—by the right route of administration. The following guideline may be helpful to a pharmacist for filling prescriptions:

(1) Make sure all the information required to fill the prescription is present. A systematic, step-by-step checking would be very helpful.
(2) Make sure that the information is correctly transferred to the prescription label.
(3) Make sure that the correct drug is being dispensed, whether generic or brand.

(4) Make sure that the DEA number is verified. The procedure for verification is provided below.

Verification of the DEA Number

The DEA number is a unique character code which can be easily verified in most cases. The first two of the nine characters are alphabets. The first alphabet is either an A or B, or alternatively, a P or R; the letters A and B designate a dispenser, while the letters P or R refer to a distributor. The second alphabet is derived from the first letter of the registrant's last name or his/her business name. These two alphabets cannot always be verified. The third to ninth positions from left represent a seven digit number which can be verified. To understand the procedure, an example of DEA #AB 0494168 verification is provided here.

(1) Add first, third, and the fifth digit of the seven-digit number following the alphabets, i.e., $0 + 9 + 1 = 10$.

(2) Add second, fourth, and the sixth number and multiply the resultant sum by two, i.e., $4 + 4 + 6 = 14$ and $14 \times 2 = 28$.

(3) Add the results of step 1 and step 2, i.e., $10 + 28 = 38$.

(4) The right most digit is eight here. The seventh or the last digit of the DEA number is also 8.

If a DEA number follows the above rule of matching the right digit, it is most likely a genuine number. If a number doesn't match the above number, it could be an illegal prescription and the pharmacist or the nurse should verify it further by contacting the appropriate authorities.

A few examples of prescription errors are provided as follows:

Example 1:

Jack Ramos, M.D.
911 Hollywood Avenue
Detroit, MI-71208
Phone No. 555-1234

Name : John Doe   Age: 70
Address: 96 Havana Blvd., MI-71208   Date: 2/28/96

Rx

Keflex 500 mg

Sig: i cap qid, 7 days

REFILL _None_

DAW _____

JRamos
DEA # AD 7973142

NORTHEAST PHARMACY
169 Hillside Avenue
Monroe, LA 71206   555-0342

R # 123456   Date: 2/28/96
Doe, John
911 Hollywood Ave
Take one capsule four times a day for
seven days
Cephalexin Caps 500 mg #40
Refill 1   J. Ramos, M.D.

Errors

1. Patient's address is wrong.
2. Number of capsules = 4 × 7 = 28 and not 40.
3. Prescription shows no refill, and the label shows one refill.
4. The DEA number is wrong.

Example 2:

```
                    Pat Moody
                 96 Alonzo Drive
                 Miami, FL-71208
                Phone No. 555-1234
──────────────────────────────────────────
  Name : Baby Starks            Age: 6 mo.
  Address: 96 Havana Blvd., FL-71208  Date: 2/29/96

  R

        Vantin 100 mg

        Sig: ss ʒ bid, 7 days


  REFILL  None

  DAW
                    PMoody
```

```
           NORTHEAST PHARMACY
              169 Hillside Avenue
           Monroe, LA 71206    555-0342

  R # 123456        Date: 2/29/95
  Starks, Baby
  96 Havana Blvd.
  Take one-half tablet twice daily for seven
  days
  Vantin 100 mg tablets
  Refill 1              P. Moody
```

Errors

1. No qualifications for Pat Moody. He is not authorized to prescribe the medication.
2. Wrong date on the label.
3. The doctor meant Vantin suspension (100 mg/5 mL) which is clear from the *signa*. Tablets are a wrong choice for an infant.
4. *Signa* should be one-half teaspoonful twice daily for seven days.
5. No refills. The label shows one.
6. Registration number or DEA is missing for Pat Moody.

Example 3:

Medication profile and a prescription

Roslyn Monroe
20 Main Street
Monroe, LA 71201   Allergy: Aspirin

Date	Dr.	R #	Patient	Drug
3/1/95	Quinn	12340	Roslyn	Synthroid 0.2 mg #100, 1 daily
5/6/95	Quinn	12350	Roslyn	Hygroton 2.5 mg #70, 1 qd
7/7/95	Quinn	12369	Roslyn	Tylenol #3 #30, ii tid, prn

Doc Rogers, M.D.
12 Desiard Street
Monroe, LA-71208
Phone No. 555-1234

Name : Roslyn Monroe   **Age**: 58 yrs
Address: 20 Main Street, Monroe   **Date**: 7/9/95

R

Fiorinal with Codeine
 # 40

Sig: ii caps, q4h daily

REFILL _1_____

DAW _✓_____

DRogers
DEA # DR1234567

Errors

1. Roslyn Monroe is allergic to aspirin. Therefore, Fiorinal® with Codeine, which contains aspirin, should not be given.
2. Roslyn Monroe is taking Tylenol® #3, which contains codeine, since 7/7/95. Probably the codeine preparation is being abused, and Dr. Rogers should be informed.

Practice Problems

Identify errors and omissions in the following prescriptions.

(1)

```
┌─────────────────────────────────────────────────────┐
│              Henry Huxtable, M.D.                    │
│              61-40 Flushing Avenue                   │
│                Monroe, LA 71208                      │
│               Phone No. 555-1234                     │
├─────────────────────────────────────────────────────┤
│  Name : John Doe              Age: 30                │
│  Address: 96 Havana Blvd., FL 31207   Date: 2/28/96 │
│                                                       │
│   R                                                   │
│   x                                                   │
│                                                       │
│          Tagamet  300 mg                             │
│                                                       │
│                                                       │
│          Sig:  i bid, 15 days                        │
│                                                       │
│                                                       │
│   REFILL _None_                                      │
│                                                       │
│   DAW ___✓_____                                      │
│                            _HHuxtable_              │
│                         DEA # AD 7973142            │
│                                                       │
└─────────────────────────────────────────────────────┘
```

```
┌──────────────────────────────────────────┐
│         NORTHEAST PHARMACY                │
│           169 Hillside Avenue             │
│        Monroe, LA 71206     555-0342      │
│                                            │
│  R # 123456         Date: 2/28/96         │
│  Doe, John                                 │
│  96 Havana Blvd.                           │
│  Take one tablet at bed time               │
│  Ranitidine 300 mg  # 40                   │
│            H. Huxtable, M.D.              │
└──────────────────────────────────────────┘
```

(2)

Henry Huxtable, M.D.
61-40 Flushing Avenue
Monroe, LA 71208
Phone No. 555-1234

Name : Baby Gore _____ Age: 8 mo. ___
Address: 96 Havana Blvd., FL 31207   Date: 2/28/96

R

V-Cillin K 250 mg/tablet

Disp. # 28

Sig: i tab q6h until finished

REFILL _____

DAW _____

HHuxtable
DEA # AD 7973142

NORTHEAST PHARMACY
169 Hillside Avenue
Monroe, LA 71206   555-0342

R # 123456   Date: 2/28/96
Gore, Baby
96 Havana Blvd.
Take one tablet every six hours until
Friday
Pen-VK 250 mg
          H. Huxtable, M.D.

(3)

Henry Huxtable, M.D.
61-40 Flushing Avenue
Monroe, LA 71208
Phone No. 555-1234

Name : Pat O'Neal   Age: 23
Address: 96 Havana Blvd., FL 31207   Date: 2/28/96

R

Neosynephrine 2.5%
10 mL

Sig: i gtt os tid

REFILL _____

DAW _____

HHuxtable
DEA # AD 7973142

NORTHEAST PHARMACY
169 Hillside Avenue
Monroe, LA 71206   555-0342

R # 123456   Date: 2/28/96
O'Neal, Pat
96 Havana Blvd.
Instill one drop in each nostril three
times daily
Neosynephrine 1.5%
          H. Huxtable, M.D.

(4)

Henry Huxtable, M.D.
61-40 Flushing Avenue
Monroe, LA 71208
Phone No. 555-1234

Name : <u>Magic Jordan</u>   Age: <u>36</u>
Address: <u>96 Havana Blvd., FL 31207</u>   Date: <u>2/28/96</u>

Rx

Xanax 0.25
#30

Sig: ss tab qd

REFILL _____

DAW _____

                          HHuxtable
            DEA # AL5052841

NORTHEAST PHARMACY
169 Hillside Avenue
Monroe, LA 71206   555-0342

R # 123456   Date: 2/28/96
Jordan, Magic
96 Havana Blvd.
Take one-half tablet daily
Zantac 0.25
            H. Huxtable, M.D.

(5)

Henry Huxtable, M.D.
61-40 Flushing Avenue
Monroe, LA 71208
Phone No. 555-1234

Name : Gill Bates　　　　**Age**: 2 yrs
Address: 96 Havana Blvd., FL 31207　**Date**: 2/28/96

R

Ampicillin 250 mg/tsp

 # f ℥ v

Sig: tsptid, 10 days

REFILL _____

DAW _____

　　　　　　　　　　HHuxtable
　　　　　　　　DEA # AD 7973142

NORTHEAST PHARMACY
169 Hillside Avenue
Monroe, LA 71206　　555-0342

R # 123456　　　Date: 2/28/96
Bates, Gill
96 Havana Blvd.
Take one tablespoonful three times daily
for 10 days
Amoxicillin 250 mg/5 mL
　　　　　H. Huxtable, M.D.

(6)

Henry Huxtable, M.D.
61-40 Flushing Avenue
Monroe, LA 71208
Phone No. 555-1234

Name : Roger Williams   **Age:** 34

Address: 96 Havana Blvd., FL 31207   **Date:** 2/28/96

R℣

Septra DS
                    #20

Sig: i bid, 7 days

REFILL _____

DAW ___✓_____

                    HHuxtable
                    DEA # AD 7973142

NORTHEAST PHARMACY
169 Hillside Avenue
Monroe, LA 71206   555-0342

R # 123456   Date: 2/28/96
Williams, Roger
96 Havana Blvd.
Take one tablet twice daily for seven
days
Sulfameth/TMP 400/80 mg # 20
          H. Huxtable, M.D.

(7)

Henry Huxtable, M.D.
61-40 Flushing Avenue
Monroe, LA 71208
Phone No. 555-1234

Name : <u>Mary Green</u>   **Age**: <u>4 mo.</u>
Address: <u>96 Havana Blvd., FL 31207</u>   **Date**: <u>2/28/96</u>

℞

APAP Suppositories 2 gr
#10

Sig: In. rect q4h, prn fever over 101°

REFILL _____

DAW _____

HHuxtable
DEA # AD 7973142

NORTHEAST PHARMACY
169 Hillside Avenue
Monroe, LA 71206   555-0342

℞ # 123456   Date: 2/28/96
Green, Mary
96 Havana Blvd.
Insert one suppository rectally four times
daily for fever over 101°
ASA Suppositories 2 gr #10
H. Huxtable, M.D.

(8) Medication profile and a prescription

| Evelyn Monroe | | | | Allergy: Penicillin, Sulfa |

Evelyn Monroe
20 Main Street
Monroe, LA 71201

Allergy: Penicillin, Sulfa

Date	Dr.	R#	Patient	Drug
3/1/95	Quinn	12340	Evelyn	Synthroid 0.2 mg #100, 1 daily
5/6/95	Quinn	12350	Evelyn	Hygroton 2.5 mg #70, 1 qd
7/7/95	Quinn	12369	Evelyn	Tylenol #3 #30, ii tid, prn

Doc Rogers, M.D.
12 Desiard Street
Monroe, LA-71208
Phone No. 555-1234

Name : Evelyn Monroe   **Age**: 18 yrs
Address: 20 Main Street, Monroe   **Date**: 7/9/95

℞

Bactrim Tablets

Sig: iqid, 7 days

REFILL 1

DAW ✓

DRogers
DEA # DR1234567

NORTHEAST PHARMACY
169 Hillside Avenue
Monroe, LA 71206   555-0342

℞ # 123456   Date: 2/28/96
Monroe, Evelyn
20 Main St
Take one tablet four times daily for
seven days
SMZ/TMP 800/160 mg # 28
            D. Rogers, M.D.

(9)

Henry Huxtable, M.D.
61-40 Flushing Avenue
Monroe, LA 71208
Phone No. 555-1234

Name : Elvis Jackson   **Age:** 52

Address: 96 Havana Blvd., FL 31207   **Date:** 2/28/96

R

Cortisporin otic solution

10 mL

Sig: iv gtt ad qid

REFILL _____

DAW __✓_____

HHuxtable
DEA # AD 0510323

NORTHEAST PHARMACY
169 Hillside Avenue
Monroe, LA 71206   555-0342

R # 123456   Date: 2/28/96
Jackson, Elvis
96 Havana Blvd.
Instill six drops in the right eye every
four hours
Cortisporin otic suspension #100 cc
H. Huxtable, M.D.

(10)

Henry Huxtable, M.D.
61-40 Flushing Avenue
Monroe, LA 71208
Phone No. 555-1234

Name : <u>Beverly Jones</u>   Age: <u>36</u>
Address: <u>96 Havana Blvd., FL 31207</u>   Date: <u>2/28/96</u>

R

Tenormin Tablets 50 mg

 # 100

Sig: i qd

REFILL _____

DAW __✓_____

HHuxtable
DEA # AD 0510323

NORTHEAST PHARMACY
169 Hillside Avenue
Monroe, LA 71206   555-0342

R # 123456   Date: 2/28/96
Jones, Beverly
96 Havana Blvd.
Tenormin 100 mg #50
          H. Huxtable, M.D.

CHAPTER 4

Principles of Weighing and Measuring

Weighing and measuring are two of the most important aspects of dispensing, compounding, and administration of medications. The present chapter deals with the fundamental operation of a prescription balance, an understanding of sensitivity requirement, an introduction to various devices used for measuring volumes of liquids, and their pertinent calculations. A knowledge of the systems of measurement, which is covered in Chapter 2, is essential to understand the material presented in this chapter.

PRESCRIPTION BALANCE AND SENSITIVITY REQUIREMENT

The successful performance of dispensing and compounding operations in a pharmacy depends on a thorough understanding of the principles of the prescription balance and strict adherence to the procedures of its care and use. Therefore, it is essential to learn proper weighing techniques, and to be conscious of the limitations of the balance to weigh certain quantities. All pharmacies are required to have a Class A prescription balance which meets the requirements of the National Bureau of Standards. It is based upon the principle of torsion. Some states may allow the use of a balance other than the Class A prescription balance, provided that their sensitivity requirement is six milligrams or less.

Solid and semi-solid substances are weighed on special weighting papers which are different from powder papers. A weighing paper has a glazed surface and is square in shape. The paper protects the pans of the prescription balance from chemical reactions and eliminates the need for repeated cleaning. It also prevents contamination. The paper for weighing should be of reasonable size to fit in the pan of the balance. It should be creased diagonally before placing

73

on the pan. It is a good practice to have a paper on each of the pans and to zero the balance before beginning the weighing operation. This zeroing is important because individual weighing papers from the same box may not be of same weight.

The balance should be arrested each time a substance is added or removed. With the balance arrested, open the balance lid and place the desired weights on the right pan. Place the material to be weighed on the left pan, then unlock the balance to observe if the material is too little or too much. Using the appropriate spatula, add or remove the material as needed. When the desired weight is obtained, the balance should be arrested, the lid closed, and the arrest is released to check the equilibrium. The arresting knob is most conveniently operated by the left hand. If the balance is not arrested, the sensitivity of the balance will be affected. For weighing liquids, small beakers or plastic weighing cups may be used after taring. A picture of the prescription balance is shown in Figure 4.1.

The Class A Prescription balance has a sensitivity requirement of 6 mg with no load and with a load of 10 g on each pan. Subject to the physical limitation of the material being weighed, the maximum amount that can be weighed on this balance is 120 g. A Class B prescription balance has a sensitivity requirement of 30 mg. The minimum amounts that can be weighed with an error of not more than 5% on Class A and Class B balances are 120

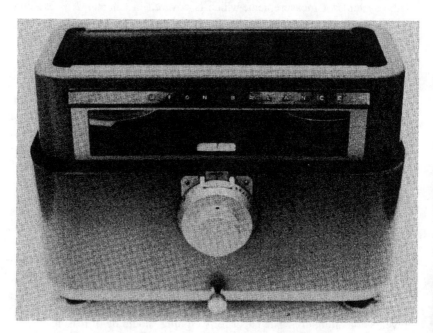

FIGURE 4.1. Class A prescription balance.

mg and 600 mg, respectively. Whenever a balance is used for the first time in a pharmacy or a laboratory, especially when the history or the condition of the balance is in doubt, four tests should be performed on the balance. They are the sensitivity requirement test, arm ratio test, shift test, and rider and graduated beam test. The procedure for these tests is beyond the scope of this text; however, it is important to know some fundamental calculations pertaining to the sensitivity requirement.

Sensitivity requirement is the minimum weight required to move the pointer by one division on the scale. The smaller the weight required to move the pointer by one division, the more sensitive is the balance. Sensitivity requirement (SR) is related to the percent error or maximum potential error by the equation,

$$\%\text{Error} = \text{SR} \times 100/\text{quantity to be weighed } (Q)$$

Percent error (%E) can also be figured by the formula given below:

$$\%E = \frac{|\text{ Actual weight or volume} - \text{Intended weight or volume }|}{(\text{Intended weight or volume})} \times 100$$

It should be remembered that if the potential for a maximum error is 5%, the percent confidence of being correct is 95. The sensitivity requirement can also be determined by finding the number of divisions a pointer moves when a 10 or 20 mg weight is added to the right pan of the prescription balance A. For example, if the pointer moves by three divisions with a weight of 20 mg, the sensitivity requirement is 20/3 = 6.67 mg.

A typical weight set used with the Class A prescription balance contains the following weights: 100 g, 50 g, 20 g (two in number), 10 g, 5 g, 2 g (two in number), 1 g, 500 mg, 200 mg (two in number), 100 mg, 50 mg, 20 mg (two in number), 10 mg, 5 mg, 2 mg (two in number), and 1 mg.

Example 1:

What is the minimum amount that can be weighed on a Class A prescription balance with a potential error of not more than 10%?

$$\%\text{Error} = 100 \times 6 \text{ mg}/Q$$

$$Q = 100 \times 6/10 = 60 \text{ mg}$$

answer: 60 mg

Note: If the sensitivity requirement for a Class A prescription balance is not provided, it should be assumed as 6 mg.

Example 2:

If a pharmacist attempts to weigh 80 mg on a prescription balance with a sensitivity requirement of 4 mg, what is the percent error associated with the weighing?

$$\%Error = 100 \times 4\ mg/80$$

$$= 400/80$$

$$= 5\%$$

answer: 5%

Example 3:

If the pointer moves two divisions when a 10 mg weight is placed on the right hand side of a prescription balance, what is its sensitivity requirement?

$$Sensitivity\ requirement = 10/2 = 5\ mg$$

answer: 5 mg

Practice Problems

(1) To achieve 92% accuracy, the amount to be weighed must be how many times greater than the sensitivity requirement of the balance?

(2) If 2 g of sulfur is weighed on a prescription balance with a sensitivity requirement of 2 mg, what would be the potential percent error?

(3) What is the smallest quantity that can be weighed with a potential error of not more than 5% on a balance with a sensitivity requirement of 4 mg?

(4) If a 10% error is observed while weighing 0.15 g, what would be the sensitivity requirement of the balance?

(5) In an attempt to weigh 200 mg on a prescription balance, a pharmacist realized that it had 8% error. What is the sensitivity requirement of that balance?

(6) For a Class B prescription balance with a sensitivity requirement of 30 mg, what would be the potential error if a pharmacist attempts to weigh 648 mg of salicylic acid?

(7) For preparing a eutectic mixture, a pharmacist needed 1/4 gr of thymol. If a pharmacist weighs that amount on a prescription balance with a sensitivity requirement of 1/10 gr, what would be the percent error?

(8) When a gr ss weight was placed on the right pan of a prescription balance, the pointer moved four divisions. What is the sensitivity requirement of the balance?

(9) A pharmacist measured 50 mL of syrup USP in a measuring cylinder, and transferred that amount to a beaker. To his surprise, he later observed that 5 mL of syrup USP was still left in the cylinder. What is the percent error in his syrup USP measurement?

(10) If one attempts to weigh 150 mg of aspirin on a balance having a sensitivity requirement of 30 mg, what would be the percent error involved?

ALIQUOT METHOD FOR SOLIDS

Frequently a health care professional has to weigh some quantity of ingredients which is beyond the limitation of a Class A prescription balance. If the quantity needed is greater than the balance's capacity, the material may be weighed in portions. For example, if 160 g of an ointment is to be measured on the Class A prescription balance (which has an upper limit of 120 g), 80 g of the ointment can be weighed twice, or 40 g can be weighed four times, depending upon the sensitivity requirement of the balance. Generally, the potential error should be 5% or less. When the desired quantity of ingredients is below the lower limits of Class A prescription balance, the aliquot method of weighing is preferred.

An aliquot is a whole number part of a given quantity. For example, five is an aliquot of ten. To be more specific, five is the second aliquot of ten, two is the fifth aliquot of ten, four is the fifth aliquot of twenty, and so on.

In the aliquot method of weighing a small quantity, the minimum weighable amount (also called the least weighable quantity or LWQ) of that compound is weighed and mixed with a certain quantity of an inert material such as lactose or starch to obtain a stock mixture. After thoroughly mixing the drug and the inert material by employing the technique of geometric dilution, weigh an aliquot of the stock mixture which provides the desired quantity of the material. The geometric dilution or mixing technique is useful for uniformly mixing ingredients of unequal amounts. For example, if 2 g of aspirin is to be mixed with 14 g of lactose, mixing should be performed by geometric dilution as follows: mix 2 g of aspirin with approximately 2 g of lactose. To this 4 g mixture, add 4 g of lactose and thoroughly mix the mixture which is now 8 g. Finally, add the remaining 8 g of lactose to the 8 g of mixture, and mix thoroughly.

Examples of Aliquot Method of Weighing[1]

Example 1:

If it is desired to weigh 60 mg of salicylic acid on a Class A prescription balance with a sensitivity requirement of 6 mg, and potential error of not more than 5%, explain how you would perform the weighing.

a. Figure out the LWQ on the given balance.

The LWQ of salicylic acid on the Class A prescription balance is:

$$5\% \text{ error} = 6 \text{ mg} \times 100/\text{LWQ}$$

$$\text{LWQ} = 600/5 = 120 \text{ mg}$$

b. Weigh 120 mg of salicylic acid. Some multiple of this quantity can also be weighed but to avoid the waste, LWQ approach is preferred.
c. Weigh a suitable amount of lactose or some other compatible inert material. The amount should be equal to or in some multiple of the LWQ. In this example, an amount of 120 mg of lactose is chosen. Therefore, weigh this amount.
d. Mix the salicylic acid and lactose thoroughly. The total mixture now is 240 mg. From this mixture, weigh an aliquot which provides 60 mg of the salicylic acid. For this calculation, the proportion is set up as follows:

$$\frac{120 \text{ mg of salicylic acid}}{240 \text{ mg of the mixture}} = \frac{60 \text{ mg of salicylic acid}}{X \text{ mg of the mixture}}$$

$$X = 240 \times 60/120 = 120 \text{ mg of the mixture}$$

answer: Instead of weighing 60 mg of salicylic acid directly, 120 mg of the mixture of salicylic acid and lactose should be weighed.

Example 2:

Explain how would you weigh gr ss of atropine sulfate on a prescription balance with a sensitivity requirement of 10 mg.

---

[1] If the percent error is not provided in a problem, it can be taken as 5%. Similarly, if the sensitivity requirement of a Class A prescription balance is not provided, it is reasonable to assume it as 6 mg.

a. LWQ equals

$$5\% = 100 \times 10 \text{ mg/LWQ}$$

$$LWQ = 1000/5 = 200 \text{ mg}$$

b. Weigh 200 mg of atropine sulfate.
c. Weigh 1031 mg of lactose. Although any quantity greater than this can be weighed, this quantity is chosen for convenience using a multiple factor of 6.154. This factor was arrived at by dividing the LWQ with the desired amount of the drug, i.e., 200/32.5 = 6.154. The multiple factor of 6.154 was chosen to obtain lactose as 200 mg × 6.154 = 1231 mg of stock mixture which contains 200 mg of atropine sulfate and the rest (1231 − 200 = 1031) is lactose. Mix the drug and lactose by geometric dilution. The total stock mixture is 200 + 1031 = 1231 mg.
d. From the stock mixture, an aliquot is calculated by setting up a proportion as follows:

$$\frac{200 \text{ mg of atropine sulfate}}{1231 \text{ mg of the stock mixture}} = \frac{32.5 \text{ mg of atropine sulfate}}{X \text{ mg of stock mixture}}$$

Note: Because of rounding off involved in multiple factor to three decimal places, 200.04 mg of the mixture is required instead of the anticipated 200 mg. Moreover, 200.04 mg can be rounded off to 200 mg.

An alternative method of aliquots is described below:

a. Weigh 200 mg of atropine sulfate.
b. Figure out the lactose amount as follows:

$$\frac{200 \text{ mg of atropine sulfate}}{X \text{ mg of the stock mixture}} = \frac{32.5 \text{ mg of atropine sulfate}}{200 \text{ mg of stock mixture}}$$

$$X = 200 \times 200/32.5 = 1231 \text{ mg of the stock mixture}$$

$$\text{Amount of lactose} = 1231 - 200 = 1031 \text{ mg}$$

c. Weigh 200 mg of atropine sulfate and mix with 1031 mg of lactose using geometric dilution.
d. From the stock mixture, weigh an aliquot of 200 mg which contains 32.5 mg or gr ss of the drug, atropine sulfate.

answer: weigh an aliquot of 200 mg

Example 3:

Show how would you weigh 20 mg of menthol on a Class A prescription balance.

a. LWQ = 120 mg
b. Multiple factor is 120/20 = 6. The amount of lactose needed is 120 × 6 = 720 mg of stock − 120 mg of menthol = 600 mg.
c. Weigh 120 mg of menthol and 600 mg of lactose. Mix them geometrically. The total weight should be 720 mg. This is the stock mixture.
d. From the stock mixture, weigh an aliquot that contains 20 mg of menthol. This is computed as follows:

$$\frac{120 \text{ mg of menthol}}{720 \text{ mg of stock mix}} = \frac{20 \text{ mg of menthol}}{X \text{ mg of stock mix}}$$

$$X = 720 \times 20/120 = 120 \text{ mg of stock mixture}$$

answer: 120 mg of stock mixture provides 20 mg of menthol

LIQUID MEASUREMENTS

Parallax error is one of the main sources of error in liquid measurements. Figure 4.2 illustrates that the liquid surface in a container is not even, and a "meniscus" is formed. For most liquids the surface is concave. The uneven surface is due to surface tension, and if not read properly, may result in an error commonly known as "parallax error." When a container with graduations for volumes has a liquid in it, the reading must always be made at the bottom of the meniscus. The parallax error is shown in Figure 4.2.

Common containers for liquid measurements include cylindrical and conical graduates for quantities of 500 mL or less, pipets for quantities of one mL or less, and a medicinal dropper for still smaller quantities. The calibration and use of medicinal droppers is explained in Chapter 2.

ALIQUOT METHOD FOR LIQUIDS

As with the weighing of solids on a prescription balance, there are limitations to liquid measuring devices as well. For example, assume that only one pipet having graduations from one to ten milliliters is available, and it is desired to measure one fluid ounce. In such a case, one ounce can be measured by measuring 10 mL three times. Measurement of volumes less than that of the

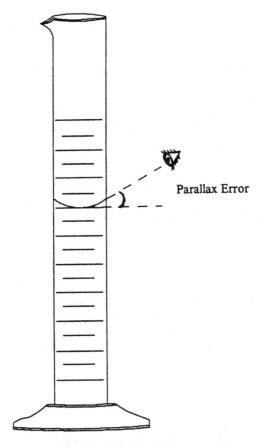

FIGURE 4.2. Parallax error.

lower limitations of the measuring device requires an aliquot approach. In the aliquot approach, a volume of liquid which can be measured would be mixed with water or a suitable liquid to obtain a stock solution. From the stock solution, an aliquot would be measured which contains the volume of liquid originally needed. The general method is outlined below following which a few examples are provided.

General Method for Aliquot Measurement of Liquids

(1) If a very small volume which cannot be measured directly is needed, measure the least measurable quantity of that liquid.

(2) Transfer that liquid to a beaker, cylinder or some large container. Find a multiple factor by dividing the volume actually measured with the volume

originally desired. By using the multiple factor, determine the amount of diluent needed as follows:

Volume of liquid measured × The multiple number = Total volume of the stock solution

Total volume of the stock solution − Volume of liquid measured initially = Volume of the diluent.

(3) Mix the liquid and diluent thoroughly to obtain the stock solution.

(4) From the stock solution, obtain an aliquot which contains the amount of liquid originally needed. This is determined by the following proportion:

$$\frac{\text{Liquid quantity measured}}{\text{Total vol of stock soln}} = \frac{\text{Liquid quantity needed}}{X = \text{Aliquot from stock soln}}$$

Example 1:

How would you measure 0.025 mL of a concentrate which is to be diluted to 60 mL following the measurement? You are provided with a 5 mL pipet with marking in units of 1 mL, a measuring cylinder, and a container to dispense the final product.

Procedure:

Before the actual product is made, it is a good idea to calibrate the final container to the required volume. In the present case, fill the container with purified water to 60 mL and mark the level of liquid from outside. Then empty the container. This process is called the calibration of container.

a. Since 0.025 mL cannot be measured and 1 mL is the minimum measurable quantity, measure one mL of the drug concentrate using the pipet and transfer this liquid to the measuring cylinder.

b. In order to make a stock solution, find the volume of water needed by making use of the multiple factor. The multiple factor in the present case is 1/0.025 = 40. The total amount of stock solution would be equal to the quantity of measured concentrate multiplied by the multiple number, i.e., 1 × 40 = 40. Therefore, the volume of water needed equals 40 − 1 = 39 mL.

c. Add 39 mL of water to the concentrate in the measuring cylinder or make up the total volume to 40 mL. Mix the solution well. From this solution, withdraw an aliquot which contains the required 0.025 mL of the concentrate and transfer to the final container. The aliquot is determined by using the following proportion:

$$\frac{1 \text{ mL of the concentrate}}{40 \text{ mL of stock soln}} = \frac{0.025 \text{ mL of the concentrate}}{X \text{ mL of the aliquot}}$$

$$X = 1 \text{ mL}$$

d. Place 1 mL of the aliquot in the final container, and add sufficient amount of purified water to fill to the calibrated mark of 60 mL.

Example 2:

FD & C dye   0.25 mg
Purified water qs. ad   90 mL

A 0.5% w/v of FD & C dye stock solution is provided. Explain how you would make this product.

Procedure:

a. Calibrate the final container to 90 mL. Determine the amount of stock solution which contains 0.25 mg of the dye as follows:

$$\frac{500 \text{ mg of the dye}}{100 \text{ mL of the stock soln}} = \frac{0.25 \text{ mg of the dye}}{X \text{ mL of stock soln}}$$

$$X = 0.05 \text{ mL}$$

b. One can either measure the 0.05 mL by a medicinal dropper after calibrating it as shown in Chapter 2 or alternatively, the stock solution can be diluted such that the diluted stock solution would provide a measurable quantity containing 0.25 mg of the dye. For dilution, measure one mL of the stock solution and add a sufficient quantity of purified water to obtain 100 mL of diluted stock solution. The concentration of diluted stock solution is

$$C_1 \times V_1 = C_2 \times V_2$$

$$0.5\% \times 1 \text{ mL} = X \times 100 \text{ mL}$$

$$X = 0.005\%$$

c. Figure out the amount of diluted solution which would provide the required 0.25 mg of the dye as follows:

$$\frac{5 \text{ mg of the dye}}{100 \text{ mL dil stock soln}} = \frac{0.25 \text{ mg of the dye}}{X \text{ mL dil stock soln}}$$

$$X = 5 \text{ mL}$$

Measure 5 mL of the diluted stock solution which contains the required 0.25 mg of the drug.

d. Transfer 5 mL of the diluted stock solution or 0.05 mL of the original stock solution to the final container and add a sufficient quantity of water to fill up to the calibrated 90-mL mark.

Example 3:

℞

Gentian violet	0.03 g
Purified water qs ad	℥ ii

Show how would you prepare this prescription using a Class A prescription balance.

Procedure:

a. Calibrate the final container to 60 mL. Since 0.03 is not weighable on Class A prescription balance, the aliquot method is required. Weigh 120 mg of gentian violet using the balance.
b. Make a stock solution such that an aliquot of stock solution will provide 0.03 g of gentian violet. Dissolve 0.12 g of gentian violet in purified water to make 20 mL (this number is arbitrarily chosen) of the stock solution.
c. From the stock solution, measure an aliquot that contains 0.03 g of the gentian violet. The aliquot amount is calculated by using the following proportion:

$$\frac{0.12 \text{ g of gentian violet}}{20 \text{ mL of the stock soln}} = \frac{0.03 \text{ g of gentian violet}}{X \text{ mL of the stock soln}}$$

$$X = 5 \text{ mL}$$

d. Transfer 5 mL of the stock solution into the final container, and add a sufficient quantity of purified water to make up to the calibrated mark of 60 mL.

Practice Problems

(1) How would you prepare the following prescription? Show stepwise procedure and all the calculations involved.

℞

    Propranolol HCl   2 mg
    D5W solution qs   fℨ iv

(2) How would you obtain 10 mg of codeine using a prescription balance
with a sensitivity requirement of 5 mg? The potential error should not
be greater than 8%.

(3) How you would prepare the following prescription?

℞

    L.C.D.   0.005 mL
    Water qs ad   50 mL

(4) Explain how would you weigh gr iss of pseudoephedrine on a prescription
balance with a sensitivity requirement of 6 mg and potential error of 2%
or less.

(5) For the above problem if 5 g of a stock mixture containing 2 g of
pseudoephedrine is provided, show how you would obtain the required
quantity of pseudoephedrine.

(6) If a pharmacist needs 0.6 mL of a drug and has a 10-mL graduated
cylinder with markings from 2 to 10 mL in units of 1 mL, explain how
you would obtain the required quantity of 0.6 mL. Use water as a diluent.

(7) If 0.75 mL of a drug is needed and a pharmacist has a 10-mL graduated
cylinder with markings from 1 to 10 mL in units of 1 mL, explain how
the required quantity of 0.75 mL can be measured. Use water as a diluent.

(8) Explain how to weigh one grain of acetaminophen on a prescription
balance having a sensitivity requirement of 1/4 grain.

(9) A prescription requires 0.015 mL of a drug concentrate. Using a pipet
with markings from one to ten in units of 1 mL and a 100-mL graduated
cylinder, explain how you would obtain the required quantity of drug
concentrate? Use water as a diluent.

(10) Explain how one can obtain 2 minims of a liquid concentrate using a 5-
mL pipet with graduations from 1–5 mL in units of 0.5 mL, and a 100-
mL measuring cylinder. Use water as a diluent.

CHAPTER 5

Calculations Involving Oral Liquids

The present chapter deals with calculations involving oral liquid dosage forms including homogenous systems such as syrups and elixirs, and heterogenous systems such as suspensions.

Syrups are oral preparations in which the vehicle is a concentrated aqueous solution of sucrose or other sugar or sugar-substitute with or without added medicinal substances and flavoring agents. Syrups are used as pleasant-tasting vehicles for disagreeable tasting drugs to be added later. Syrups, in addition to purified water and any drug substance(s), contain a sugar, antimicrobial preservatives, colorants, and flavorants. The sugar content may vary from 60 to 85%. For example, *Syrup, USP* (also referred to as "simple syrup") contains 85 g of sucrose per 100 mL of syrup, and it has a specific gravity of about 1.313. Simple syrup is resistant to microbial growth, due to the unavailability of the water required for the growth of microorganisms, and, therefore, contains no preservative.

Elixirs are clear oral solutions in which the vehicle is a hydroalcoholic mixture containing potent or nauseating drugs. Elixirs are pleasantly flavored and attractively colored. The presence of hydroalcoholic vehicle in an elixir makes it possible to include both water-soluble and alcohol-soluble substances in solution. In comparison to syrups, elixirs are less sweet and less viscous because of lower sugar content. From the manufacturing aspects and from the stability standpoint, elixirs are favored over syrups.

Suspensions are two-phase systems consisting of finely divided particles of drug(s) dispersed in a vehicle in which the drug is insoluble or poorly soluble. The particle size of the dispersed solid is typically greater than 0.5 µm. Most of the suspensions of pharmaceutical interest are aqueous dispersions, available either in ready-to-use form or as dry powders to circumvent the

87

instability of aqueous dispersions of certain drugs, such as antibiotics. At the time of dispensing, the latter type of preparations are reconstituted with water to complete the suspension. These preparations are designated in the USP as "... for Oral Suspension." Calculations involving reconstitution of powdered drugs are presented in Chapter 10. The preparations that are already available as ready-to-use suspensions are designated simply as "... Oral Suspension."

Oral preparations including syrups, elixirs, and suspensions are supplied in liquid form (with the exception of powders for reconstitution) and contain a specific amount of drug in a given amount of liquid. The solution strength, stated on the label, may indicate the amount (in microgram, milligram, or gram) of drug per 1 mL or multiple milliliters of solution, such as 10 mg per 1 mL, 1.2 g per 20 mL, etc. The strength may also be expressed as gram or milligram per teaspoonful (or 5 mL). The strength of certain biological products may be expressed as units of activity per milliliter or milliequivalents per liter.

CALCULATIONS ASSOCIATED WITH BULK PREPARATIONS

Certain oral medications may be prepared in bulk to be dispensed later or to be used as stock solutions. Official formulas for manufacturing, in general, are based on the preparation of one liter or one kilogram of product. The quantities of active ingredients required to prepare in bulk can be determined by the method of proportions which is outlined in Chapter 1.

Example 1:

An elixir of aprobarbital contains 40 mg of aprobarbital in each 5 mL. How many milligrams would be used in preparing 1 L of the elixir?

$$\frac{40 \text{ mg}}{5 \text{ mL}} = \frac{X \text{ mg}}{1000 \text{ mL}}$$

answer: $X = 8000$ mg

Example 2:

If pentobarbital elixir contains 18.2 mg of pentobarbital per 5 mL, how many grams of pentobarbital would be used in preparing a pint of the elixir?

$$1 \text{ pint} = 473 \text{ mL}$$

$$\frac{18.2 \text{ mg}}{5 \text{ mL}} = \frac{X \text{ mg}}{473 \text{ mL}}$$

answer: $X = 1722$ mg or 1.72 g

Example 3:

A formula for a cough syrup contains 1/8 gr of codeine phosphate per tea-spoonful. How many grams of codeine phosphate should be used in preparing two pints of the cough syrup?

$$1 \text{ pint} = 473 \text{ mL}$$

$$2 \text{ pints} = 473 \times 2 = 946 \text{ mL}$$

$$\frac{5 \text{ mL}}{1/8 \text{ gr}} = \frac{946 \text{ mL}}{X \text{ gr}}$$

$$X = 23.65 \text{ gr}$$

$$1 \text{ gr} = 0.065 \text{ g}$$

$$\frac{1 \text{ gr}}{0.065 \text{ g}} = \frac{23.65 \text{ gr}}{X}$$

answer: $X = 1.54$ g

Practice Problems

(1) A syrup contains the equivalent of 32 gr of active ingredient in each fluidounce (480 minims) of the syrup. How many minims would provide the equivalent of 20 gr of the active ingredient?

(2) If a pharmacist had four one-liter stock bottles of each of the ingredients, how many times could the following prescription be filled?

℞

Actifed® Syrup   60 mL
Robitussin® Syrup ad   120 mL
Sig. 5 mL as required for cough

(3) How many mL of Decadron® Elixir would be taken in the initial dose of the prescription?

℞

Decadron® Elixir
Benadryl® Elixir aa (of each)   20 mL

Triple Sulfas Suspension   80 mL
Sig. 10 mL stat., then 5 mL t.i.d.

(4) How many grams of potassium thiocyanate should be used in compounding the following prescription?

℞

Potassium Thiocyanate
Aromatic Elixir   aa   q.s.
Make a solution to contain 0.2 g/tsp
Disp. 150 mL
Sig. 5 mL in water daily

(5) How many milliliters of paregoric and how many grams of pectin are present in each 15-mL dose?

℞

Paregoric	15.0 mL
Pectin	0.5 g
Kaolin	20.0 g
Ethanol	1.0 mL
Purified water ad	100.0 mL

Mix and make a suspension
Sig. 15 mL p.r.n. for diarrhea

(6) How many grains of dihydrocodeinone should be used in compounding the prescription?

℞

Dihydrocodeinone   gr 1/12/tsp
Hydriodic Acid Syrup
Cherry Syrup   aa   ℥iii
Sig. Tsp. every 2 hr. for cough

(7) A physician prescribes tetracycline suspension for a patient to be taken in doses of two teaspoonfuls four times a day for four days, and then one teaspoonful four times a day for two days. How many milliliters of the suspension should be dispensed to provide the quantity for the prescribed dosage regimen?

(8) A medication order for theophylline oral suspension for a patient to be taken in doses of one teaspoonful three times a day for five days, and then one teaspoonful two times a day for two days. How many milliliters of the suspension should be dispensed to provide the quantity for the prescribed dosage regimen?

(9) The pediatric dose of cefadroxil is 30 mg/kg/day. A child is receiving a daily dose of 2 tsp of a pediatric cefadroxil suspension based on the body weight. If the child's weight is 18.3 lb, how many milligrams of the drug is the child receiving in each dose?

(10) A patient has been instructed to take 15 mL of Vistaril® (hydroxyzine pamoate) oral suspension every six hours for four doses daily. How many days will two 6 fluidounce bottles of the suspension last?

CALCULATION OF DOSES

For oral medications supplied in solution form, one can calculate the quantity of liquid which contains the prescribed dosage of the drug by using the method of proportion.

Example 1:

A cough syrup contains 48 mg of brompheniramine maleate in 120 mL. How many mg of brompheniramine maleate would be contained in each 5-mL dose?

$$\frac{48 \text{ mg}}{120 \text{ mL}} = \frac{X \text{ mg}}{5 \text{ mL}}$$

answer: $X = 2$ mg

Example 2:

Amobarbital Elixir contains 4 g of amobarbital/liter. How many milligrams of amobarbital are contained in a teaspoonful dose of the elixir?

$$4 \text{ g} = 4000 \text{ mg}$$

$$\frac{4000 \text{ mg}}{1000 \text{ mL}} = \frac{X \text{ mg}}{5 \text{ mL}}$$

answer: $X = 20$ mg

Doses Based on Body Weight

The doses of oral liquids may, sometimes, be calculated on the basis of body weight. This type of problem can also be solved by the method of proportion.

Example 3:

A child weighing 28 lb is to receive 4 mg of phenytoin per kilogram of body weight daily as an anticonvulsant. How many milliliters of pediatric phenytoin suspension containing 30 mg per 5 mL should the child receive?

By setting up appropriate proportions, this type of a problem may be solved in two steps:

Step 1. Find the dose for the child.

4 mg/kg or 4 mg/2.2 lb

If the dose is 4 mg/lb, a 28-lb child should receive:

$$\frac{4 \text{ mg}}{2.2 \text{ lb}} = \frac{X \text{ mg}}{28 \text{ lb}}$$

answer: X = 50.9 or 51 mg

Step 2. Find how many milliliters would contain that dose.

If 30 mg are contained in 5 mL, 51 mg would be contained in:

$$\frac{30 \text{ mg}}{5 \text{ mL}} = \frac{51 \text{ mg}}{X \text{ mL}}$$

answer: X = 8.5 mL

Practice Problems

(1) Codeine Elixir contains 1 gr of codeine/fluidounce. How much additional codeine should be added to 4 fluidounces of the elixir so that each teaspoonful will contain 15 mg of codeine?

(2) How many mg each of noscapine and guaifenesin would be contained in each dose of the following prescription?

R̨

Noscapine	0.60 g
Guaifenesin	4.80 g

```
Alcohol                        15.00 mL
Cherry Syrup    ad            100.00 mL
Sig. 5 mL t.i.d. p.r.n. cough
```

(3) If 2 fluidounces of a cough syrup contain 20 gr of sodium citrate, how many milligrams are contained in 5 mL?

(4) An elixir of ferrous sulfate contains 220 mg of ferrous sulfate in each 5 mL. If each mg of ferrous sulfate contains the equivalent of 0.2 mg of elemental iron, how many milligrams of elemental iron would be presented in each 5 mL of the elixir?

(5) How many mL of Maalox Suspension would be contained in each dose?

℞

```
Alurate® Elixir        10 mL
Maalox® Susp.    ad    60 mL
Sig. 5 mL t.i.d.
```

(6) How many milligrams of dextromethorphan should be used in filling the prescription?

℞

```
Dextromethorphan              15 mg/5 mL
Guaifenesin Syrup    ad       f℥viii
Sig. 5 mL q. 4h. p.r.n. cough
```

(7) If a cough syrup contains 0.24 g of codeine in 120 mL, how many milligrams of codeine are contained in each teaspoonful dose?

(8) If a potassium chloride elixir contains 40 milliequivalents of potassium ion in each 30 mL of elixir, how many milliliters will provide fifteen milliequivalents of potassium ion to the patient?

(9) The dose of digoxin for rapid digitalization is a total of 1 mg in two divided doses at intervals of six to eight hours. How many milliliters of digoxin elixir containing 50 μg/mL would provide this dose?

(10) A physician ordered 1.5 mg of theophylline to be administered orally to a baby. How many milliliters of theophylline elixir containing 30 mg of theophylline per 10 mL should be used in dispensing the medication order?

PERCENTAGE STRENGTH CALCULATIONS OF ORAL LIQUIDS

Alligation Medial

When two or more liquid medications of known quantities and concentrations are mixed, the resulting strength is the "weighted average" of the percentage strengths of all the individual components used. The percentage strength of the mixture may be calculated by dividing the sum of the products of percentage strength of each constituent of the mixture multiplied by its corresponding quantity by the sum of the quantities mixed. This method is referred to as "alligation medial."

By the method of alligation medial, the percentage strength of a mixture may be calculated using the following steps:

- Step 1: Add up the quantity of each component used in the mixture.
- Step 2: Multiply the quantity of each component used in the mixture by its corresponding percentage strength, and add up the products.
- Step 3: Divide the value obtained in Step 2 by the value obtained in Step 1.

The method of *alligation medial* may be best explained by the following examples.

Example 1:

What is the percentage of alcohol in the following prescription?

℞

Chloroform Spirit	50.0 mL (90% alcohol)
Aromatic Elixir	150.0 mL (21% alcohol)
Terpin Hydrate Elixir	300.0 mL (45% alcohol)
Sig. 5 mL for cough	

Step 1. 50 + 150 + 300 = 500 mL

Step 2

$$
\begin{aligned}
50 \times 90 &= 4500 \\
150 \times 21 &= 3150 \\
300 \times 45 &= \underline{13,500} \\
&21,150
\end{aligned}
$$

Step 3. answer: 21,150/500 = 42.3%

Example 2:

What is the percentage strength (v/v) of alcohol in a mixture of 100 mL of 10% v/v alcohol, 60 mL of 15% v/v alcohol, and 40 mL of 20% v/v alcohol?

Step 1. 100 + 60 ÷ 40 = 200 mL

Step 2.

$$
\begin{aligned}
100 \times 10 &= 1000 \\
60 \times 15 &= 900 \\
40 \times 20 &= \underline{800} \\
& 2700
\end{aligned}
$$

Step 3. answer: 2700/200 = 13.5%

Example 3:

What is the percentage of alcohol in the following prescription?

℞

Phenobarbital Elixir	30 mL (15% alcohol)
Aromatic Elixir	120 mL (22% alcohol)
Belladonna Tincture	50 mL (65% alcohol)
Purified Water	ad 250 mL
Sig. Teaspoonful t.i.d.	

Step 1. Total quantity is 250 mL.

Step 2. Quantity of water used in the preparation

$$= 250 - (30 + 120 + 50) = 50 \text{ mL}$$

$$
\begin{aligned}
30 \times 15 &= 450 \\
120 \times 22 &= 2640 \\
50 \times 65 &= 3250 \\
50 \times 0 &= \underline{0} \\
& 6340
\end{aligned}
$$

Step 3. answer: 6340/250 = 25.36 or 25.4%

DILUTION AND CONCENTRATION

When a liquid medication of a given strength is diluted, its strength will be reduced. For example, 10 mL of a solution containing 1 g of a substance has a strength of 1:10 or 10% w/v. If this solution is diluted to 20 mL, i.e., the volume of the solution is doubled by adding 10 mL of solvent, the original strength will be reduced by one-half to 1:20 or 5% w/v (refer to Chapter 1 for more information on this topic).

To calculate the strength of a solution prepared by diluting a solution of known quantity and strength, a proportion may be set up as follows:

$$\text{(known quantity)} \times \text{(known concentration)}$$
$$= \text{(final quantity after dilution)} \times \text{(final concentration after dilution)}$$

The above expression can simply be reduced to:

$$C_1 \times V_1 = C_2 \times V_2$$

From this expression, strength (or final concentration) of the solution can be determined. To calculate the volume of solution of desired strength that can be made by diluting a known quantity of a solution, a similar expression may be used.

Example 1:

If 5 mL of a 20% w/v aqueous solution of furosemide is diluted to 10 mL, what will be the final strength of furosemide?

$$5 \text{ (mL)} \times 20 \text{ (\%)} = 10 \text{ (mL)} \times X \text{ (\%)}$$

answer: $X = 5 \times 20/10 = 10\%$ w/v

Example 2:

If a phenobarbital elixir containing 4% w/v phenobarbital is evaporated to 90% of its volume, what is the strength of phenobarbital in the remaining solution?

$$100 \text{ (mL)} \times 4 \text{ (\%)} = 90 \text{ (mL)} \times X \text{ (\%)}$$

answer: $X = 400/90 = 4.44\%$ w/v

Example 3:

How many milliliters of a 1:20 v/v solution of methyl salicylate in alcohol can be made from 100 mL of 2% v/v solution?

$$1:20 = 1/20 = 0.05 \text{ or } 5\%$$

$$100 \text{ (mL)} \times 2 \text{ (\%)} = X \text{ (mL)} \times 5 \text{ (\%)}$$

$$\text{answer: } X = 200/5 = 40 \text{ mL}$$

Alligation Alternate

A pharmacist may mix two or more liquid preparations of known strength to prepare a mixture of desired strength. The desired strength should be somewhere in between the individual strengths of the components used. The strength of the mixture obtained is the "weighted" average of the individual strengths of the components used in the mixture. One can calculate the quantity of each component to be used to obtain a mixture of desired strength by the method of *alligation alternate.*

The following steps may be used to find out the proportional parts of each component to be used in a two-component mixture to obtain the desired strength:

(1) Make three columns. In column 1, write down the concentrations of the components to be mixed.
(2) In column 2, write down the desired percentage strength of the mixture to be prepared.
(3) In column 3, write down the difference in strength by reading diagonally (as illustrated in Example 1).
(4) Find the relative proportions of the components (as illustrated in Example 1).

Example 1:

How many milliliters of phenytoin suspensions containing 30 mg per 5 mL and 100 mg per 5 mL should be used in preparing 500 mL of a suspension containing 10 mg of phenytoin per mL?

30 mg per 5 mL is the same as 6 mg/mL or 0.6%.

100 mg per 5 mL is the same as 20 mg/mL or 2.0%.

10 mg per 1 mL or 1.0%.

Column 1   Column 2   Column 3

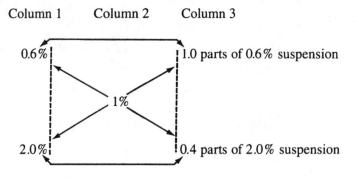

0.6%   1.0 parts of 0.6% suspension

1%

2.0%   0.4 parts of 2.0% suspension

1.4 parts in total

The quantities of each component to be used to obtain the specified quantity can be determined by the method of proportion as follows:

$$\frac{1.4}{1.0} = \frac{500}{X}$$

$$X = 357 \text{ mL of } 0.6\%$$

$$\frac{1.4}{0.4} = \frac{500}{X}$$

answer: $X = 143$ mL of 2.0%

Example 2:

How many milliliters of a syrup having a specific gravity of 1.30 should be mixed with 2000 mL of a syrup having specific gravity of 1.22 to obtain a product having a specific gravity of 1.25?

Column 1   Column 2   Column 3

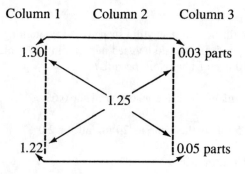

1.30   0.03 parts

1.25

1.22   0.05 parts

The quantity of the syrup with the specific gravity of 1.22 is specified as 2000 mL. This is equal to 0.05 proportional parts. The proportional parts required for the syrup having a specific gravity of 1.30 is 0.03. The quantity of the syrup with the specific gravity of 1.30 can be determined by the method of proportion as follows:

$$\frac{0.05 \text{ parts}}{2000 \text{ mL}} = \frac{0.03 \text{ parts}}{X}$$

answer: $X = 1200$ mL of syrup with specific gravity of 1.30

Example 3:

A physician prescribes an ophthalmic suspension to contain 100 mg of cortisone acetate in 8 mL of normal saline solution (NSS). The pharmacist has a 2.5% suspension of cortisone acetate in NSS. How many milliliters of this and how many milliliters of NSS should be used in preparing the medication order?

If 100 mg are contained in 8 mL, the percentage strength may be calculated as follows:

$$\frac{0.1 \text{ g}}{8 \text{ mL}} = \frac{X \text{ g}}{100 \text{ mL}}$$

$X = 1.25$ g/100 mL or 1.25%

Column 1   Column 2   Column 3

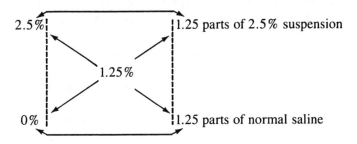

Thus, a suspension of cortisone acetate of desired strength can be obtained by mixing equal parts (i.e., 1.25 parts or 4 mL each) of 2.5% suspension and normal saline.

This may be confirmed by $C_1 \times V_1 = C_2 \times V_2$ method as follows:

$$8 \text{ mL} \times 1.25\% = X \text{ mL} \times 2.5\%$$

$$X = \frac{8 \times 1.25}{2.5}$$

$$= 4 \text{ mL}$$

answer: Thus, 4 mL of 2.5% suspension and 4 mL of NSS may be mixed to contain 100 mg/8 mL

Practice Problems

(1) What is the percentage of alcohol in the following prescription?

℞

Chloroform Spirit	110.0 mL (88% alcohol)
Armoatic Elixir	85.0 mL (22% alcohol)
Terpin Hydrate Elixir	255.0 mL (40% alcohol)
Sig. 5 mL for cough	

(2) What is the percentage strength (v/v) of alcohol in a mixture of 200 mL of 12% v/v alcohol, 150 mL of 18% v/v alcohol, and 250 mL of 25% v/v alcohol?

(3) If a phenobarbital elixir containing 5% w/v phenobarbital is evaporated to 65% of its volume, what is the strength of phenobarbital in the remaining solution?

(4) If Benadryl® Elixir containing 25 mg diphenhydramine hydrochloride per 10 mL is evaporated to 70% of its volume, what is the strength of diphenhydramine hydrochloride in the remaining solution?

(5) How many milliliters of a 1:500 v/v solution of methyl salicylate in alcohol can be made from 100 mL of 5% v/v solution?

(6) If 50 mL of a Choledyl® Elixir containing 100 mg/5 mL active ingredient (oxtriphylline) is diluted to 250 mL, what will be the final strength of oxtriphylline?

(7) How many milliliters of phenobarbital elixir containing 20 mg per 5 mL and 30 mg per 5 mL should be used in preparing a liter of phenobarbital elixir containing 4.8 mg of phenobarbital per mL?

(8) How many milliliters of methenamine mandelate oral suspension containing 250 mg and 500 mg per 5 mL should be used in preparing a liter of a suspension containing 60 mg of methenamine mandelate per mL?

(9) How many milliliters of griseofulvin oral suspension containing 100 mg and 125 mg per mL should be used in preparing 100 mL of a suspension containing 12% of griseofulvin?

(10) A physician order calls for a theophylline oral suspension to contain 100 mg of theophylline in 5 mL of aqueous vehicle. The pharmacist has on hand a 5% aqueous suspension of theophylline. How many mL of aqueous vehicle should be added to the preparation on hand in preparing the prescribed suspension?

MILLIEQUIVALENT CALCULATIONS OF ORAL ELECTROLYTE SOLUTIONS

The concentrations of electrolyte solutions are generally expressed in chemical units known as milliequivalents (mEq). The milliequivalent weight represents the amount, in milligrams, of a solute equal to 1/1000 of its gram equivalent weight. A milliequivalent is a unit of measurement of the amount of chemical activity of an electrolyte. A milliequivalent unit is related to the total number of ionic charges in solution and it takes the valence of the ions into consideration. Table 5.1 provides valence, atomic and milliequivalent weights, and formulae of selected ions.

TABLE 5.1. Valance, Atomic and Milliequivalent Weights, and Formulae of Selected Ions

Ion	Valence	Atomic Weight	Milliequivalent Weight	Formula
Lithium	1	7	7	Li^+
Ammonium	1	18	18	NH_4^+
Sodium	1	23	23	Na^+
Chloride	1	35.5	35.5	Cl^-
Potassium	1	39	39	K^+
Acetate	1	59	59	$C_2H_3O_2^-$
Bicarbonate	1	61	61	HCO_3^-
Lactate	1	89	89	$C_3H_5O_3^-$
Gluconate	1	195	195	$C_6H_{11}O_7^-$
Phosphate	1	97	97	$H_2PO_4^-$
	2	96	48	HPO_4^{--}
Magnesium	2	24	12	Mg^{++}
Calcium	2	40	20	Ca^{++}
Ferrous	2	56	28	Fe^{++}
Carbonate	2	60	30	CO_3^{--}
Sulfate	2	96	48	SO_4^{--}
Aluminum	3	27	9	Al^{+++}
Ferric	3	56	18.7	Fe^{+++}
Citrate	3	189	63	$C_6H_5O_7^{---}$

Under normal conditions, plasma contains 155 mEq of cations and 155 mEq of anions. The total concentration of cations always equals the concentration of anions. Any number of milliequivalents of Na^+, K^+, Ca^{++}, Mg^{++}, or any cation always reacts with precisely the same number of mEq of Cl^-, HCO_3^-, SO_4^{2-}, or any other cation.

Concentrations of electrolytes in body fluids and in pharmaceutical solutions are usually expressed as mEq/L or Eq/L. In institutional practice, various electrolyte solutions are administered to correct electrolyte imbalances. The doses of electrolytes are calculated either in milliequivalents or in metric weights.

The relationship between mEq and mg quantities of a substance can be expressed in one of the following ways:

Weight of the substance in mg = Number of milliequivalents
× Milliequivalent weight

Weight of the substance in g = Number of milliequivalents
× Equivalent weight

The milliequivalent concentration of a solute may be quickly calculated using the following expression:

$$mEq/L = \frac{\text{Weight of the solute (g/L)}}{\text{Molecular weight (g)}} \times \text{Valence} \times 1000$$

Equivalent weights may be calculated for molecules as well as atoms using the following expression:

Equivalent weight = Atomic weight ÷ Valence

The equivalent weight of monovalent ions (such as sodium and chlorine) is identical to its molecular weight. The equivalent of NaCl is the sum of the equivalent weights of sodium (23 g/Eq) and chlorine (35.5 g/Eq), i.e., 58.5 which is identical to its molecular weight. However, the equivalent weight of a molecule having atoms that are not monovalent is different from its molecular weight. For example, the equivalent weight of Na_2CO_3 is 53 g/Eq, or half its molecular weight of 106. This can be explained as follows.

The sodium ion has two sodium atoms, each with an atomic weight of 23 (23 × 2 = 46); these have a total valence of two and an equivalent weight of 23 g/Eq. The carbonate ion has a molecular weight of 60 and a valence of 2, and, therefore, an equivalent weight of 30 g/Eq. The equivalent weight of Na_2CO_3 molecule is sum of the equivalent weights of both ions in the molecule, i.e., 53 (23 + 30) g/Eq. The equivalent weight of a bivalent compound, thus,

can be determined by dividing the sum of molecular or atomic weights of all atoms in the radical by the total valence of the positive or negative radical.
Some basic milliequivalent calculations are as follows:

Example 1:

What is the milliequivalent weight of potassium chloride?

Molecular weight of KCl = 74.5
Potassium chloride has a valence of 1

Equivalent weight of KCl = 74.5/1 = 74.5 g

mEq KCl = 1/1000 × 74.5 = 0.0745 g or 74.5 mg

answer: 74.5 mg

Example 2:

What is the milliequivalent weight of calcium chloride?

Molecular weight of $CaCl_2 \cdot 2H_2O$ = 147
Calcium chloride has a valence of 2

Equivalent weight of $CaCl_2 \cdot 2H_2O$ = 147/2 = 73.5 g
mEq $CaCl_2 \cdot 2H_2O$ = 1/1000 × 73.5 = 0.0735 g or 73.5 mg

answer: 73.5 mg

Example 3:

How many milliequivalents of calcium are present in a liter of a solution containing 150 mg/dL of calcium?

Molecular weight of Ca^{2+} = 40
Calcium has a valence of 2

Equivalent weight of Ca^{2+} = 40/2 = 20 g

Milliequivalent weight of Ca^{2+} = 20/1000 = 0.02 g or 20 mg

A solution containing 150 mg/dL of Ca^{2+} would have 1500 mg Ca^{2+}/L

$$\frac{1500 \text{ mg/L}}{20 \text{ mg/mEq}} = 75 \text{ mEq/L}$$

answer: 75 mEq/L

DOSAGE CALCULATIONS INVOLVING MILLIEQUIVALENTS

Example 1:

How many grams of potassium citrate should be used in preparing 500 mL of a potassium ion elixir so as to supply 15 mEq of K$^+$ in each 5-mL dose? If 5 mL contain 15 mEq, 500 mL contain 1500 mEq

Mol. wt. of potassium citrate ($C_6H_5K_3O_7 \cdot H_2O$) = 324

Equivalent weight of potassium citrate = 324/3 = 108

Milliequivalent weight = 108 g/1000 = 0.108 g or 108 mg

Weight of potassium citrate required = 1500 × 108 = 162,000 mg

answer: = 162 g

Example 2:

How many milliequivalents of potassium chloride are represented in each prescribed dose of the following prescription?

℞

Potassium chloride 10%
Cherry Syrup ad 480 mL
Sig. Tablespoonful b.i.d.

KCl 10% = 10 g/100 mL

1 tbsp = 15 mL

$$\frac{10 \text{ g}}{100 \text{ mL}} = \frac{X}{15 \text{ mL}}$$

$$X = 1.5 \text{ g or } 1500 \text{ mg}$$

Mol. wt. of KCl = 74.5, Eq. wt. of KCl = 74.5

mEq of KCl = (1 × 74.5)/1000 = 74.5 mg

$$\text{Number of mEq} = \frac{\text{Weight in mg}}{\text{mEq weight}}$$

$$X = \frac{1500 \text{ mg}}{74.5 \text{ mg}}$$

answer: X = 20.1 mEq

Example 3:

A patient is to receive 10 mEq of potassium gluconate four times a day for three days. The dose is a teaspoonful.

a. How many milligrams of potassium gluconate should be used in compounding the prescription?
b. What is the volume, in milliliters, to be dispensed to provide the prescribed dosage regimen?

Molecular weight of potassium gluconate ($C_6H_{11}KO_7$) = 234

10 mEq of $C_6H_{11}KO_7$ given 4 times a day for 3 days = 10 × 4
× 3 = 120 mEq

Eq. wt. of $C_6H_{11}KO_7$ = 234

a. Weight in mg = mEq weight × Number of mEq

= 234 × 120

= 28,080 mg = 28.08 g

b. A proportion can be set to calculate the volume, in milliliters, to be dispensed to provide the prescribed dosage regimen as follows:

$$\frac{10 \text{ mEq}}{5 \text{ mL}} = \frac{120 \text{ mEq}}{X \text{ mL}}$$

answer: X = (5 × 120)/10 = 60 mL

Practice Problems

Refer to Table 5.1 as needed.

(1) Twenty milliequivalents of K^+ are ordered. Calculate the amount of KCl needed.

(2) How many grams of NaCl should be used to prepare a solution containing 156 mEq/L?

(3) How many milligrams of calcium are required to prepare a solution containing 12.5 mEq/L?

(4) What is the concentration, in milligrams per milliliter, of a solution containing 2.75 mEq of KCl per milliliter?

(5) An electrolyte preparation contains 74 mg% of Fe^{++} ions. Express this concentration in terms of milliequivalents/liter.

(6) How many grams of sodium bicarbonate are needed to provide 25 mEq of bicarbonate ion?

(7) The normal potassium level in the blood plasma is 17 mg%. Express this concentration in terms of milliequivalents/liter.

(8) How many grams of NaCl should be used in preparing 10 liters of a solution containing 125 milliequivalents per liter?

(9) Five milliliters of lithium citrate syrup contain the equivalent of 8 milliequivalents of Li^+. Calculate the equivalent, in terms of milligrams, of lithium carbonate (Li_2CO_3 M.W. = 74) in each 5-mL dose of the syrup.

(10) Two and a half milliequivalents of Ca^{++} are ordered. Calculate the amount, in milligrams, of calcium dihydrate (molecular weight of $CaCl_2 \cdot 2H_2O$ = 147) needed.

CHAPTER 6

Calculations Involving Capsules, Tablets, and Powder Dosage Forms

STRENGTH OF DOSAGES

Many dosage forms including capsules and tablets are available in more than one strength. If a capsule or a tablet of higher strength is prescribed but unavailable, two capsules or tablets of one-half the strength may be dispensed. Thus, a pharmacist or a health care professional may need to administer one-half or some other portion of the tablet. For example, if 300-mg tablets of ibuprofen are prescribed, and only 600-mg ibuprofen tablets are available. In such a case, one-half of the total number of tablets required should be dispensed to the patients with clear instructions to take ½ tablet. A few helpful tips for such calculations are provided below:

(1) Do not break the tablets that are not scored.

(2) Enteric coated tablets are designed to resist the acidic environment in the stomach and release the medication in the small intestine. If such tablets are broken, their enteric properties may be lost. Therefore, do not break them.

(3) As a general rule, do not divide sustained/controlled release medications as they may lose their controlled release properties. However, there may be some exceptions to this rule. For example, Calan SR 240 tablets which are to be given once daily can be split to administer 120 mg (or ½ tablet) twice daily. Therefore, unless specifically suggested by the manufacturer, controlled release tablets should not be crushed or broken.

Example 1:

If a prescription is received with the instructions of providing gr x of

APAP to a patient, and the pharmacist has 325 mg tablets, how many tablets should the patient be instructed to take?

$$325 \text{ mg} = 5 \text{ gr}$$

answer: two tablets should be taken by the patient

Example 2:

Tenormin® is available in a strength of 50 mg. If a prescription is written for 100 mg daily for three weeks as directed, how many tablets should be dispensed?

Two 50 mg tablets should be given in one day

answer: for 21 days, 42 tablets should be dispensed

Example 3:

℞

Motrin® 600 mg
#21
Sig. I tab tid, pc

Assume that the patient has a stock of Advil® (ibuprofen 200 mg) at home and he decides to take them instead of getting the prescription filled by a pharmacist. How many Advil® tablets should the patient take in one day?

$$1 \text{ Motrin}® \text{ 600 mg} = 3 \text{ Advil}®$$

answer: the patient should take 9 Advil® (3 × 3) every day

Practice Problems

(1) If a prescription requires a stat dose of 0.375 mg of Lanoxin and the

pharmacist has digoxin tablets of strength, 0.125 mg, how many digoxin tablets should the patient take if generic tablets are authorized?

(2) If a pharmacist dispenses cephalexin 250 mg capsules, what directions should be provided to the patient?

℞

Cephalexin Caps 500 mg

Sig. i cap tid, 10 days

(3) In the above problem, how many cephalexin 250 mg capsules should be dispensed totally?

(4) Spironolactone tablets are available in 25 mg strength, but a drug order comes for 150 mg dose. How many tablets should be dispensed?

(5) How many 20 mEq tablets should be dispensed for the prescription?

℞

K-Dur® (Extended Release) 10 mEq
#20

Sig: 10 mEq bid

(6) A pharmacist had 12 tablets of phenobarbital 32 mg. After notifying the physician, he dispensed those tablets to the patient. How long would the medication last?

℞

Phenobarbital gr i
#21 tablets

Sig: i tablet tid, finish all

(7) If a pharmacist dispensed Synthroid® 25 mcg tablets, how many tablets would the patient take every day?

℞

Synthroid® 100 mcg
    30 tablets

Sig: i qd

(8) If the available tablets have a strength of 250 mg, how many tablets should be dispensed? It is known that one mg of penicillin K = 1600 units.

℞
V-Cillin K®
800,000 units tid, 5 days

(9) How many 500 milligram Gantrisin® tablets should be dispensed?

℞

Gantrisin® gr L
    #14

Use as directed.

(10) If the pharmacist dispensed 25 mg tablets of Phenergan®, how many tablets should the patient take at bedtime?

℞

Phenergan® tablets 12.5 mg

Dispense 14 tablets

Sig: ss qhs

EXTEMPORANEOUS FILLING OF CAPSULES

Capsules are of two types: hard and soft gelatin capsules. The present chapter will focus on the extemporaneous filling of hard gelatin capsules. Generally, the soft gelatin capsules are not compounded extemporaneously. Therefore, they are not discussed in this chapter.

Hard gelatin capsules are available in a range of sizes such as 00, 0, 1, 2, 3, 4, and 5 which represent a gradual decrease in size from 00 to 5. The largest capsule size, symbolized as "000," is rarely used. The hard gelatin capsules consist of a cylindrical body and a cap. The cap is slightly larger and broader but shorter, and the body is narrower and longer. The medication is filled in the body, following which the cap is fitted over it. For the compounding of capsules, powdered ingredients are accurately weighed, mixed by the geometric dilution method, and filled in appropriate size capsules. Sometimes if the powdered ingredients are not readily available, they can be obtained by crushing available tablets. Lactose or some other diluent may be needed to make up the volume of powder to fill in the capsules. Capsules of smallest size that will hold the quantity of powdered material should be selected. To figure the size of the capsule needed, accurately weighed powdered material is usually filled in one or two capsules as a trial. If the size is appropriate, then the rest of the material is filled in capsules of the same size.

As an approximate method for getting an idea about the size of capsule needed, a simple "rule of six" is very useful. Although not very accurate, the rule of six serves as an initial guide for the capsule size selection. When the bulk density of the powdered material is 0.6 g/cc, this rule helps in obtaining the capsule size which is fairly accurate. However, since the bulk density of pharmaceutical powders is different, it is always a good idea to verify the capsule size by actually filling the material. This rule will certainly narrow down the choice of capsule size selection for initial trials. The rule of six is given below:

Number six	6	6	6	6	6	6
Capsule size	0	1	2	3	4	5
Weight of powder in grains	6–7	5	4	3	2	½–1

The above table shows that with the exception of capsule size #0 and #5, the amount of powder in grains that can be filled in the capsules can be obtained by subtracting capsule size from the number six. As an example, five grains or $65 \times 5 = 325$ mg of powdered drug can be filled in capsule size #1. In capsule size #4, 2 gr or approximately 130 mg of the powder can be filled. Capsule size #5 is an exception because it can be filled with one-half to a grain instead of just 1 gr. Similarly, capsule size #0 can be filled with 6–7 gr instead of just the 6 gr.

Compounding Tips and Calculations for Filling Capsules

In order to fill capsules as a dosage form, the following steps may provide a helpful guide.

- Step 1: Determine whether the prescription is based upon one unit or upon a bulk formula to be subdivided into individual units. *Subscription* of the prescriptions is very important for this determination. For example, *M et Div* suggests that the prescription is written for some bulk formula which is to be subdivided into individual capsules. On the other hand, *D.T.D.* in the *subscription* suggests that the formula is given for one capsule, and depending upon the number of capsules needed in the prescription, the formula quantities should be multiplied. Sometimes, there are some errors in the prescription, and extreme care is needed to fill the prescription correctly. One such example is D.T.D. instead of *M et. Div.* Example #3 in this section will illustrate this problem.
- Step 2: Determine the weight of each ingredient in the formula, weigh them accurately, and mix by the geometric mixing technique. If the ingredients are to be obtained from commercial tablets, determine the appropriate number of tablets needed, crush them, and weigh out the material. Then proceed as with powders.
- Step 3: Determine the capsule size by using the rule of six. If the amount of powder is less than the required amount to fill the capsules whose size has been determined, add suitable amount of diluent, preferably lactose, to make up the volume. As a confirmation of the size, fill one or two capsules and determine the appropriateness. If the capsule size is correct "punch" out the remaining capsules after forming a cake on a powder paper or an ointment tile.
- Step 4: Wipe all the capsules from outside with a clean tissue paper, and dispense the capsules in appropriate container after affixing the label. Contents of the label and the need for any auxiliary label will depend upon the contents of the prescription, and the nature of the medication.

Example 1:

How would you fill the following prescription? Show all the calculations, procedure, and the label for the product.

Henry Huxtable, M.D.
61-40 Flushing Avenue
Monroe, LA 71208
Phone No. 555-1234

Name : Sonya Burns   **Age:** 36
Address: 96 Havana Blvd., FL 31207   **Date:** 3/18/96

R̶x̶

Hydrochlorothiazide	20 mg
Triamterene	40 mg
Lactose q.s.	

M. ft caps. DTD # 10

Sig: i cap bid, UD

REFILL 1 x

DAW _____

HHuxtable
DEA # AD 7973142

Tablets available: HCTZ 50 mg and Triamterene 50 mg.

Procedure:

Step 1: The prescription is based upon one capsule and Dr. Huxtable wants ten such capsules for his patient, Ms. Burns.

Step 2: 20 mg × 10 = 200 mg of hydrochlorthiazide and 40 mg × 10 = 400 mg of triamterene are needed for the ten capsules that are required for the prescription. Since bulk powders are not provided, the available tablets of hydrochlorthiazide and triamterene should be used. The number of tablets to be crushed are determined by using the following proportion:

$$\frac{50 \text{ mg of HCTZ}}{1 \text{ tablet}} = \frac{200 \text{ mg of HCTZ}}{X \text{ tablets}}$$

$$X = 4 \text{ tablets of HCTZ}$$

$$\frac{50 \text{ mg of triamterene}}{1 \text{ tablet}} = \frac{400 \text{ mg of triamterene}}{X \text{ tablets}}$$

$$X = 8 \text{ tablets of triamterene}$$

Weigh four tablets of hydrochlorthiazide and eight tablets of triamterene. Assume that the four tablets of hydrochlorthiazide weigh 800 mg and eight tablets of triamterene weigh 1200 mg. Crush the four and eight tablets, respectively. Mix these two powders geometrically. The total powder now weighs 2000 mg.

Step 3: Determine the capsule size by using the rule of six. Capsule size #3 can hold 3 grains or 195 mg. Weigh 200 mg of the tablet mixture (which is obtained as 2000 mg of total powder/10 capsules) and try to fill in capsule size #3. If the capsule is not filled or it is too full, go for the next capsule size, i.e., #2 which holds approximately 4 grains or 260 mg of powder. Verify the appropriateness by filling one or two capsules of size #2. If appropriate, select this size. For 10 capsules, the total powder should be 2600 mg. Therefore add 600 mg of lactose in the tablet mixture of 2000 mg by geometric dilution. Transfer the 2600 mg of powder on a clean paper or an ointment tile, compress as a cake, and fill all the capsules by a sliding motion.

Step 4: Wipe all the capsules from outside with a clean dry tissue paper, and submit the capsules in a suitable container with the following label:

NORTHEAST PHARMACY
169 Hillside Avenue
Monroe, LA 71206   555-0342

R # 123456   Date: 3/18/96
Burns, Sonya
96 Havana Blvd.
Take one capsule twice daily as directed
Compounded capsules #10
Refill: 1
          H. Huxtable, M.D.

Example 2:

Show the detailed method of compounding the following prescription along with all the calculations.

Henry Huxtable, M.D.
61-40 Flushing Avenue
Monroe, LA 71208
Phone No. 555-1234

Name : Frank Smith   Age: 32

Address: 142 Garden Street, LA 71201   Date: 3/16/96

℞

Ephedrine Sulfate	0.30 g
Phenobarbital	0.18 g
Lactose qs	

Ft. caps. M et Div. #12

Sig: i cap bid

REFILL _None_

DAW _____

HHuxtable

DEA # AD 7973142

Powdered ingredients are available.

Procedure:

Step 1: The prescription is based upon twelve capsules, i.e., the ingredient quantities given (ephedrine sulfate 0.3 g and phenobarbital 0.18 g) are for twelve capsules.

Step 2: Weigh 300 mg of ephedrine sulfate and 180 mg of phenobarbital and mix thoroughly. The total quantity of the mixture of these two powders is 480 mg. The amount of ephedrine sulfate needed for one capsule is 25 mg (300 mg of powder/twelve capsules) and that of phenobarbital is 15 mg (180 mg of powder/twelve capsules). The total amount of powdered drugs in each capsule is 40 mg. The minimum weight that can be weighed on a Class A prescription balance with a potential error of not more than 5% is 120 mg. Therefore, the weight of powder for each capsule has to be increased to a quantity equal to or greater than 120 mg.

Step 3: By the *rule of six* capsule size #4 can hold a total powder quantity of about 130 mg. Considering this amount, the total amount of powder for twelve capsules of size #4 is 1560 mg. The amount of lactose that should be added for twelve capsules is 1080 mg (calculated as 1560 mg − 480 mg = 1080 mg). Therefore, weigh 1080 mg of lactose and add to the drug mixture by geometric dilution. As a confirmation of the size, fill one or two capsules of size #4 with 130 mg of the mixture and determine the appropriateness. If the capsule size is correct, punch out the remaining capsules after forming a cake on a powder paper or an ointment tile.

Step 4: Wipe all the capsules from outside with a clean and dry tissue paper, and submit in an appropriate container after affixing the following label:

NORTHEAST PHARMACY
169 Hillside Avenue
Monroe, LA 71206   555-0342

℞ # 123645   Date: 3/16/96
Smith, Frank
142 Garden St
Take one capsule twice daily
Compounded Capsules #12
                    H. Huxtable, M.D.

Example 3:

How would you dispense the following prescription? Show all the calculations involved.

Patrick Mills, M.D.
61-40 Flushing Avenue
New York, NY 12345
Phone No. 555-1234

Name : Samuel Doe   Age: 32
Address: 96 Main St., NY 12345   Date: 3/9/96

R

    ASA   0.30 g
    Phenobarb.   0.03 g
    Lactose   qs

    Ft. caps. *M et. Div.* # 15

    Sig: i cap q8h

REFILL None

DAW _____
                      PMills
                 Lic # 333444

Tablets available: ASA 5 gr (325 mg) and Phenobarbital 0.5 gr (32 mg).

Procedure:

Step 1: There is an error in the signa because if 300 mg of aspirin is divided into 15 capsules, the 32-year-old patient would get only 20 mg which is much lesser than the usual dose of aspirin. Similarly phenobarbital would also be an under-dose. Therefore, the *subscription* should be *D.T.D* #15 instead of *M et. Div.*

Step 2: For 15 capsules the amount of aspirin needed is 4.5 g (calculated as 0.3 g × 15 = 4.5 g) and the amount of phenobarbital needed is 0.45 g (calculated as 0.03 g × 15 = 0.45 g). Since the available source for these chemicals are tablets containing 325 mg of aspirin and 32 mg of phenobarbital, the number of tablets required to obtain the desired amount of chemicals are calculated by using the following proportions:

$$\frac{0.325 \text{ g of ASA}}{1 \text{ tablet}} = \frac{4.5 \text{ g of ASA}}{X \text{ tablets}}$$

$$X = 13.85 \text{ or } 14 \text{ tablets of ASA}$$

$$\frac{0.032 \text{ g of phenobarb.}}{1 \text{ tablet}} = \frac{0.45 \text{ g of phenobarb.}}{X \text{ tablets}}$$

$$X = 14.06 \text{ tablets}$$

Weigh fourteen tablets of aspirin and crush them. Assume that the fourteen tablets weigh 5.6 g. Find the amount of powder needed for 13.85 tablets by using the following proportion:

$$\frac{5.6 \text{ g of ASA powder}}{14 \text{ tablets of ASA}} = \frac{X \text{ g of ASA powder}}{13.85 \text{ tablets of ASA}}$$

$$X = 5.54 \text{ g}$$

Since it is difficult to weigh 14.06 tablets of phenobarbital, weigh fifteen tablets and crush them. Assume that the powder from fifteen tablets of phenobarbital weighs three grams. By setting up a proportion, find the amount of powder that is equivalent to 14.06 tablets as follows:

$$\frac{3 \text{ g of phenobarb. powder}}{15 \text{ tablets of phenobarb.}} = \frac{X \text{ g of phenobarb. powder}}{14.06 \text{ tablets of phenobarb.}}$$

$$X = 2.81 \text{ g}$$

Weigh 5.54 g of acetyl salicylic acid powder and 2.81 g of phenobarbital powder and mix them thoroughly.

Step 3: The total powder mixture weighs 5.54 + 2.81 g = 8.35 g. Therefore, the weight of each capsule will be 8.35 g/15 = 0.557 g. Determine the size of the capsule that can hold 0.557 g or 557 mg of the powder. It is known from the rule of six that size #0 can hold up to 7 gr, i.e., 7 × 65 = 455 mg. Obviously, the next capsule size #00 appears to be the right choice. Therefore, fill one or two capsules with 557 mg of the medication powder and determine the appropriateness. If appropriate, transfer all the powder to a clean paper or an ointment tile, form a cake by compressing the powder, and fill the capsules with 557 mg each by punching them. If 557 mg of powder is less for capsule size #00, appropriate amount of lactose can be added to make up the required volume.

Step 4: Wipe all the capsules from outside with a clean and dry tissue paper, and submit in an appropriate container after affixing the following label:

NORTHEAST PHARMACY
169 Hillside Avenue
Monroe, LA 71206   555-0342

℞ # 654321   Date: 3/9/96
Doe Samuel
96 Main St
Take one capsule every eight hours
Compounded Capsules #15
P. Mills, M.D.

Practice Problems

The following ten prescriptions are for capsules that are to be prepared either from bulk chemicals or tablets, the information about which is provided following each prescription. For all the prescriptions, check if the *subscription* is correct and provide all the steps to be followed to fill the prescription. Make sure that all the calculations involved, the capsule size selected, and the label for final container are shown.

(1)

Patrick Mills, M.D.
61-40 Flushing Avenue
New York, NY 12345
Phone No. 555-1234

Name : Samuel Doe   Age: 32
Address: 96 Main St., NY 12345   Date: 3/9/96

℞

   Aldomet   1.2 g
   Hydralazine   0.1 g
   Lactose   qs   3.25 g

   Ft. caps. # 10

   Sig: i cap qid

REFILL None

DAW

                 PMills
          Lic # 333444

Available tablets: Methyldopa 500 mg weighing 1 g each, and Hydralazine tablets 50 mg weighing 200 mg each.

(2)

Patrick Mills, M.D.
61–40 Flushing Avenue
New York, NY 12345
Phone No. 555-1234

Name : Magic Jordan   Age: 32
Address: 96 Main St., NY 12345   Date: 3/9/96

R

Hydralazine HCl 10 mg
HCTZ   20 mg
Lactose   qs

Ft. caps. # xiv

Sig: i 8 A.M., and 4 P.M.

REFILL _None_

DAW _____
                                        PMills
                              Lic # 333444

Available tablets: Hydralazine HCl 50 mg weighing 200 mg each, and HCTZ 20 mg tablets weighing 160 mg each.

(3)

Patrick Mills, M.D.
61–40 Flushing Avenue
New York, NY 12345
Phone No. 555-1234

Name : Michael Johnson   Age: 32
Address: 96 Main St., NY 12345   Date: 3/9/96

R

CPM   5 mg
Pseudoephedrine HCl   40 mg
ASA   300 mg
Lactose qs ad

Ft. caps. DTD # 12

Sig: i cap q6h

REFILL _None_

DAW _____
                                        PMills
                              Lic # 333444

Available: Bulk powders of all the ingredients.

(4)

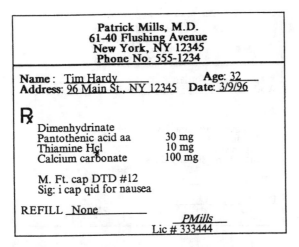

Patrick Mills, M.D.
61-40 Flushing Avenue
New York, NY 12345
Phone No. 555-1234

Name : Tim Hardy   Age: 32
Address: 96 Main St., NY 12345   Date: 3/9/96

℞

Dimenhydrinate
Pantothenic acid aa   30 mg
Thiamine Hcl   10 mg
Calcium carbonate   100 mg

M. Ft. cap DTD #12
Sig: i cap qid for nausea

REFILL None
                                             PMills
                                   Lic # 333444

Available: Bulk powder of dimenhydrinate and pantothenic acid, 25 mg tablets of thiamine HCl weighing 200 mg each, and 500 mg tablets of calcium carbonate weighing 1 g each.

(5)

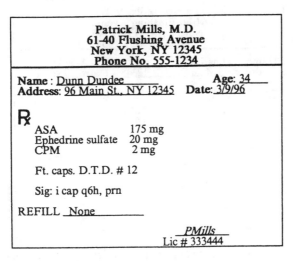

Patrick Mills, M.D.
61-40 Flushing Avenue
New York, NY 12345
Phone No. 555-1234

Name : Dunn Dundee   Age: 34
Address: 96 Main St., NY 12345   Date: 3/9/96

℞

ASA   175 mg
Ephedrine sulfate   20 mg
CPM   2 mg

Ft. caps. D.T.D. # 12

Sig: i cap q6h, prn

REFILL None

                                             PMills
                                   Lic # 333444

Available: 325 mg aspirin tablets weighing 0.7 g each, 60 mg ephedrine sulfate weighing 200 mg each, and 4 mg cpm weighing 150 mg each.

(6)

```
┌─────────────────────────────────────────────────┐
│               Patrick Mills, M.D.                │
│               61-40 Flushing Avenue              │
│               New York, NY 12345                 │
│               Phone No. 555-1234                 │
├─────────────────────────────────────────────────┤
│ Name : Vicky Jordan           Age: 23            │
│ Address: 96 Main St., NY 12345  Date: 3/9/96     │
│                                                  │
│ Rx                                               │
│     Diphenhydramine HCl     20 mg                │
│     Prednisone              2. 5 mg              │
│     Lactose qs ad           300 mg              │
│     Sig: i cap q8h for 5 days                    │
│                                                  │
│ REFILL _None_____                              │
│                                                  │
│ DAW _____                                  │
│                                   PMills         │
│                               Lic # 333444       │
└─────────────────────────────────────────────────┘
```

Available: 50 mg Benadryl® capsules weighing 200 mg, and 4 mg predni-sone tablets weighing 180 mg each.

(7)

```
┌─────────────────────────────────────────────────┐
│               Patrick Mills, M.D.                │
│               61-40 Flushing Avenue              │
│               New York, NY 12345                 │
│               Phone No. 555-1234                 │
├─────────────────────────────────────────────────┤
│ Name : Latina David           Age: 21            │
│ Address: 96 Main St., NY 12345  Date: 3/9/96     │
│                                                  │
│ Rx                                               │
│     Simethicone          0.02 g                  │
│     Phenobarb.           0.075 g                 │
│     Magnesium carbonate  0.05 g                  │
│                                                  │
│     M. Ft caps D.T.D. # 12                       │
│     Sig: ii caps tid & HS                        │
│                                                  │
│ REFILL _None_____                              │
│                                                  │
│ DAW _____                                  │
│                                   PMills         │
│                               Lic # 333444       │
└─────────────────────────────────────────────────┘
```

Available: 20 mg simethicone tablets weighing 150 mg each, pheno-barbital powder, and 500 mg magnesium carbonate tablets weighing 1 g each.

(8)

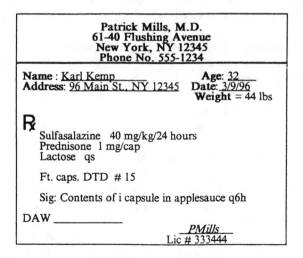

Patrick Mills, M.D.
61-40 Flushing Avenue
New York, NY 12345
Phone No. 555-1234

Name : Hill Grant_____   **Age:** 24___
Address: 96 Main St., NY 12345   **Date:** 3/9/96

R

   Warfarin sodium   1.5 mg
   Lactose qs ad   300 mg

   M.Ft. Cap D.T.D. # xii

   Sig: i qAM

REFILL _None_____

DAW _____
                          PMills
                    Lic # 333444

Tablets available: 5 mg warfarin sodium tablets weighing 150 mg each.

(9)

Patrick Mills, M.D.
61-40 Flushing Avenue
New York, NY 12345
Phone No. 555-1234

Name : Karl Kemp_____   **Age:** 32___
Address: 96 Main St., NY 12345   **Date:** 3/9/96
                             Weight = 44 lbs

R

   Sulfasalazine   40 mg/kg/24 hours
   Prednisone 1 mg/cap
   Lactose qs

   Ft. caps. DTD # 15

   Sig: Contents of i capsule in applesauce q6h

DAW _____
                          PMills
                    Lic # 333444

Bulk powders for all the ingredients are available.

(10)

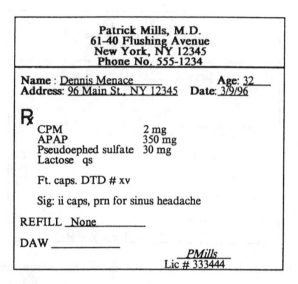

Patrick Mills, M.D.
61-40 Flushing Avenue
New York, NY 12345
Phone No. 555-1234

Name : Dennis Menace   Age: 32
Address: 96 Main St., NY 12345   Date: 3/9/96

℞

CPM   2 mg
APAP   350 mg
Pseudoephed sulfate 30 mg
Lactose   qs

Ft. caps. DTD # xv

Sig: ii caps, prn for sinus headache

REFILL _None_

DAW _____
                        PMills
                  Lic # 333444

Bulk powders are available for all the ingredients.

COMPOUNDING TIPS AND CALCULATIONS FOR FILLING POWDER PRESCRIPTIONS

These prescriptions appear rarely in a pharmacy practice, but are important from an examination point of view. Moreover, even for rare prescriptions, it is the pharmacist's responsibility as an expert to fill those prescriptions. Therefore, a brief introduction and a few examples are provided in this section for calculations involving the powder prescriptions.

Pharmaceutical powder is a mixture of finely divided drugs and/or chemicals in dry form. They are dispensed as bulk powders or divided powders. When the prescription is received for powders, first determine whether it is based upon one unit or upon a bulk formula to be subdivided into individual units. Bulk powders are provided as multiple doses in a container and the patient measures the dose as instructed at the time of administration. Some examples of bulk powders include Tolnaftate Powder USP and Nystatin Topical Powder USP as antifungals, and Desitin® Powder for diaper rash. Divided powders are meant to be provided as single dose units in individually wrapped powder papers. Such single dose packets are stacked in a powder box, and the label is placed on the box. The procedure for folding the divided papers is shown in Figure 6.1.

After determining the type of dispensing, i.e., bulk or divided powders, determine the weight of each ingredient required: Reduce all the ingredients to a fine powder. Then by the geometric dilution method, mix all the ingredients with trituration. If bulk dispensing is required, fill the powder in a wide mouthed bottle. If divided powder papers are needed, weigh single doses and fill in the powder papers. Fold the powder papers as shown in the figure. Finally, stack the papers in the powder box and affix the label.

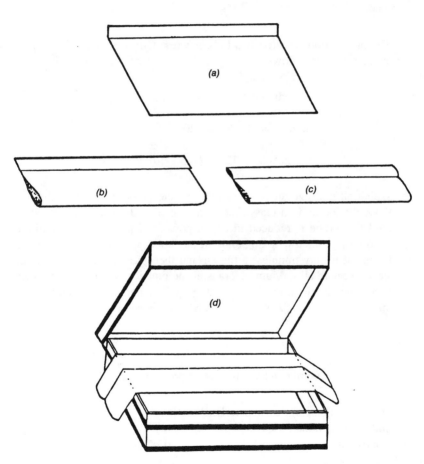

FIGURE 6.1. (a) Single fold on top, (b) single fold down, (c) double fold up, (d) use of powder box to mark for the crease to fold the packet on back side.

Example 1:

Show how you will prepare the following prescription.

℞
  Iodine 1%
  Boric acid 10 g
  Lactose qs 30 g
  Ft. ℈-iv

Sig: AAbid, UD

Procedure:

The preparation required is a bulk powder. Quantity of the ingredients is calculated as follows:

$$\text{Iodine } (1/100) \times 120 = 1.2 \text{ g}$$

$$\text{Boric acid} = (10/30) \times 120 = 40 \text{ g}$$

$$\text{Lactose} = 120 - (1.2 + 40) = 78.8 \text{ g}$$

Weigh all the ingredients separately. Iodine must be finely subdivided. Place the iodine in a glass mortar, add alcohol drop wise, and triturate until the iodine is reduced to a fine powder. Then add boric acid and lactose by geometric mixing until the alcohol evaporates. Dry the powder for about twenty minutes in the air and then pass through a #40 mesh sieve to break all the lumps. Transfer the powder into a wide-mouthed, four-ounce bottle. Label appropriately as "Compounded Powder" with the instructions of "Apply to affected area twice daily as directed."

Example 2:

Explain how to compound the following preparation.

Precipitated calcium carbonate USP	0.6 g
Sodium bicarbonate USP	1.0 g
Lactose qs	3.0 g

M. Ft. chart DTD #12

Available information: Turns® tablets (containing 0.5 g of calcium carbonate) and bulk powder sodium carbonate are available for this prescription.

Procedure

The preparation is for a single powder and twelve such powder packets are needed. Quantity of the ingredients are calculated as follows:

Precipitated calcium carbonate: 0.6×12 powders = 7.2 g needed

(0.5 g/1 Tums® tablet) = (7.2 g/X Tums® tablet)

$X = 14.4$ or 15 Tums® tablets

The exact amount of precipitated calcium carbonate is calculated as follows: each Tums® tablet containing 0.5 gram of calcium carbonate weighs one gram totally. Therefore fifteen tablets weigh 15 g and contain $15 \times 0.5 =$ 7.5 g of calcium carbonate.

$$\frac{7.5 \text{ g of calcium carbonate}}{15 \text{ g of Tums® powder}} = \frac{7.2 \text{ g of calcium carbonate}}{X \text{ g of Tums® powder}}$$

$X = 14.4$ g of Tums® powder

Sodium bicarbonate USP: $1 \text{ g} \times 12$ powders = 12 g of the powder

Lactose: $3 \text{ g} \times 12$ powders = 36 g of total powder for the twelve capsules. Therefore the lactose needed is 36 g $-(14.4 + 12) = 9.6$ g.

Crush 15 Tums® tablets and weigh out 14.4 g of the resultant powder. Weigh 12 g of sodium bicarbonate USP powder and 9.6 g of the lactose. Mix all the three powders in a wedgewood mortar by the geometric dilution method. Make sure that there are no lumps in the preparation. If there are lumps, pass the powder through some sieve, preferably USP Standard Sieve #40. Weigh three grams of the powder each time and fill in the powder paper as shown earlier. Make twelve such packets and arrange them in the powder paper box. Finally, label the box.

Calculations Involving Ointments, Creams, and Other Semisolids

The present chapter deals with calculations involving topical semisolid dosage forms, which include ointments, creams, and pastes.

Ointments are semisolid preparations that are intended for external use. Ointments may contain either finely powdered drugs or their mixtures, liquids, and other drug forms incorporated into appropriate bases. They are applied to the skin for their physical effects as emollients (which make the skin more pliable), protectants, lubricants, and drying agents. Ointment bases are also used as vehicles in which to incorporate topical medications which exert specific effect. There are four types of ointment bases, namely, oleaginous, absorption, water removable, and water soluble bases.

Creams are semisolid preparations meant for external application as emollients or as topical medications. They are semisolid emulsions of either the oil-in-water or the water-in-oil type.

Pastes are also semisolid preparations intended for external application to the skin, and differ from ointments and creams in that they contain a high solid content. Pastes are made stiff by the addition of powders such as starch, zinc oxide, calcium carbonate or their mixtures.

Amongst the various types of semisolid preparations, ointments represent the type of extemporaneous preparations most likely to be prepared by a pharmacist. A variety of ingredients may be included in the formula of semisolid dosage forms.

COMPOUNDING TIPS

The following general guidelines are useful for the preparation of ointments or creams:

(1) Menthol, camphor, or similar substances can be mixed to form a eutectic mixture, which can be absorbed onto wool fat (anhydrous lanolin), and then incorporated into the intended base. If such ingredients are not provided as mixtures, they can be dissolved in warm liquid petrolatum or vegetable oil before being incorporated into the base.

(2) Vegetable drug extracts may be softened with alcohol before they are incorporated into ointment bases.

(3) Small amounts of levigating agents facilitate the formation of uniform preparation. To incorporate insoluble powders, such as calamine, sulfur, and zinc oxide into oleaginous bases, mineral oil or warm petrolatum may be used. Glycerin may be used as a levigating agent when incorporating the drug into water washable or water removable bases.

(4) For soluble drugs, dissolve them in water and absorb into aquaphor base approximately double its quantity (for example, take 20 g of the base for a 10-mL liquid), and then mix in the intended base.

(5) For the preparation of creams, heat the aqueous phase containing all of the water soluble ingredients to about 70°C, and add this phase to the oil phase which has been similarly heated to 70°C. Mix the two liquids at high temperatures for a few minutes, and cool while stirring. If some volatile ingredients or perfumes are to be added, wait until the cream has cooled to at least 37°C.

CALCULATIONS ASSOCIATED WITH BULK PREPARATIONS

The practicing pharmacists may be called upon to prepare a semisolid dosage form in large quantity. The formulae for such preparations, in general, indicate *proportional parts* (or relative quantities) of ingredients to be used in compounding the desired total quantity.

The following steps may be used to find the quantity of each ingredient to be used for the desired bulk quantity:

(1) Find the total number of parts (by volume or weight).
    Note: (A) When parts by volume or weight are specified, make sure that all the quantities are expressed in the common denomination (or same units), such as milliliter, gram, pound, etc. (B) When parts by volume are provided, one can convert only to volumes and not to weights. Similarly, when parts by weight are provided, one can convert only to weights.

(2) Write down the desired quantity of the product to be prepared.

(3) The quantity of each ingredient to be used for the desired quantity (X) may be found by the method of proportion:

$$\frac{\text{Total number of parts specified in the formula}}{\text{Number of parts of each ingredient in the formula}} = \frac{\text{Desired quantity of the product to be prepared}}{X}$$

(4) Add up the quantities of all the ingredients from Step 3. The total should equal the desired quantity of the product to be prepared.

Example 1:

From the following formula, calculate the number of grams of each ingredient required to make 1000 grams of the ointment:

Salicylic acid	1.5 parts
Precipitated sulfur	3.5 parts
Hydrophilic ointment	45.0 parts

Step 1: 1.5 + 3.5 + 45.0 = 50.0 total parts

Step 2: Desired quantity of the product to be prepared = 1000 g

Step 3:

$$\text{Salicylic acid: } \frac{50}{1.5} = \frac{1000}{X}$$

$$X = 30.0 \text{ g}$$

$$\text{Precipitated sulfur: } \frac{50}{3.5} = \frac{1000}{X}$$

$$X = 70.0 \text{ g}$$

$$\text{Hydrophilic oint.: } \frac{50}{45} = \frac{1000}{X}$$

$$X = 900 \text{ g}$$

Step 4: answer: total = 30 + 70 + 900 = 1000 g

Example 2:

From the following formula, calculate the amount, in g, of each ingredient required to make 1 lb (avoir.) of cold cream.

Mineral Oil	50.0 parts
Cetyl Esters Wax	15.0 parts
White Wax	12.0 parts
Sodium Borate	1.0 parts
Water	22.0 parts

Step 1: 50 + 15 + 12 + 1 + 22 = 100 total parts

Step 2: Desired quantity of the product to be prepared = 1 lb (avoir.) = 454 g

Step 3:

$$\text{Mineral oil: } \frac{100}{50} = \frac{454}{X}$$

$$X = 227 \text{ g}$$

$$\text{Cetyl esters wax: } \frac{100}{15} = \frac{454}{X}$$

$$X = 68.1 \text{ g}$$

$$\text{White wax: } \frac{100}{12} = \frac{454}{X}$$

$$X = 54.48 \text{ g}$$

$$\text{Sodium borate: } \frac{100}{1} = \frac{454}{X}$$

$$X = 4.54 \text{ g}$$

$$\text{Water: } \frac{100}{22} = \frac{454}{X}$$

$$X = 99.88 \text{ g}$$

Step 4: answer: total = 227 + 68.1 + 54.48 + 4.54 + 99.88 = 454.0 g or 1 lb (avoir.)

Example 3:

From the following formula, calculate the quantity of each ingredient required to prepare 5 lb (avoir.) of the ointment:

Benzoic acid	6 parts
Salicylic acid	4 parts
PEG ointment	90 parts

Step 1: 6 + 4 + 90 = 100 total parts

Step 2: Desired quantity of the product to be prepared = 5 lb (avoir.) =
5 × 454 = 2270 g

Step 3:

$$\text{Benzoic acid: } \frac{100}{6} = \frac{2270}{X}$$

$$X = 136.2 \text{ g}$$

$$\text{Salicylic acid: } \frac{100}{4} = \frac{2270}{X}$$

$$X = 90.8 \text{ g}$$

$$\text{PEG ointment: } \frac{100}{90} = \frac{2270}{X}$$

$$X = 2043.0 \text{ g}$$

Step 4: answer: total = 136.2 + 90.8 + 2043.0 = 2270 g or 5 lb

PERCENTAGE STRENGTH CALCULATIONS OF SEMISOLID PREPARATIONS

Percentage by weight (% weight-in-weight) of a drug may be defined as
the number of parts by weight of active medicinal agent that are contained
in 100 parts by weight of the mixture. If the weight of the active ingredient
in a given quantity of mixture is known, one can calculate the percentage
strength.

Example 1:

Two triamcinolone acetonide ointment preparations are available: one containing 1 mg/g (i.e., 1 mg of triamcinolone acetonide per 1 gram of the ointment) and the other 5 mg/g. Express these concentrations as percentage strengths (% w/w).

a. If 1 g of the ointment contains 1 mg of drug, 100 g contain 100 mg, i.e., 100 mg/100 g

$$= 0.1 \text{ g/100g}$$

$$\text{answer:} = 0.1\% \text{ w/w}$$

b. If 1 g of the ointment contains 5 mg of drug, 100 g contain 500 mg, i.e., 500 mg/100 g

$$= 0.5 \text{ g/100 g}$$

$$\text{answer:} = 0.5\% \text{ w/w}$$

When weight of any mixture of solids and the amount of active ingredient in that mixture are known, one can calculate the percentage strength of active ingredient (% w/w) by the method of proportion. These calculations are explained best by following Examples 2 and 3.

Example 2:

If Efudex® Cream contains 5% of fluorouracil, calculate the percentage (w/w) of fluorouracil in the prescription.

R	
Fluorouracil	20 g
Efudex Cream	60 g
White Petrolatum ad	300 g
Sig. Apply as directed.	

Fluorouracil present in Efudex® Cream can be found by the method of proportion:

$$\frac{100 \text{ g}}{5 \text{ g}} = \frac{60 \text{ g}}{X \text{ g}}$$

$$X = (5 \times 60) \times 100 = 3 \text{ g}$$

$$\text{Total fluorouracil} = 20 + 3 = 23 \text{ g}$$

If 23 g are present in a total of 300 g, the percentage of fluorouracil can be found by the method of proportion:

$$\frac{23 \text{ g}}{300 \text{ g}} = \frac{X \text{ g}}{100 \text{ g}}$$

$$\text{answer: } X = 7.67\%$$

Example 3:

Calculate the percentage (w/w) of coal tar in the finished product when 8 grams of coal tar is mixed with 120 g of a 4% coal tar ointment.

By the method of proportion, 120 g of 4% coal tar ointment contains:

$$\frac{100 \text{ g}}{4 \text{ g}} = \frac{120 \text{ g}}{X \text{ g}}$$

$$X = 4.8 \text{ g}$$

$$\text{Total coal tar} = 8 + 4.8 = 12.8 \text{ g}$$

If 12.8 g are present in a total of 128 g, the percentage of coal tar can be found by the method of proportion:

$$\frac{12.8 \text{ g}}{128 \text{ g}} = \frac{X \text{ g}}{100 \text{ g}}$$

$$\text{answer: percent of coal tar, } X = 10\%$$

Alligation Medial

When two or more substances of known quantities and concentrations are mixed, the percentage strength of the final product may be calculated by the method of *alligation medial.* The following steps may be used to calculate the percentage strength of a mixture that has been prepared by mixing two or more components:

(1) Add up the quantity of each component used in the mixture.
(2) Multiply the quantity of each component used in the mixture by its corresponding percentage strength, and add them up.
(3) Divide the value obtained in Step 2 by the value obtained in Step 1.

Example 1:

What is the percentage of ophthalmic hydrocortisone ointment prepared by mixing 10 grams of 2.5% hydrocortisone ointment, 8 g of 2% hydrocortisone ointment, and 14 g of ointment base (diluent)?

Step 1: 10 + 8 + 14 = 32 g

Step 2:

$$
\begin{array}{r}
10 \times 2.5 = 25 \\
8 \times 2.0 = 16 \\
14 \times 0 = \underline{0} \\
41
\end{array}
$$

Step 3: answer: 41/32 = 1.28%

Example 2:

What is the percentage of ichthammol in the finished product when 100 g of 10% ichthammol ointment, 400 g of 5% ichthammol ointment, and 100 g of petrolatum (diluent) are mixed?

Step 1: 100 + 400 + 1000 = 1500

Step 2:

$$
\begin{array}{r}
100 \times 10 = 1000 \\
400 \times 5 = 2000 \\
1000 \times 0 = \underline{0} \\
3000
\end{array}
$$

Step 3: answer: 3000/1500 = 2%

Example 3:

What is the percentage of zinc oxide in an ointment prepared by mixing 2 lb (avoir.) of a 10% zinc oxide ointment, 900 g of a 20% zinc oxide ointment, and 3 lb (avoir.) of white petrolatum (diluent)?

Step 1: 2 lb = 2 × 454 = 908 g
        3 lb = 3 × 454 = 1362 g

        Total quantity = 908 + 900 + 1362 = 3170 g
Step 2:

        10 × 908 =   9080
        20 × 900 = 18,000
         0 × 1362 = _____0
                   27,080

Step 3: answer: 27080/3170 = 8.54%

Practice Problems

(1) From the following formula, calculate the quantity of each ingredient required to make 5 lb (avoir.) of the ointment.

Vioform® powder	0.1 g
Hydrocortisone powder	0.5 g
Cold cream ad	15.0 g

(2) From the following formula, calculate the quantity of each ingredient required to prepare 1 lb (avoir.) of the ointment base.

Cetyl alcohol	15 partsl
white wax	1 part
Glycerin	10 parts
Sodium lauryl sulfate	2 parts
Water	72 parts

(3) Two betamethasone valerate (Valisone®) creams are available: one containing 1 mg/g and the other 0.1 mg/g. Express these concentrations as percentage strengths (% w/w).

(4) Four anthralin (Anthra-Derm®) ointments are available which contain:

   a. 1000 μg/g

    b. 2500 μg/g

    c. 5000 μg/g

    d. 10,000 μg/g

Express these concentrations as percentage strengths (% w/w).

(5) What is the percentage (w/w) of coal tar in the finished product when 12 g of coal tar is mixed with 360 g of a 5% coal tar ointment?

(6) What is the percentage (w/w) of hydrocortisone in the finished product when 500 mg of hydrocortisone is mixed with 10 g of Cortril® ointment containing 1% hydrocortisone?

(7) What is the percentage of ophthalmic hydrocortisone ointment prepared by mixing 75 g of 5% hydrocortisone ointment, 150 g of 1.5% hydrocortisone ointment, and 180 g of ointment base (diluent)?

(8) What is the percentage of ichthammol in the finished product when 20 g of 10% ichthammol ointment, 40 g of 8% ichthammol ointment, and 80 g of petrolatum (diluent) are mixed?

(9) What is the percentage of zinc oxide in an ointment prepared by mixing 200 g of an 8% zinc oxide ointment, 150 g of a 12% zinc oxide ointment, and 300 g of white petrolatum (diluent)?

(10) What is the percentage (w/w) of hydrocortisone in the finished product when 50 g of hydrocortisone is mixed with 5 lb (avoir.) of Cortril® ointment containing 1% hydrocortisone?

DILUTION AND CONCENTRATION

When semisolid preparations of certain strength are diluted with ointment bases (also referred to as diluents), the strength of the mixture will be lowered. The percentage strength decreases as the quantity increases. To calculate the *percent by weight* strength of a semisolid mixture, an equation may be used as follows:

$$Q_1 \times C_1 = Q_2 \times C_2$$

where

Q_1 = known quantity
C_1 = known concentration
Q_2 = final quantity of the mixture
C_2 = final concentration of the mixture

Example 1:

How many grams of the ointment base (diluent) should be used to make an ointment containing 5% of boric acid?

R		
Boric Acid Oint.	(8%)	20 g
Ointment Base		q.s.
M. ft. 5% ungt.		
Sig. Apply.		

$$20 \text{ g} \times 8\% = X \text{ g} \times 5\%$$

$$X = \frac{20 \times 8}{5} = 32 \text{ g, total}$$

answer: ointment base needed = 32 − 20 = 12 g

Example 2:

How many grams of petrolatum (diluent) should be added to 250 g of a 20% ichthammol ointment to make a 6% ointment?

$$250 \text{ g} \times 20\% = X \text{ g} \times 6\%$$

$$X = \frac{250 \times 20}{6} = 833.3 \text{ g}$$

answer: diluent needed = 833.3 − 250 = 583.3 g

Example 3:

How many grains of 20% benzocaine ointment and how many grains of white petrolatum (diluent) should be used in compounding the following prescription?

R	
Benzocaine Oint. f℥ iii	
	2.0%
Sig. Apply p.r.n.	

$$3 \text{ oz (ounce; apoth)} = 3 \times 480 = 1440 \text{ grains}$$

$$1440 \text{ gr} \times 2.0\% = X \text{ gr} \times 20\%$$

$$X = \frac{1440 \times 2}{20} = 144 \text{ gr}$$

answer: 144 gr of benzocaine ointment, and $1440 - 144 = 1296$ gr of white petrolatum are needed.

Alligation Alternate

A practicing pharmacist may mix two or more components of known strength to prepare a mixture of desired strength. The strength that is desired should be somewhere in between the individual strengths of the components employed. The strength of the mixture obtained is the "weighted" average of the individual strengths of the components used. One can calculate the number of parts of each component used to obtain a mixture of desired strength by the method of *alligation alternate.*

When using the method of alligation alternate to find out the quantity of each component used in a binary mixture to obtain the desired strength, one may use the following steps:

(1) Make three columns. In column 1, write down the concentrations of the components to be mixed.

(2) In column 2, write down the desired percentage strength of the mixture to be prepared.

(3) In column 3, write down the difference in strength by reading diagonally (as illustrated in Example 1).

(4) Find the relative proportions of the components (as illustrated in Example 1).

The calculations involving the method of alligation alternate are explained best by the following examples.

Example 1:

In what proportion should a 20% coal tar ointment be mixed with white petrolatum (diluent) to produce a 2% coal tar ointment?

Column 1   Column 2   Column 3

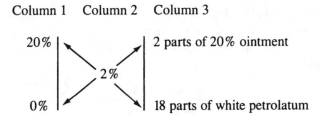

20%   2 parts of 20% ointment

                2%

0%   18 parts of white petrolatum

answer: 2:18

Example 2:

In what proportion should a 10% and 4% zinc oxide ointments be mixed to prepare a 6% ointment?

Column 1   Column 2   Column 3

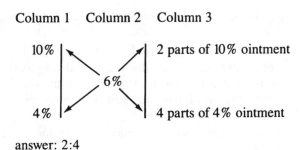

10%   2 parts of 10% ointment

                6%

4%   4 parts of 4% ointment

answer: 2:4

Example 3:

How many grams of salicylic acid should be added to 1200 g of a 1% salicylic acid ointment to prepare a product containing 2.5% of salicylic acid?

Salicylic acid = 100%
Salicylic acid ointment = 1%

Column 1   Column 2   Column 3

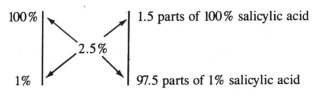

100%   1.5 parts of 100% salicylic acid

                2.5%

1%   97.5 parts of 1% salicylic acid

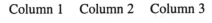

1.5:97.5 parts

Since the quantity of 1% salicylic acid ointment and the individual parts of the two components to be used in the ointment product are known, one can calculate the quantity of salicylic acid to be used by the method of proportion:

$$\frac{97.5 \text{ parts}}{1200 \text{ g}} = \frac{1.5 \text{ parts}}{X \text{ g}}$$

answer: $X = 18.46$ g

The examples above involve mixing two components. The method of alligation alternate may also be employed to find out the relative amounts of more than two components to be mixed to obtain a product of the desired percentage.

When three components are used to obtain the desired strength, one may use the following steps:

(1) Select any two components; one stronger and one weaker than the desired strength.

(2) Follow the steps as explained above for two component mixtures.

(3) Select one of the two components that has been already used, and pair it up with the remaining component. In pairing up the components, one must make sure that one of the components is stronger and the other one is weaker than the desired strength.

(4) Follow the steps, once again, as explained above for two component (binary) system.

(5) Find the relative proportions of each component used (as illustrated in Example 1).

Example 1:

A physician ordered 20% monobenzone (Benoquin®) ointment to be used for the temporary bleaching of hyperpigmented skin. In what proportion may 25%, 10%, and 5% monobenzone ointments be mixed in order to prepare an ointment of the desired concentration?

Column 1   Column 2   Column 3

$$
\begin{array}{lll}
\ulcorner 25\% & & \mid 10 + 15 = 25 \\
\llcorner 10\% & 20\% & \mid 5 = 5 \\
\llcorner 5\% & & \mid 5 = 5 \\
\end{array}
$$

25:5:5

The above answer can be further reduced to 5:1:1. Thus, to obtain alcohol of 20% strength, the three components are mixed according to the following proportion:

> 5 parts of 25% ointment
> 1 parts of 10% ointment
> 1 parts of 5% ointment

Alternatively, the problem can be solved as follows. In the above example, two concentrations are less than required concentration of 20%, and only one is higher. To balance this, the higher concentration (i.e., 25%) may be used twice. This is explained as follows:

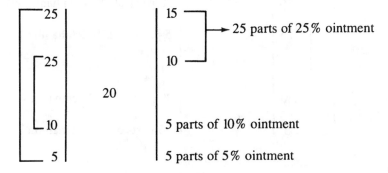

answer: 25:5:5 or 5:1:1

Example 2:

A 25% sulfacetamide sodium ointment is needed for certain topical antibiotic activity. In what proportion may 40%, 30%, and 10% sulfacetamide sodium ointments be mixed in order to prepare a mixture of 25% concentration?

Column 1   Column 2   Column 3

40%		15 parts of 40% ointment
30%	25%	15 parts of 30% ointment
10%		5 + 15 = 20 parts of 10% ointment

answer: 15:15:20 or 3:3:4

When four components are used to obtain the desired strength, each of the weaker components is paired with one of the stronger to give the desired strength. *Note:* Since it is possible to pair the components in two ways, there may be two sets of correct answers for these problems.

Example 3:

Four lots of ichthammol ointment, containing 5%, 10%, 25% and 40% of ichthammol are available. How many grams of each may the pharmacist use to prepare 5 kg of a 15% ichthammol ointment?

Column 1   Column 2   Column 3

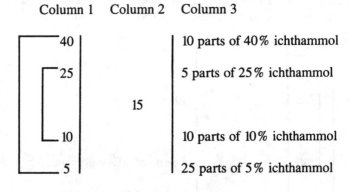

40   10 parts of 40% ichthammol

25   5 parts of 25% ichthammol

              15

10   10 parts of 10% ichthammol

5   25 parts of 5% ichthammol

Total parts = 10 + 5 + 10 + 25 = 50

answer: quantity of ointment to be prepared = 5 kg or 5000 g

By the method of proportion, the quantity of each component to be used can be found as follows:

40% ichthammol:

$$\frac{50 \text{ parts}}{10} = \frac{5000 \text{ g}}{X}$$

answer: $X = 1000$ g

25% ichthammol:

$$\frac{50 \text{ parts}}{5} = \frac{5000 \text{ g}}{X}$$

answer: $X = 500$ g

10% ichthammol:

$$\frac{50 \text{ parts}}{10} = \frac{5000 \text{ g}}{X}$$

answer: $X = 1000$ g

5% ichthammol:

$$\frac{50 \text{ parts}}{25} = \frac{5000 \text{ g}}{X}$$

answer: $X = 2500$ g

or

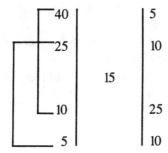

5:10:25:10, or the answer can further be reduced to: 1:2:5:2 for a total parts of 10.

By the method of proportion, the quantity of each component to be used can be found as follows:

40% ichthammol:

$$\frac{10 \text{ parts}}{1} = \frac{5000 \text{ g}}{X}$$

answer: $X = 500$ g

25% ichthammol:

$$\frac{10 \text{ parts}}{2} = \frac{5000 \text{ g}}{X}$$

answer: $X = 1000$ g

10% ichthammol:

$$\frac{10 \text{ parts}}{5} = \frac{5000 \text{ g}}{X}$$

answer: $X = 2500$ g

5% ichthammol:

$$\frac{10 \text{ parts}}{2} = \frac{5000 \text{ g}}{X}$$

answer: $X = 1000$ g

Practice Problems

(1) In what proportions 3%, 12%, and 15% sulfur ointments must be mixed to prepare 8% sulfur ointment?

(2) How many grams of the ointment base (diluent) should be used to make an ointment containing 2% boric acid?

℞

Boric Acid Ointment (3%)   16 g
Ointment Base   q.s.
M. ft. 2% ungt.
Sig. Apply as directed

(3) How many grams of coal tar should be added to 925 g of zinc oxide paste to prepare an ointment containing 6% of coal tar?

(4) How many grams of 2% ophthalmic hydrocortisone acetate ointment and how many grams of ophthalmic base (diluent) should be used in compounding the prescription?

℞

Hydrocortisone Acetate Ointment   20 g
    0.50%
Sig. Apply to the eye

(5) How much zinc oxide should be added to the product in order to make an ointment containing 8% of zinc oxide?

℞

Zinc Oxide	2.0
Hydrophilic Petrolatum	2.5
Purified Water	5.0
Hydrophilic Ointment ad	40.0

Sig. Apply to affected areas

(6) How many grams of coal tar should be added to 420 g of zinc oxide paste to prepare an ointment containing 5% of coal tar?

(7) How many grams of coal tar should be added to a mixture of 1000 g of zinc oxide paste and 500 g of wool fat to make an ointment containing 10% of coal tar?

(8) In what proportion should 5% and 20% zinc oxide ointments be mixed to prepare an 8% ointment?

(9) A pharmacist has on hand one kg of a 5% coal tar ointment and 4 lb (avoir) of a 10% coal tar ointment. (A) What is the concentration of coal tar in the finished product, if the two ointments are mixed? (B) How many grams of coal tar should be added to the product to obtain an ointment containing 20% of coal tar?

(10) Four lots of ichthammol ointment containing 5%, 12%, 20% and 25% of ichthammol are available. How many grams of each may the pharmacist use to prepare 5 lb (avoir.) of a 15% ichthammol ointment? (Use all four lots.)

CHAPTER 8

Calculations Involving Topical Ophthalmic, Nasal, and Otic Preparations

A variety of pharmaceutical dosage forms are applied topically to the eye, nose, and ear which include solutions, suspensions, and ointments. In general, drugs are applied to the eye for the local effects of the medication, either on the surface of the eye or its interior. Amongst the various types of dosage forms for the eye, aqueous solutions are the most frequently used. In the extemporaneous preparation of ophthalmic formulations, one should consider sterility, preservation, isotonicity, pH and buffering, and viscosity. Nasal preparations are generally used for their decongestant activity on the nasal mucosa. Important considerations in the preparation of nasal solutions include isotonicity, pH and buffering, and viscosity. Ear preparations are also referred to as *otic* or *aural* preparations. Most of the official ear preparations are aqueous solutions of medications. They are used for treating mild infections, softening wax, cleansing after infections, drying wet surfaces, and as antiseptics. The important considerations in the formulation of otic products include pH and buffering. For example, an otic product with a pH value of less than 4 may cause burning and stinging sensation in the ear canal.

The present chapter deals with calculations involving isotonicity, pH, and buffering of topical preparations. The discussion presented here is also relevant to the dosage forms for other routes of administration including parenteral routes.

ISOTONICITY

Whenever a solution is separated from a solvent by a membrane permeable only to solvent molecules but impermeable to solutes (referred to as a "semi-

149

permeable membrane''), the solvent passes across the membrane into the solution. This is the phenomenon of osmosis, which may be defined as the passage of solvent molecules across a semipermeable membrane against the concentration gradient. Osmosis can also occur when a concentrated solution is separated from a less concentrated solution by a semipermeable membrane. The pressure differential that develops across the membrane is called ''osmotic pressure.''

Osmotic pressure is a colligative property and is dependent on the number of particles of solute(s) in a solution. The total number of particles of a solute in a solution is the sum of the undissociated molecules and the number of ions into which the molecule dissociates. The number of ions, in turn, depends on the degree of ionization. Thus, a chemical that is highly ionized contributes a greater number of particles to the solution than the same amount of a poorly ionized chemical. When a chemical is a nonelectrolyte such as sucrose or urea, the concentration of the solution depends only on the number of molecules present. The values of the osmotic pressure and other colligative properties are approximately the same for equal concentrations of different nonelectrolyte solutions.

Body fluids, including blood and tears, have the same osmotic pressure as that of a 0.9% w/v sodium chloride solution. Solutions having the same osmotic pressure as that of 0.9% w/v NaCl solution are said to be *isotonic* with blood. Solutions with a higher osmotic pressure than body fluids are called *hypertonic* and those with a lower osmotic pressure are called *hypotonic*.

Osmotic effects are very important from a physiological standpoint. This is because biological membranes including the membrane of red blood cells behave like semipermeable membranes. Consequently, when red blood cells are immersed in a hypertonic solution (e.g., D_5 $\frac{1}{2}$ NS or D_5NS), they shrink as water leaves the blood cells in an attempt to dilute and establish a concentration equilibrium across the blood cell membrane. Thus, when hypertonic solutions are administered into the blood stream, the fluid moves from interstitial and cellular space into the intravascular space. Conversely, when cells are placed in hypotonic environment (e.g., $\frac{1}{2}$ NS), they swell because of the entry of fluid from the intravascular compartment, and may eventually undergo lysis.

In the eye, hypertonic solutions may cause drawing of water towards the site of application; whereas hypotonic solutions may cause water to move from the topical application site through the tissues of the eye. When instilled into the eye, isotonic solutions cause no contraction or swelling of the tissues with which they come in contact, and cause no discomfort. Therefore, it is very important to adjust the isotonicity of topical ophthalmic products. Isotonic adjustments are also important for nasal and aural preparations, parenteral products, and irrigating solutions. In a given product, all the additives including the active and inactive ingredients, contribute to the osmotic pressure of the solution.

CALCULATION OF DISSOCIATION (*i*) FACTOR

Since osmotic pressure depends upon the number of particles of solute(s) in solution, the osmotic pressure of an electrolyte is directly proportional to the degree (or extent) of dissociation. The dissociation factor, symbolized by the letter *i*, can be calculated by dividing the total number of particles (which include undissociated molecules and ions) in a solution by the number of particles before dissociation, i.e.,

$$i = \frac{\text{Total number of particles of solute in a solution after dissociation}}{\text{Number of particles before dissociation}}$$

Example 1:

What is the dissociation factor of NaCl, having 80% dissociation in water?

Assume that we have 100 particles of NaCl prior to dissociation. Upon 80% dissociation, 100 molecules of sodium chloride yield:

80	sodium ions
80	chloride ions
20	undissociated sodium chloride particles
180	total particles in solution

answer: $i = 180/100 = 1.8$

Note: About 80% of NaCl is dissociated in water. Thus, the dissociation factor, *i*, of NaCl is assumed to be 1.8.

Example 2:

What is the dissociation factor of zinc sulfate, having 40% dissociation in water?

Assume that we have 100 particles of zinc sulfate prior to dissociation. Upon 40% dissociation, 100 molecules of zinc sulfate yield:

$$
\begin{array}{rl}
40 & \text{zinc ions} \\
40 & \text{sulfate ions} \\
\underline{60} & \text{undissociated zinc sulfate particles} \\
140 & \text{total particles in solution}
\end{array}
$$

answer: $i = 140/100 = 1.4$

Example 3:

What is the dissociation factor of zinc chloride, having 80% dissociation in water?

Assume that we have 100 particles of zinc chloride prior to dissociation. Upon 80% dissociation, 100 molecules of zinc chloride yield:

$$
\begin{array}{rl}
80 & \text{zinc ions} \\
160 & (2 \times 80) \text{ chloride ions} \\
\underline{20} & \text{undissociated zinc chloride particles} \\
260 & \text{total particles in solution}
\end{array}
$$

answer: $i = 260/100 = 2.6$

SODIUM CHLORIDE EQUIVALENTS OF DRUG SUBSTANCES

The sodium chloride equivalent of a chemical is defined as the amount of sodium chloride (in grams or grains) that has the same osmotic pressure as that of 1 g of the chemical. The sodium chloride equivalents are symbolized by the letter E. The quantities of two substances that are isotonic equivalents are proportional to the molecular weight of each multiplied by the i value of the other. Thus, if the molecular weight and i value of a given chemical are known, one can calculate the sodium chloride equivalent, E, of that chemical as follows:

$$
E = \frac{\text{MW of NaCl}}{i \text{ value of NaCl}} \times \frac{i \text{ value of the chemical}}{\text{MW of the chemical}}
$$

Example 1:

Calculate the sodium chloride equivalent of a 1% solution of pilocarpine nitrate.

Pilocarpine nitrate has a molecular weight of 271 and i of 1.8.

$$E = \frac{\text{MW of NaCl}}{i \text{ value of NaCl}} \times \frac{i \text{ value of pilocarpine nitrate}}{\text{MW of pilocarpine nitrate}}$$

$$E = \frac{58.5}{1.8} \times \frac{1.8}{271}$$

$$= 105.3/487.8$$

$= 0.22$., i.e., 1 g of pilocarpine nitrate is equivalent to 0.22 g of NaCl

answer: $E = 0.22$

Example 2:

Calculate the sodium chloride equivalent of a 1% zinc chloride.

Zinc chloride has a molecular weight of 136 and i of 2.6.

$$E = \frac{\text{MW of NaCl}}{i \text{ value of NaCl}} \times \frac{i \text{ value of zinc chloride}}{\text{MW of zinc chloride}}$$

$$E = \frac{58.5}{1.8} \times \frac{2.6}{136}$$

$$= 152.1/244.8$$

$= 0.62$, i.e., 1 g of zinc chloride is equivalent to 0.62 g of NaCl

answer: $E = 0.62$

Example 3:

Calculate the sodium chloride equivalent of a 1% boric acid.

Boric acid has a molecular weight of 62 and i of 1.

$$E = \frac{\text{MW of NaCl}}{i \text{ value of NaCl}} \times \frac{i \text{ value of boric acid}}{\text{MW of boric acid}}$$

$$E = \frac{58.5}{1.8} \times \frac{1}{62}$$

$$= 58.5/111.6$$

$= 0.52$, i.e., 1 g of boric acid is equivalent to 0.52 g of NaCl

answer: $E = 0.52$

TABLE 8.1. *Number of Ions, Dissociation Factor (I), and Molecular Weight (MW) of Selected Compounds.*

	Ions	i	MW
Boric acid	1	1.0	62
Chlorobutanol	1	1.0	177
Dextrose, anhydrous	1	1.0	180
Dextrose, H_2O	1	1.0	198
Mannitol	1	1.0	182
Benzalkonium chloride	2	1.8	360
Cocaine HCl	2	1.8	340
Cromolyn sodium	2	1.8	512
Dipivefrin HCl	2	1.8	388
Ephedrine HCl	2	1.8	202
Epinephrine bitartrate	2	1.8	333
Eucatropine HCl	2	1.8	328
Homatropine HBr	2	1.8	356
Oxymetazoline HCl	2	1.8	297
Oxytetracycline HCl	2	1.8	497
Phenylephrine HCl	2	1.8	204
Procaine HCl	2	1.8	273
Scopolamine HBr·$3H_2O$	2	1.8	438
Silver nitrate	2	1.8	170
Sodium chloride	2	1.8	58
Sodium phosphate, monobasic, anhydrous	2	1.8	120
Sodium phosphate, monobasic·H_2O	2	1.8	138
Tetracaine HCl	2	1.8	301
Zinc sulfate·$7H_2O$	2	1.8	288
Atropine sulfate, H_2O	3	2.6	695
Ephedrine sulfate	3	2.6	429
Sodium phosphate, dibasic, anhydrous	3	2.6	142
Sodium phosphate, dibasic·$7H_2O$	3	2.6	268

Table 8.1 lists number of ions produced upon dissociation, dissociation factor (i), and molecular weight of selected compounds.

ISOTONICITY ADJUSTMENTS BY SODIUM CHLORIDE EQUIVALENT METHOD

The sodium chloride equivalent method is the most frequently used method in the calculation of the amount of sodium chloride needed to prepare isotonic drug solutions. The sodium chloride equivalent of any drug substance, as discussed earlier, is the amount (in grams) of sodium chloride that is osmotically equivalent to 1 g of the drug. The sodium chloride equivalents for selected compounds are listed in Table 8.2.

Any hypotonic solution containing one or more drugs can be rendered isotonic by adding appropriate quantity of sodium chloride. Following is a sample prescription that requires isotonic adjustments:

R	
Atropine Sulfate	1%
Sodium Chloride	q.s.
Purified Water ad	100
Make isoton. sol.	
Sig. Gtt. i.o.u.	

TABLE 8.2. *Sodium Chloride Equivalents (E) and Freezing Point Depression ($\Delta T_f^{\%}$) Values of Selected Compounds.*

Substance	E	$\Delta T_f^{\%}$
Ammonium chloride	1.08	0.64
Apomorphine hydrochloride	0.14	0.08
Atropine sulfate	0.13	0.07
Boric acid	0.52	0.29
Chlorobutanol	0.18	0.14
Cocaine hydrochloride	0.16	0.09
Dextrose monohydrate	0.16	0.09
Ephedrine hydrochloride	0.30	0.18
Ephedrine sulfate	0.23	0.14
Epinephrine bitartrate	0.18	0.11
Epinephrine hydrochloride	0.29	0.17
Eucatropine hydrochloride	0.18	0.11
Fluorescein sodium	0.31	0.18
Glycerin	0.34	0.20
Naphazoline hydrochloride	0.27	0.16
Neomycin sulfate	0.11	0.06
Oxymetazoline	0.20	0.11
Phenol	0.35	0.2
Phenylephrine hydrochloride	0.32	0.18
Pilocarpine nitrate	0.22	0.14
Procaine hydrochloride	0.21	0.11
Scopolamine hydrobromide	0.12	0.07
Silver nitrate	0.33	0.19
Sodium chloride	1.00	0.58
Sulfacetamide sodium	0.23	0.14
Tetracaine hydrochloride	0.18	0.11
Zinc chloride	0.62	0.37
Zinc sulfate·$7H_2O$	0.15	0.09

E = Sodium chloride equivalent.
$\Delta T_f^{\%}$ = Freezing point depression of 1% solution.

In the prescription above, 1% atropine sulfate is ordered. The sodium chloride equivalent of atropine sulfate is 0.13 (refer to Table 8.2). This means that 1% solution of atropine sulfate has same osmotic pressure as that of 0.13% solution of sodium chloride. This solution is hypotonic. Addition of 0.77 g (i.e., 0.9 − 0.13 = 0.77) of sodium chloride per 100 mL of the 1% solution of atropine sulfate results in an isotonic solution. To determine the amount of sodium chloride required to render a given solution isotonic, the following steps may be used:

- Step 1: Find how much sodium chloride is needed to render the formulation isotonic with body fluids. (Remember isotonicity refers to 0.9% or 0.9 g/100 mL).
- Step 2: Find the amount of sodium chloride represented by the ingredients in the prescription by multiplying the quantity of each ingredient by its E value. Add up all the values obtained. This is the total amount of sodium chloride represented by all the ingredients in the prescription.
- Step 3: Subtract the total value obtained in Step 2 from the amount of sodium chloride required to render the formulation isotonic (i.e., the value obtained in Step 1). The value obtained in this step represents the amount of sodium chloride required to render the solution isotonic.

Example 1:

Find the quantity of sodium chloride required in compounding the following prescription. The sodium chloride equivalent of cocaine HCl is 0.16.

R	
Cocaine Hydrochloride	0.2
Sodium Chloride	q.s.
Purified Water ad	30.0
Make isoton. sol.	
Sig. One drop in each eye.	

Step 1: $(0.9/100) \times 30 = 0.27$ g

Step 2: $0.20 \times 0.16 = 0.032$ g

Step 3: answer: $0.27 − 0.032 = 0.238$ or 0.24 g

Example 2:

Find the quantity of sodium chloride to be used in compounding the following prescription. The sodium chloride equivalent of ephedrine sulfate is 0.23.

R
Ephedrine Sulfate	0.5
Sodium Chloride	q.s.
Purified Water ad	50
Make isoton. sol.	
Sig. Use as directed.	

Step 1: Sodium chloride needed to render the prescribed volume isotonic

$$(0.9/100) \times 50 = 0.45 \text{ g}$$

Step 2: $0.50 \times 0.23 = 0.115$ g

Step 3: answer: grams of sodium chloride needed to make the solution isotonic = $0.45 - 0.115 = 0.335$ or 0.34 g

Example 3:

Find the quantity of sodium chloride to be used in compounding the following prescription. The values of sodium chloride equivalent of epinephrine HCl and scopolamine HBr are 0.29 and 0.12, respectively.

R
Epinephrine Hydrochloride	1%
Scopolamine Hydrobromide	0.5%
Sodium Chloride	q.s.
Purified Water ad	60.0
Make isoton. sol.	
Sig. Use in the eye.	

Step 1: Sodium chloride needed to render the prescribed volume isotonic

$$(0.9/100) \times 60 = 0.54 \text{ g}$$

Step 2: (a) Epinephrine HCl:

$$(1/100) \times 60 = 0.60$$

$$0.60 \times 0.29 = 0.174 \text{ g}$$

(b) Scopolamine HCl:

$$(0.5/100) \times 60 = 0.30$$

$$0.30 \times 0.12 = 0.036 \text{ g}$$

The total of sum of the weights (in grams) of epinephrine HCl and scopolamine HCl multiplied by their E values, i.e., the total of (a) + (b)

$$= 0.174 + 0.036 \text{ g} = 0.21 \text{ g}$$

Step 3: answer: sodium chloride required to make the solution isotonic

$$0.54 - 0.21 = 0.33 \text{ g}$$

TONICITY AGENTS OTHER THAN SODIUM CHLORIDE

If one desires to use a chemical other than sodium chloride, such as dextrose or boric acid, the quantity of that chemical can be calculated by dividing the value obtained in Step 3 (i.e., the amount of sodium chloride needed to render the solution isotonic with body fluids) with the E value of that chemical. A proportion can be set up which can be treated as Step 4 in addition to the three steps described earlier.

Example 1:

Find the quantity of boric acid (in grams) to be used in compounding the following prescription.

R	
Atropine Sulfate	1%
Boric Acid	q.s.
Purified Water ad	30.0
Make isoton. sol.	
Sig. One drop in each eye.	

Step 1: $(0.9/100) \times 30 = 0.27$ g

Step 2: $(1/100) \times 30 = 0.3$ g

$$0.3 \times 0.13 = 0.039 \text{ g}$$

Step 3: $0.27 - 0.039 = 0.231$ g

Step 4: From Step 3, 0.231 g of sodium chloride is required to make the preparation isotonic. But the prescription calls for boric acid as the tonicity agent. Boric acid has an *E* value of 0.52. This means that 1% boric acid is osmotically equivalent to 0.52% NaCl or 1 g of boric acid is equivalent to 0.52 g of NaCl.

$$\frac{1 \text{ g}}{0.52 \text{ g}} = \frac{X}{0.231 \text{ g}}$$

where *X* is grams of boric acid equivalent to 0.231 g of sodium chloride.

answer: solving for *X*, we get: $(0.231 \times 1) \div 0.52 = 0.444$ grams

Example 2:

Find the quantity of boric acid (in grams) to be used in compounding the following prescription.

R	
Tetracaine Hydrochloride	0.1
Zinc Sulfate	0.05
Boric Acid	q.s.
Purified Water ad	30.0
Make isoton. sol.	
Sig. Drop in eye.	

Sodium chloride equivalents are as follows:

Tetracaine HCl = 0.18
Zinc sulfate = 0.15
Boric Acid = 0.52

Step 1: $(0.9/100) \times 30 = 0.27$

Step 2: (a) Tetracaine HCl:

$$0.1 \times 0.18 = 0.018 \text{ g}$$

(b) Zinc Sulfate:

$$0.05 \times 0.15 = 0.0075 \text{ g}$$

$$(a) + (b) = 0.018 + 0.0075 \text{ g} = 0.0255 \text{ g}$$

Step 3: $0.27 - 0.0255 = 0.2445$ or 0.245 g

Step 4: From Step 3, 0.245 g of sodium chloride is required to make the preparation isotonic. But the prescription calls for boric acid as the tonicity agent. Boric acid has an E value of 0.52. To find the quantity of boric acid equivalent to 0.245 grams of sodium chloride, a proportion can be set up as follows:

$$\frac{1 \text{ g}}{0.52 \text{ g}} = \frac{X}{0.245 \text{ g}}$$

answer: solving for X, we get: $(0.245 \times 1) \div 0.52 = 0.471$ grams

Example 3:

How many grams of dextrose should be used in compounding the prescription?

R	
Ephedrine Hydrochloride	0.5
Chlorobutanol	0.25
Dextrose	q.s.
Rose Water ad	50.0
Make isoton. sol.	
Sig. Nose drops.	

Sodium chloride equivalents are as follows:

Ephedrine HCl = 0.30
Chlorobutanol = 0.18
Dextrose = 0.16

Step 1: $(0.9/100) \times 50 = 0.45$ g

Step 2: (a) Ephedrine HCl:

$$0.50 \times 0.30 = 0.15 \text{ g}$$

(b) Chlorobutanol:

$$0.25 \times 0.18 = 0.045 \text{ g}$$

$$(a) + (b) = 0.15 + 0.045 \text{ g} = 0.195 \text{ g}$$

Step 3: $0.45 - 0.195 = 0.255$ g

Step 4:

$$\frac{1 \text{ g}}{0.16 \text{ g}} = \frac{X}{0.255 \text{ g}}$$

answer: $X = 1.59$ g

Practice Problems

When solving these problems, refer to Tables 8.1 and 8.2 as needed.

(1) Calculate the dissociation factor of pilocarpine hydrochloride dissociating 80% (2 ions) in a certain concentration.

(2) Calculate the E values of the following aqueous solutions at 1% concentration:

(a) Chlorobutanol
(b) Tetracaine hydrochloride
(c) Ephedrine sulfate

(3) How many grams of sodium chloride should be used in compounding the prescription?

℞

Procaine Hydrochloride	1%
Sodium Chloride	q.s.
Sterile Water for Injection ad	100
Make isoton. sol.	
Sig. For injection.	

(4) How many grams of sodium chloride should be used in compounding the prescription?

℞

Cocaine Hydrochloride	0.6
Eucatropine Hydrochloride	0.6
Chlorobutanol	0.1
Sodium Chloride	q.s.
Purified Water ad	30.0

Make isoton. sol.
Sig. For the eye.

(5) How many grams of boric acid should be used in compounding the prescription?

℞

Zinc Sulfate	0.06
Boric Acid	q.s.
Purified Water ad	30.0

Make isoton. sol.
Sig. Drop in eyes.

(6) How many milliliters of a 0.9% solution of sodium chloride should be used in compounding the prescription?

℞

Phenylephrine Hydrochloride	1.0
Chlorobutanol	0.5
Sodium Chloride	q.s.
Purified Water ad	100.0

Make isoton. sol.
Sig. Use as directed.

(7) How many grams of sodium chloride should be used in preparing the solution?

Dextrose, Monohydrate	2.0%
Sodium Chloride	q.s.
Sterile Water for Injection ad	1000 mL

Label: Isotonic Dextrose and Saline Solution.

(8) How many milliliters of a 5% solution of boric acid should be used in compounding the prescription?

℞

Oxymetazoline Hydrochloride	2%
Boric Acid Solution	q.s.
Purified Water ad	15.0

Make isoton. sol.
Sig. For the nose, as decongestant.

(9) How many grams of dextrose monohydrate should be used in preparing a liter of a ½% isotonic ephedrine sulfate nasal spray?

(10) How many grams of boric acid should be used in compounding the prescription?

℞

Tetracaine Hydrochloride	1.0
Boric Acid	q.s.
Purified Water ad	30.0

Make isoton. sol.
Sig. Eye drops.

ISOTONICITY ADJUSTMENTS BY CRYOSCOPIC METHOD

Since osmotic pressure of a solution is not a readily measurable quantity, other easily measurable colligative properties such as the *freezing point depression* is used in the isotonicity calculations. The normal freezing (or melting) point of a pure compound is the temperature at which the solid and the liquid phases are in equilibrium at a pressure of 1 atm. Pure water has a freezing point of 0°C. When solutes are added to water, its freezing point is lowered. The freezing point depression (or lowering) of a solvent is dependent *only* on the number of particles in the solution. Blood plasma has a freezing point of −0.52 {or freezing point depression of 0.52, i.e., (− [−0.52])}. If freezing point depression value of a chemical in certain concentration is known, one can calculate the concentration of that chemical required for isotonicity by setting a proportion as follows:

$$\frac{\text{Known percentage conc. of a given chemical}}{\text{Freezing point depression of the chemical at that concentration}} = \frac{X}{\text{Freezing point depression of blood plasma}}$$

where X = percentage concentration of the chemical required to be isotonic with blood plasma.

Since *freezing point depression* of a series of compounds at 1% concentration is readily available from standard references, the above expression can be represented as:

$$\frac{1\% \text{ chemical}}{\Delta T_f^{1\%} \text{ of the chemical}} = \frac{X}{\Delta T_f \text{ of blood plasma or tears}}$$

where X = percentage concentration of the chemical required to be isotonic with blood plasma or tears.

Example 1:

1% NaCl solution has a freezing point depression of 0.576°C. What is the percentage concentration of NaCl required to make isotonic saline solution?

One can calculate the percentage concentration of NaCl by setting up the following proportion and solving for X:

$$\frac{1\%}{0.576} = \frac{X}{0.52}$$

$$X = (0.52 \times 1)/0.576$$

$$= 0.903 \text{ or } 0.9\% \text{ w/v}$$

Thus, 0.9% sodium chloride has the same osmotic pressure and the same freezing point depression of 0.52 as that of blood plasma, red blood cells, and tears. Drug solutions which have a freezing point depression of 0.52 are, therefore, isotonic with blood. A list of freezing point depression values of selected compounds at 1% concentration is presented in Table 8.2. These ΔT_f values may be used to calculate the concentration of tonicity agents, such as sodium chloride or boric acid, needed to render a hypotonic drug solution isotonic with blood plasma. The following steps may be used to find the percentage concentration of NaCl required to render hypotonic drug solutions isotonic with blood plasma:

Step 1: Find the value of freezing point depression of the drug at 1% concentration, $\Delta T_f^{1\%}$ from Table 8.2.

Step 2: Subtract $\Delta T_f^{1\%}$ of the drug from the value of freezing point depression of 0.9% sodium chloride solution, i.e., 0.52. This difference may be symbolized as $\Delta T'_f$, which is the freezing point lowering needed for isotonicity.

Step 3: Since 0.9% sodium chloride has a freezing point depression of 0.52, one can calculate the percentage concentration of sodium chloride required to lower the difference in freezing points, i.e., the value obtained in Step 2, $\Delta T'_f$, by the method of proportion. The calculations involved in this method are explained best by following examples.

Example 2:

Compound the following prescription.

R	
Atropine Sulfate	1%
Sodium Chloride	q.s.
Purified Water ad	100
Make isoton. sol.	
Sig. One drop in each eye.	

Step 1: Freezing point depression (ΔT_f) of 1% atropine solution (from Table 8.2) is 0.07.

Step 2: Find $\Delta T'_f$ by subtracting the ΔT_f value of 1% atropine sulfate from the ΔT_f of blood plasma, i.e., $0.52 - 0.07 = 0.45$. This means, sufficient sodium chloride must be added to lower the freezing point by an additional 0.45°.

Step 3: Find the percentage concentration of sodium chloride required by setting up the proportion as follows:

$$\frac{0.9\%}{0.52} = \frac{X}{0.45}$$

In Table 8.2, it is observed that 1% solution of sodium chloride has a freezing point lowering of 0.58. Therefore, one can also express the proportion as:

$$\frac{1\%}{0.58} = \frac{X}{0.45}$$

answer: solving for X, we get: $(0.45/0.58) \times 1 = 0.78\%$

0.78% sodium chloride will render the above preparation isotonic. Thus, the isotonic solution will be prepared by dissolving 1.0 g of atropine sulfate and 0.78 g of sodium chloride in sufficient water to make 100 mL of solution.

Example 3:

Compound the following prescription.

R	
Apomorphine Hydrochloride	1%
Sodium Chloride	q.s.
Purified Water ad	100
Ft isoton. sol.	
Sig. gtts ii OD T.I.D.	

Step 1: Freezing point depression (ΔT_f) of 1% apomorphine HCl solution (from Table 8.2) is 0.08.

Step 2: Find $\Delta T_f'$ by subtracting the ΔT_f value of 1% atropine sulfate from the ΔT_f of blood plasma, i.e., $0.52 - 0.08 = 0.44$. This means, sufficient sodium chloride must be added to reduce the freezing point by an additional 0.44°.

Step 3: Find the percentage concentration of sodium chloride required by setting up the proportion as follows:

$$\frac{0.9\%}{0.52} = \frac{X}{0.44}$$

or

$$\frac{1\%}{0.58} = \frac{X}{0.44}$$

solving for X, we get: $(0.44/0.58) \times 1 = 0.76\%$

answer: $X = 0.76\%$

0.76% sodium chloride will render the above preparation isotonic. Thus, the isotonic solution will be prepared by dissolving 1.0 g of apomorphine hydrochloride and 0.76 g of sodium chloride in sufficient water to make 100 mL of solution.

VOLUMES OF ISO-OSMOTIC SOLUTIONS

White-Vincent Method

White and Vincent[2] provided a method for readily finding the correct volume of water in which to dissolve a drug to produce a solution iso-osmotic with tears, followed by the addition of an isotonic vehicle to bring the solution to the final volume. The volume (V) of isotonic solution that can be prepared from any given drug is obtained by the equation:

$$V = \omega \times E \times 111.1$$

where

ω = weight of the drug in grams
E = sodium chloride equivalent

If more than one ingredient is contained in an isotonic preparation, the volumes of isotonic solution, obtained by mixing each drug with water, are additive. If that is the case, V can be calculated as follows:

$$V = [(\omega_1 \times E_1) + (\omega_2 \times E_2) + \ldots (\omega_n \times E_n)] \times 111.1$$

Example 1:

Make the following solution isotonic with tears.

Procaine Hydrochloride	1%
Sodium Chloride	q.s.
Purified Water ad	60

The weight of procaine hydrochloride = (60/100) × 1 = 0.6 g.

The E value of procaine hydrochloride = 0.21.

The volume (V) of isotonic solution that can be prepared from 0.6 g of the drug:

$$V = \omega \times E \times 111.1$$

$$= 0.6 \times 0.21 \times 111.1$$

$$= 13.99 \text{ or } 14 \text{ mL}$$

[2]White A. I. and Vincent H. C. *J. Am. Pharm. Assoc. Pract. Ed.*, 8, 406, 1947.

In order to make isotonic solution, 0.6 g of procaine hydrochloride is dissolved in purified water to make 14 mL of an isotonic solution, and the preparation is adjusted to a volume of 60 mL by adding isotonic vehicle such as NSS (normal saline solution).

Example 2:

Make the following prescription isotonic with tears.

℞

Ephedrine Sulfate	0.5
Boric Acid	0.2
Ammonium Chloride	0.25
Purified Water ad	60.0

The E values of ephedrine sulfate, boric acid, and ammonium chloride are 0.23, 0.52, and 1.08, respectively.

The volume (V) of isotonic solution that can be prepared from the three ingredients can be calculated from the following equation:

$$V = [(\omega_1 \times E_1) + (\omega_2 \times E_2) + (\omega_3 \times E_3)] \times 111.1$$

$$= [(0.5 \times 0.23) + (0.2 \times 0.52) + (0.25 \times 1.08)]$$

$$\times 111.1$$

$$= 54.3 \text{ mL}$$

In order to make isotonic solution, the three ingredients are dissolved in purified water to make 54.3 mL of an isotonic solution, and the preparation is adjusted to a volume of 60 mL by adding isotonic vehicle.

U.S.P. Method

On the basis of freezing point depression values, the USP includes a method for rapidly adjusting isotonicity of ophthalmic solutions. Since depression of freezing point depends upon the number of particles of solute(s) in solution, a proportion can be set up to solve for the volume of isotonic solution produced by 1 g of a given drug substance. This is illustrated by the following example.

Example 3:

Freezing point depression of 1% atropine sulfate is 0.074°C. Calculate the volume of iso-osmotic solution produced by 1 g of atropine sulfate. Since a freezing point depression of 0.074°C is caused by 1 g of atropine sulfate in 100 mL of water, a depression of 0.52°C will be produced by a solution containing 1 g in X mL can be calculated by as follows:

$$\frac{0.074}{0.52} \times 100 = 14.23 \text{ mL}$$

Thus, when 1 g of drug is dissolved in q.s. sterile water and the solution is adjusted to 14.23 mL, the resulting solution is iso-osmotic with tears.

The volumes of isotonic solutions prepared in milliliters from a gram of selected drug substances are listed in Table 8.3.

TABLE 8.3. *Volume of Isotonic Solutions Prepared (in Milliliters) from 1 g of Drug Substance.*

Compound	Volume
Atropine sulfate	14.3
Boric acid	55.7
Chlorobutanol	26.7
Cocaine hydrochloride	17.7
Ephedrine sulfate	25.7
Epinephrine bitartrate	20.0
Eucatropine hydrochloride	20.0
Fluorescein sodium	34.3
Homatropine hydrobromide	19.0
Neomycin sulfate	12.3
Phenylephrine hydrochloride	35.7
Procaine hydrochloride	23.3
Scopolamine hydrobromide·$3H_2O$	13.3
Silver nitrate	36.7
Sodium phosphate, dibasic·$7H_2O$	32.3
Sulfacetamide sodium	25.7
Tetracaine hydrochloride	20.0
Tetracycline hydrochloride	15.7
Zinc sulfate·$7H_2O$	16.7

Adapted from USP XXII.

Practice Problems

When solving these problems, refer to Tables 8.1 and 8.2 as needed.

(1) 1% boric acid solution has a freezing point depression of 0.29°. What is the percentage concentration of boric acid required to make the solution isotonic?

(2) 1% silver nitrate solution has a freezing point depression of 0.19°. What is the percentage concentration of silver nitrate required to make an isotonic solution?

(3) The freezing point of a 5% solution of boric acid is −1.55°. How many grams of boric acid should be used in preparing 100 mL of an isotonic solution?

(4) Determine if the following preparations are hypotonic, isotonic, or hypertonic:

a. A 5.5% atropine sulfate solution
b. A parenteral infusion containing 20% (w/v) of dextrose
c. A solution containing 2% ephedrine sulfate and 0.5% chlorobutanol
d. A 5% phenol solution

Compound the following two prescriptions using White-Vincent method.
(5) ℞

Ephedrine sulfate	1%
Sodium chloride	q.s.
Isotonic solution	40 mL
Sig. gtt ii each nostril q6h	

(6) ℞

Phenylephrine HCl	0.5
Boric acid	q.s.
Water q.s.	50 mL
Sig. UD	
Make isotonic solution	

(7) How much NaCl is required to render the above prescription isotonic?

(8) How much NaCl is required to render 100 mL of a 2% solution of epinephrine bitartrate isotonic with tears?

(9) Freezing point depression of 1% pilocarpine nitrate is 0.14°. Calculate the volume of iso-osmotic solution produced by 1 gram of pilocarpine nitrate by U.S.P. method.

(10) Freezing point depression of 1% fluorescein sodium is 0.18°. Calculate the volume of iso-osmotic solution produced by 1 g of fluorescein by U.S.P. method.

pH ADJUSTMENT

The pH is defined as the *logarithm of the reciprocal of the hydrogen ion concentration.* The pH value of topical dosage forms is adjusted for various reasons including minimization of discomfort, maintenance of chemical stability, and improvement of therapeutic response. The values of hydronium ion concentration are very small and are therefore expressed in exponential notations as pH.

$$pH = \log \frac{1}{[H^+]}$$

Since a bare proton does not exist by itself in water but is hydrated, the above expression can also be written as:

$$pH = \log \frac{1}{[H_3O^+]}$$

where $[H^+]$ or $[H_3O^+]$ indicates the molar concentration of hydrogen or hydronium ion.

Thus, $pH = -\log [H^+]$ or $[H_3O^+]$ and, therefore, the pH may be defined as the *negative logarithm of the hydrogen ion concentration.* This expression may also be represented as:

$$[H^+] \text{ or } [H_3O^+] = 10^{-pH}$$

Note: The connotations "hydrogen" and "hydronium ion" are used synonymously.

CONVERSION OF HYDROGEN ION CONCENTRATION TO pH

Example 1:

The hydronium ion concentration of a 0.05 M solution of HCl is 0.05 M. The pH value may be calculated as follows:

$$pH = -\log (0.05)$$

$$= -(-1.30)$$

answer: $= 1.30$

or 0.05 can be represented as: 5×10^{-2}

$$\therefore pH = -\log (5 \times 10^{-2})$$

$$= \log 10^2 - \log 5$$

$$\text{answer: } = 2 - 0.699 = 1.30$$

Example 2:

The hydronium ion concentration of a 0.1 M solution of barbituric acid is 3.24×10^{-3} M. The pH value may be calculated as follows:

$$pH = -\log (3.24 \times 10^{-3})$$

$$= \log 10^3 - \log 3.24$$

$$\text{answer: } = 3 - 0.51 = 2.49$$

Example 3:

The hydronium ion concentration of a solution is 1.32×10^5 M. The pH value may be calculated as follows:

$$pH = -\log (1.32 \times 10^{-5})$$

$$= \log 10^5 - \log 1.32$$

$$\text{answer: } = 5 - 0.12 = 4.88$$

CONVERSION OF pH TO HYDROGEN ION CONCENTRATION

When the pH of a given solution is known, one can calculate hydrogen ion concentration. The following examples illustrate the method of converting pH to hydrogen ion concentration.

Example 1:

The pH of a solution is 4.75. The hydrogen ion concentration of this solution may be calculated as follows:

$$pH = -\log [H^+] = 4.75$$

$$= \log [H^+] = -4.75$$

Note: One can solve the above expression in two ways:

(1) Simply take the antilog of -4.75

$$= \text{antilog of } -4.75 \text{ is } 0.0000178$$

By moving the decimal to the right, one can conveniently express the above answer as: 1.78×10^{-5}.

(2) Round the number (-4.75) to the next highest digit and express as:

$$-4.75 = -5.00 + 0.25$$

$$\therefore \log [H^+] = -4.75 = -5.00 + 0.25$$

$$[H^+] = \text{antilog } 0.25 \times \text{antilog } (-5)$$

$$[H^+] = 1.78 \times 10^{-5}$$

This method is recommended as the chances of computational errors are very less.

Example 2:

The pH of a solution is 3.72. The hydrogen ion concentration of this solution may be calculated as follows:

$$pH = -\log [H^+] = 3.72$$

$$\log [H^+] = -3.72 = -4.00 + 0.28$$

$$[H^+] = \text{antilog } 0.28 \times \text{antilog } (-4)$$

$$[H^+] = 1.91 \times 10^{-4}$$

Example 3:

The pH of a solution is 6.80. The hydrogen ion concentration of this solution may be calculated as follows:

$$pH = -\log [H^+] = 6.80$$

$$\log [H^+] = -6.80 = -7.00 + 0.20$$

$$[H^+] = \text{antilog } 0.20 \times \text{antilog } (-7)$$

$$[H^+] = 1.58 \times 10^{-7}$$

Alternatively, pH problems may be solved in one step as follows:

$$H^+ = 10^{-pH}$$

$$= 10^{-6.8} = 1.58 \times 10^{-7}$$

BUFFERS

Buffers are compounds or mixtures of compounds that, when present in solution, resist changes in pH upon the addition of small amounts of acids or alkali. In essence, they are capable of maintaining the pH values relatively constant and, therefore, are insensitive towards addition of small quantities of acids and/or bases. The ability to resist changes in pH is called *buffer action*. Buffers are added to topical formulations to control the pH that provides an acceptable balance between chemical stability, therapeutic activity, and comfort.

Buffers contain mixtures of weak acids and their salts (i.e., the conjugate bases of acids), or mixtures of weak bases and their conjugate acids. Typical buffer systems used in pharmaceutical dosage forms include mixtures of boric acid and sodium borate, acetic acid and sodium acetate, and sodium acid phosphate and disodium phosphate. The reason for the buffering action of a weak acid, HA (e.g., acetic acid) and its ionized salt, A⁻ (e.g., sodium acetate) is that A⁻ ions from the salt combine with the added hydrogen ions, removing them from solution as undissociated weak acid.

$$A^- + H_3O^+ \rightleftharpoons H_2O + HA$$

When OH⁻ ions are added, they are neutralized by the weak acid present in the buffer to form undissociated water molecules.

$$HA + OH^- \rightleftharpoons H_2O + A^-$$

Similarly, the buffering action of a mixture of a weak base and its salt is the result of neutralizing the H⁻ ions by reacting with a base to form the salt and neutralizing OH⁻ ions by the salt to form undissociated water:

$$B + H_3O^+ \rightleftharpoons H_2O + BH^+$$

$$BH^+ + OH^- \rightleftharpoons H_2O + B$$

The concentration of buffer components needed to maintain a solution at the desired (or required) pH may be calculated by using buffer equations derived by Henderson Hasselbalch as follows:

For weak acids

$$pH = pK_a + \log \frac{[salt]}{[acid]}$$

For weak bases

$$pH = pK_a + \log \frac{[base]}{[salt]}$$

$$pH = pK_w - pK_b + \log \frac{[base]}{[salt]}$$

where pK_a is the logarithm of the reciprocal of the *acid dissociation constant* or *acidity constant, K_a*:

$$pK_a = \log \frac{1}{K_a}$$

$$pK_a = -\log K_a \qquad (\text{or } K_a = 10^{-pK_a})$$

Similarly, pK_b is the logarithm of the reciprocal of the *basicity constant, K_b.*

$$\therefore pK_b = -\log K_b \qquad (\text{or } K_b = 10^{-pK_b})$$

The ion product (also referred to as "autoprotolysis constant") of water is symbolized by pK_w. The values of pK_w, pK_a, and pK_b are interrelated by the expression:

$$pK_w = pK_a + pK_b$$

Using appropriate buffer equations, one can calculate: (a) the pH value of a buffer system when pK and molar ratio (or concentration) of buffer components are known, and (b) the molar ratio of buffer components required to prepare a buffer with a desired pH value.

CALCULATIONS INVOLVING pH VALUE OF A BUFFER

Example 1:

What is the pH of a solution containing 0.1 mole of ephedrine and 0.001 mole of ephedrine hydrochloride per liter of solution?

pK_a of ephedrine is 9.36 at 25°C.

Ephedrine is a weakly basic drug. Therefore one can use:

$$pH = pK_a + \log [base]/[salt]$$

$$pH = 9.36 + \log [0.1]/[0.001]$$

$$pH = 9.36 + \log 100$$

$$answer: pH = 9.36 + 2 = 11.36$$

Example 2:

What is the pH of a buffer solution containing 0.55 M concentration of sodium acetate and 0.1 M concentration of acetic acid in 1 liter of solution. The pK_a of acetic acid is 4.76 at 25°C.

$$pH = pK_a + \log [salt]/[acid]$$

$$pH = 4.76 + \log [0.55]/[0.10]$$

$$answer: pH = 4.76 + 0.74 = 5.50$$

Example 3:

What is the pH of a buffer solution containing 0.05 M of sodium benzoate and 0.50 M of benzoic acid in 1 L of solution. The pK_a of benzoic acid is 4.20 at 25°C.

$$pH = pK_a + log\ [salt]/[acid]$$

$$pH = 4.20 + log\ [0.05]/[0.50]$$

answer: $pH = 4.20 - 1.0 = 3.20$

MOLAR RATIO OF BUFFER COMPONENTS IN A BUFFER

Using the buffer (Henderson Hasselbalch) equation, one can calculate the molar ratio of buffer components needed to prepare a buffer of desired pH. This is explained in the following examples.

Example 1:

What is the molar ratio of salt/acid needed to prepare an acetic acid buffer having a pH of 5.

The pK_a of acetic acid is 4.76 at 25°C.

The buffer equation for weak acids is:

$$pH = pK_a + log\ [salt]/[acid]$$

$$5 = 4.76 + log\ [salt]/[acid]$$

$$5 - 4.76 = 0.24 = log\ [salt]/[acid]$$

$[salt]/[acid]$ = antilog $0.24 = .1.74$ or 1.74:1, answer

Note: 1.74:1 is to be expressed as 1:0.575 by setting up a proportion and solving for *X*:

$$\frac{1.74}{1} = \frac{1}{X}$$

answer: $X = 1/1.74 = 0.575$

Example 2:

What molar ratio of acid to salt is required to adjust the pH of a solution to 8.8 using boric acid-sodium borate buffer?

pK_a of boric acid is 9.24 at 25°C.

$$pH = pK_a + \log [\text{salt}]/[\text{acid}]$$

To get the acid to salt ratio, the above equation can be rearranged as:

$$\log [\text{acid}]/[\text{salt}] = pK_a - pH$$

$$\log [\text{acid}]/[\text{salt}] = 9.24 - 8.80 = 0.44$$

$$[\text{acid}]/[\text{salt}] = \text{antilog } 0.44 = 2.75 \text{ or } 2.75{:}1$$

answer: 2.75:1

Example 3:

What is the molar ratio of base to salt required to prepare a buffer solution having a pH of 10? Assume that the pK_b of the base is 4.62 at 25°C.

$$pH = pK_a + \log [\text{base}]/[\text{salt}]$$

$$6.20 = 14 - 4.62 + \log [\text{base}]/[\text{salt}]$$

$$10 - 9.38 = 0.62 = \log [\text{base}]/[\text{salt}]$$

$$[\text{base}]/[\text{salt}] = \text{antilog } 0.62 = 4.17$$

answer: 4.17:1

Following are useful equations pertaining to pH and buffer calculations:

$$K_w = [H_3O^+] \times [OH^-]$$

$$K_w = K_a \times K_b$$

$$pH = -\log [H^+] \text{ or } -\log [H_3O^+]$$

$$pK_a = -\log K_a$$

$$pK_w = pK_a + pK_b$$

$$pK_w = pH + pOH$$

For weak acids:

$$pH = pK_a + \log [salt]/[acid]$$

For weak bases:

$$pH = pK_a + \log [base]/[salt]$$

$$pH = pK_w - pK_b + \log [base]/[salt]$$

Practice Problems

(1) Calculate the pH of the following solutions having a hydronium ion concentration (at 25°C) of:

    a. 2.77×10^{-5}
    b. 9.20×10^{-2}
    c. 3.40×10^{-8}
    d. 5.76×10^{-4}

(2) Calculate the hydronium ion concentration of the following solutions (at 25°C) at a pH value of:

    a. 4.70
    b. 9.20
    c. 3.40
    d. 11.5

(3) A buffer solution contains 0.05 M concentration of sodium acetate and 0.5 M concentration of acetic acid in 1 L of solution. The pK_a of acetic acid is 4.76 at 25°C. What is the pH of the solution?

(4) What is the pH of a solution containing 0.01 mole of ephedrine and 0.1 mole of ephedrine hydrochloride per liter of solution? The pK_b of ephedrine is 4.64.

(5) A buffer solution contains 0.05 M concentration of disodium phosphate and 1 M sodium acid phosphate in 1 L of solution. The pK_a of sodium acid phosphate is 7.21 at 25°C. What is the pH of the solution?

(6) What is the molar ratio of bicarbonate to carbonic acid at pH 6.8? The pK_a of the carbonic acid is 6.1 at 25°C.

(7) What molar ratio of salt/acid (sodium borate to boric acid) is required to prepare a buffer solution having a pH of 9.6? The pK_a of boric acid is 9.24 at 25°C.

(8) At a pH value of 5.76, the molar ratio of sodium acetate to acetic acid in a given buffer is 10:1 at 25°C. Calculate the pK_a of the acid?

(9) A buffer solution contains 0.001 M concentration of disodium phosphate and 0.05 M sodium acid phosphate in 1 liter of solution. The pK_a of sodium acid phosphate is 7.21 at 25°C. What is the pH of the solution?

(10) What molar ratio of salt/acid (sodium borate to boric acid) is required to prepare a buffer solution having a pH of 8.9? The pK_a of boric acid is 9.24 at 25°C.

CHAPTER 9

Calculations Involving Suppositories

Suppositories are solid dosage forms of various weights and shapes that are designed to be inserted into rectal, vaginal, or urethral orifices of the human body. Upon insertion, these suppositories melt, soften, or dissolve at body temperature. A suppository may act as a protectant or palliative to the local tissues at the point of insertion or as a carrier of therapeutic agents for systemic or local action. While rectal suppositories are generally inserted with the fingers, some vaginal suppositories may be inserted with the help of a special insertion appliance. Suppositories are convenient for use in patients who are children, uncooperative, or in a coma, and for patients with some local infections. Because suppositories can be extemporaneously prepared, tailoring of the dose of a drug should be easier as compared to other solid dosage forms. Some of the common, commercially available suppositories include Glycerin, Indocin®, Thorazine®, Cafergot®, Anusol®-HC, Phenergan®, Gyne-Lotrimin®, Sultrin®, Terazol-3®, Flagyl®, and Monistat®-7.

The rectal suppositories for adults are about 1½ inch long and weigh 2 g with cocoa butter. They are usually cylindrical with a tapered end that provides a bullet-like shape. When inserted gently, the rectum contracts and pulls the suppositories inside rather than expelling them. Rectal suppositories are used locally in the treatment of hemorrhoids, constipation, pain, and itching. The antihemorrhoidal suppositories such as Anusol® and Preparation-H® may contain ingredients that have vasoconstrictor, astringent, analgesic, local anesthetic, emollient, and protectant properties. Rectal suppositories are also used systemically in the control of nausea, vomiting, migraine, and other types of pain. The vaginal suppositories (also known as ''pessaries'') are of various sizes and weigh 5 g. They are usually cone-shaped or oval and are locally used as contraceptives, antiseptics, or antifungals. The urethral suppositories for men are about 6 inches long, 3–6 mm in diameter, and weigh 4 g. For women, the urethral suppositories are 3 inches long, 3–6 mm in diameter, and weigh 3 g. The urethral suppositories are used rarely as antiseptics or for the preparation of urethral exam.

Suppositories contain active medication in a diluent, which is called a suppository base. An ideal suppository base is nontoxic, nonirritating, nonsensitizing, compatible with drugs, has a melting point below body temperature, is solid at room temperature, and is chemically stable. A suppository base may be oleaginous (e.g., cocoa butter), water miscible (e.g., glycerinated gelatin), water soluble (polyethylene glycol), or an emulsion base (e.g., tween in combination with methylcellulose or hydroxypropyl cellulose). Among these bases, cocoa butter is commonly used in rectal suppositories. Most of the suppository calculations pertain to cocoa butter suppositories. Cocoa butter, also known as theobroma oil or theobroma cocoa, is a triglyceride with a melting point of 34.5°C, and it exhibits polymorphism. When inserted into the rectum, cocoa butter releases the medication by melting. It should be heated slowly and allowed to solidify by cooling to obtain physically stable suppositories. A major problem with cocoa butter is the reduction of its melting point when additives such as chloral hydrate are added. This may cause leakage from the rectal area. However, this problem can be overcome by the addition of stiffening agents such as white beeswax. Water miscible bases such as glycerinated gelatin are commonly used for pessaries and bougies. Glycerinated gelatin contains 60% glycerin, 20% gelatin, and 20% water. This base softens and releases the drug slowly. Therefore, it is an ideal choice for controlled release formulations. Glycerinated gelatin is humectant and draws water from surrounding tissues to cause irritation. Suppositories prepared with glycerinated gelatin base should, therefore, be dipped in water prior to insertion into body orifices. Polyethylene glycol which is a water soluble base is available in different molecular weight grades such as PEG 200, 300, 400, 600, 1000, 1500, 1540, 3000, 4000, 8000, etc. PEGs with molecular weights from 200–600 are liquids at room temperature and from 1000 and above are waxy solids. Various combinations of PEG grades can be combined to obtain suppositories of desired consistency. However, PEG bases are incompatible with drugs such as sulfas, aspirin, and tannic acid.

In addition to the active ingredients and base, suppositories may also contain stiffening agents, suspending agents, emulsifying agents, and preservatives. They are usually prepared by first melting the base followed by incorporating the powdered medication and then pouring this mixture in suppository molds after lubrication. They can also be prepared by mixing the active ingredients with the base followed by compressing it.

In the preparation of suppositories, the proportion of base may be varied to maintain a suitable consistency under different climatic conditions, provided the concentration of active ingredients is not changed. The size of mold is fixed depending upon the weight and shape of the suppositories. The weight of suppositories made with cocoa butter is one or two grams and that of vaginal suppositories made with glycerinated gelatin is five grams. If the amount of active ingredients is large, the cocoa butter amount has to be calculated and adjusted such that the total volume of suppositories is not changed. The density difference between the active ingredients and cocoa butter should be taken into consideration and appropriate allowance has to be made for the change in density of the total mass.

The main calculations involved in preparing suppositories pertain to the determination of displacement values, calculation of cocoa butter amounts by making use of displacement values, and the reduction and enlargement of formulae.

DISPLACEMENT VALUE

The displacement value is defined as the number of parts of suppository ingredients that displace one gram of cocoa butter base. These values are summerized in Table 9.1. The following examples will illustrate the displacement value calculations:

Example 1:

If a prescription requires 400 mg of bismuth subgallate per suppository weighing two grams, what would be the displacement value if it is known that six suppositories with required bismuth subgallate weigh 13.6 g?

Theoretical weight of six cocoa butter suppositories without bismuth subgallate = 12 g

Given weight of six cocoa butter suppositories with bismuth subgallate = 13.6 g

Amount of bismuth subgallate in the suppositories = 0.4 × 6 = 2.4 g

Amount of cocoa butter in the bismuth subgallate suppositories = 13.6 − 2.4 = 11.2 g

Cocoa butter displaced by 2.4 g of bismuth subgallate = 12 − 11.2 = 0.8

The displacement value of bismuth subgallate is 2.4/0.8 = X/1, or X = 3

Example 2:

If 12 cocoa butter suppositories containing 40% zinc oxide weigh 17.6 grams, what is the displacement value of zinc oxide? Assume that the suppositories are made in a 1-g mold.

TABLE 9.1.   Approximate Cocoa Butter
Displacement Values of Certain Drugs in
Suppositories.

Drug	Displacement Value
Aminophylline	1.5
Aminopyrine	1.3
Aspirin	1.1
Belladonna Extract	1.2
Bismuth Subgallate	3.0
Bismuth Subnitrate	6.0
Boric Acid	1.5
Chloral Hydrate	1.5
Cocaine Hydrochloride	1.5
Codeine Phosphate	1.1
Digitalis Leaf	1.6
Dimenhydrinate	1.3
Diphenhydramine HCl	1.3
Gallic Acid	2.0
Hamamelis Dry Extract	1.5
Hydrocortisone	1.5
Hydrocortisone Acetate	1.5
Ichthammol	1.0
Menthol	0.7
Morphine Hydrochloride	1.5
Peru Balsam	1.0
Phenobarbital Sodium	1.2
Potassium Bromide	2.2
Quinidine HCl	3.0
Resorcinol	1.0
Salicylic Acid	1.3
Secobarbital Sodium	1.2
Tannic Acid	1.6
Zinc Oxide	5.0
Zinc Sulfate	2.8

Given weight of 12 suppositories with zinc oxide = 17.6 grams

Weight of zinc oxide in the suppositories = $(40/100) \times 17.6 = 7.04$ g

Weight of cocoa butter in the suppositories = $(60/100) \times 17.6 = 10.56$ g

Theoretical weight of 12 suppositories without zinc oxide = 12 g

Cocoa butter displaced by 7.04 g of zinc oxide = $12 - 10.56 = 1.44$

Displacement value of zinc oxide = $(7.04/1.44) = (X/1)$; $X = 4.89$

Example 3:

From the information provided below, find the displacement value of phenobarbital sodium:

Six phenobarbital sodium suppositories, each containing 60-mg of drug, weigh 12 g.

The mold of suppository used was 2 g.

Given weight of six suppositories with phenobarbital sodium = 12 g

Weight of phenobarbital sodium = 60 mg × 6 = 360 mg or 0.36 g

Weight of cocoa butter in the suppositories = 12 − 0.36 = 11.64 = 0.36 g

Theoretical weight of six suppositories without phenobarbital sodium = 12 g

Cocoa butter displaced by 0.36 g of phenobarbital sodium = 12 − 11.64 = 0.36 g

Displacement value of phenobarbital sodium = (0.36/0.36) = (X/1); X = 1

Practice Problems

(1) What would be the displacement value of hydrocortisone acetate if it is known that ten suppositories containing 250 mg each of the drug weigh 20.83 g?

(2) What would be the displacement value of belladonna extract if it is known that six suppositories containing 60 mg each of the drug weigh 12.08 g?

(3) If a prescription requires 360 mg of bismuth subgallate per suppository of two grams, what would be the displacement value if it is known that six suppositories with required bismuth subgallate weigh 13.44 g?

(4) From the information provided below, find the displacement value of phenobarbital sodium:

Twelve phenobarbital sodium suppositories containing 60 mg of drug each weigh 24 g. The mold of suppository used was 2 g.

(5) From the information provided below, find the displacement value of quinidine hydrochloride:

Ten quinidine hydrochloride suppositories containing 600 mg of drug each weigh 24 g. The mold of suppository used was 2 g.

(6) If 24 cocoa butter suppositories containing 40% zinc oxide weigh 35.2 grams, what is the displacement value of zinc oxide? Assume that the suppositories are made in a I-g mold.

(7) From the information provided below, find the displacement value of zinc sulfate:

Ten zinc sulfate suppositories containing 200 mg of drug each weigh 21.29 g. The mold of suppository used was 2 g.

(8) If a prescription requires 325 mg of aspirin per suppository of two grams, what would be the displacement value if it is known that 12 suppositories with required aspirin weigh 24.35 g?

(9) What would be the displacement value of belladonna extract if it is known that 12 suppositories containing 60 mg each of the drug weigh 24.16 g?

(10) If a prescription requires 360 mg of bismuth subgallate per suppository of two grams, what would be the displacement value if it is known that 12 suppositories with required bismuth subgallate weigh 26.88 g?

PREPARATION OF SUPPOSITORIES WITH COCOA BUTTER

The calculations involved here include determination of the amount of cocoa butter needed by using the displacement values as well as the amount of other ingredients. The calculations are shown in Examples 1–3. In this section, a brief overview is provided for the method of suppository preparation with cocoa butter. The first step is to decide whether cocoa butter is appropriate for the suppositories that are required to be prepared. If the use of cocoa butter is justified, the second step is to determine the weight of the suppository. Usually the adult rectal suppository with cocoa butter is 2 g, the children's suppository is 1 g, and the glycero-gelatin suppository for vagina is 5 g. The final step involves calculation of the amounts of all ingredients needed.

Suppositories are prepared by hand rolling, compression, and by fusion methods. Since fusion is the most commonly used method for preparing suppositories containing cocoa butter, glycero-gelatin, and polyethylene glycol bases, a brief discussion is presented here. Drug(s) and other ingredients are weighed accurately and are finely powdered. The appropriate quantity of cocoa butter is grated, and a small amount of grated cocoa butter is melted at about 34°C. The finely powdered drug mixture is then mixed with molten cocoa butter, and the remaining cocoa butter is added by keeping the entire contents at 34°C or less. The contents are stirred until a creamy liquid is formed, which is poured in lubricated molds and is allowed to congeal. Because the suppository mass generally shrinks upon cooling, it is a good practice to slightly overfill and then to trim after congealing. If the ingredients lower the melting point of the cocoa butter base, stiffening agents should be added in order to obtain suppositories that are solid at room temperature and melt when inserted in the body. The lowering of the melting point is common with soluble ingredients. If semisolid ingredients are used, liquefy them first by triturating before adding to the base. When the ingredients are liquid, emulsify them before use and add stiffening agents.

Example 1:

Aspirin gr-v

Cocoa butter qs

Ft. Supp. DTD #12

Since the amount of aspirin in each suppository is 325 mg, it is an adult suppository. Therefore, 2 g mold should be used. The displacement value of aspirin as seen in Table 9.1 is 1.1. Therefore, the amounts of cocoa butter and aspirin are calculated as follows:

Amount of aspirin needed = 325 × 12 = 3900 mg or 3.9 g

Theoretical amount of cocoa butter needed (without aspirin) = 2 × 12 = 24 g

Cocoa butter displaced by aspirin = (3.9/1.1) = 3.55 g

Cocoa butter needed for aspirin suppositories = 24 − 3.55 = 20.45 g

Therefore, weigh out 3.9 g of aspirin and 20.45 g of cocoa butter. By following the appropriate procedure, prepare 12 suppositories.

Example 2:

Zinc oxide 30%

Cocoa butter qs

Make six suppositories

In this problem, the active ingredient, zinc oxide, is prescribed as a percentage. If the displacement value is used and the cocoa butter amount is varied, the zinc oxide percent will not be 30%. Therefore, in situations like this, prepare a 30% zinc oxide - cocoa butter mixture and fill in the molds to obtain the desired suppositories. There is no need to vary the cocoa butter amount.

Example 3:

Zinc oxide 300 mg

Cocoa butter qs

Ft. Supp. DTD #12

Use a 2-g mold. The displacement value of zinc oxide as seen in Table 9.1 is 5. Therefore, the amounts of cocoa butter and zinc oxide are calculated as follows:

Amount of zinc oxide needed = $300 \times 12 = 3600$ mg or 3.6 g

Theoretical amount of cocoa butter needed when there is no zinc oxide = $2 \times 12 = 24$ g

Cocoa butter displaced by zinc oxide = $3.6/5 = 0.72$ g

Cocoa butter needed for zinc oxide suppositories = $24 - 0.72 = 23.28$ g

Therefore, weigh out 3.6 g of aspirin and 23.28 g of cocoa butter. By following the appropriate procedure, prepare 12 suppositories.

Practice Problems

(1) Show how you would prepare 15 prochlorperazine suppositories containing 30 mg of the drug in each suppository. Assume that you are required to use cocoa butter and that the displacement value of prochlorperazine is 2.

(2) Show how you would prepare 12 promethazine hydrochloride suppositories containing 20 mg of the drug in each suppository. Assume that you are required to use cocoa butter and that the displacement value of promethazine hydrochloride is 2.5.

(3) Zinc oxide 250 mg
Cocoa butter qs
Ft. Supp. DTD #15

(4) Zinc oxide 40%
Cocoa butter qs
Make 12 suppositories

(5) Phenobarbital sodium 30 mg
Cocoa butter qs
Make 10 suppositories

(6) Show how you would prepare 10 dimenhydrinate suppositories containing 400 mg of the drug in each suppository. Assume that you are required to use cocoa butter base.

(7) Show how you would prepare 15 morphine hydrochloride suppositories containing 25 mg of the drug in each suppository. Assume that you are required to use cocoa butter base.

(8) Bismuth subgallate 300 mg
Cocoa butter qs
Ft. suppositories. DTD #12

(9) Hamamelis Extract 250 mg
Zinc oxide 400 mg
Cocoa butter qs
Ft. suppositories, DTD #10

(10) Show how you would prepare 12 promethazine hydrochloride suppositories containing 30 mg of the drug in each suppository. Assume that you are required to use cocoa butter and that the displacement value of promethazine hydrochloride is 2.5.

CHAPTER 10

Calculations Involving Injectable Medications

The present chapter deals with different calculations associated with parenteral medications which include rate of flow of intravenous fluids, parenteral insulin and heparin administration, reconstitution of powdered medications, and milliequivalent and milliosmole calculations pertinent to injectable medications.

RATE OF FLOW OF INTRAVENOUS FLUIDS

Intravenous fluids must be precisely regulated to ensure adequate hydration of the patient. Generally, the packaging of the solution administration equipment will state the drop factor (drops per milliliter) that the set delivers. Intravenous administration sets are commercially available that deliver 10, 12, 15, 20, 60, and other numbers of drops per mL. Standard IV solution administration sets deliver 10 gtt (drops) per mL. Blood administration sets deliver 15 gtt/mL. Microdrop (sometimes referred to as "minidrop") sets deliver 60 gtt/mL. The large volume parenteral solutions are administered by either allowing the solution to drip slowly into a vein by gravity flow or through the use of an electrical or battery-operated volumetric infusion pumps.

Medicated IV Drips

Medicated IV drips are solutions that have potent medications added. When administered, these infusions require extreme care and meticulous observation so that exactly the prescribed amount of medication in solution is administered to the patient. Generally, infusion pump or a controlled volume chamber and a microdrip set are used to administer medicated IV drips.

To calculate the rate of flow (rate of infusion) of IV solutions, one can use either the method of proportion (which generally involves two steps) or the formula method. In the formula method, the rate of infusion can be calculated as follows:

No. of drops per minute (or gtt/min) =

$$= \frac{\text{Number of mL of solution to be infused} \times \text{Number of drops per mL (or Drop factor)}}{\text{Number of hours for adm.} \times 60 \text{ (minutes per hour)}}$$

The above formula can be simplified and memorized as follows:

$$R = \frac{V \times D}{T}$$

where

R = rate of flow (gtt/min)
V = total volume to be infused (in mL)
D = drop factor (gtt/mL)
T = total time of infusion (in minutes)

Example 1:

An intravenous fluid of 1000 mL of Ringer's Injection was started in a patient at 8:00 A.M. and was scheduled to run for 12 hours. At 3:00 P.M. it was found that 800 mL of the fluid remained in the bottle. At what rate of flow should the remaining fluid be regulated using an IV set that delivers 15 drops per mL in order to complete the administration of the fluid in the scheduled time?

Fluid remaining = 800 mL

Time remaining = 5 hr or 300 min

By formula method:

Number of drops per minute (or gtt/min) =

$$\frac{800 \times 15}{5 \times 60}$$

$$= 40 \text{ drops/min}$$

By the method of proportion:

a. If 800 mL are infused in 300 minutes, how many milliliters will be infused in 1 minute?

$$\frac{800 \text{ mL}}{300 \text{ min}} = \frac{X \text{ mL}}{1 \text{ min}}$$

$$X = 2.67 \text{ mL}$$

b. If 15 drops are contained in 1 mL, how many drops would be contained in 2.67 mL?

$$\frac{15 \text{ drops}}{1 \text{ mL}} = \frac{X \text{ drops}}{2.67 \text{ mL}}$$

$$X = 40 \text{ drops}$$

answer: rate of flow = 40 drops per minute

Example 2:

The physician's order reads "1000 cc D5W IV in 24 hours." How many drops per minute should the IV infusion run if a microdrop administration set is used? The microdrop set delivers 60 gtt/mL.

By formula method:

Number of drops per minute (or gtt/min) =

$$\frac{1000 \times 60}{24 \times 60}$$

answer: = 41.66 or 42 gtt/min

By the method of proportion:

a. If 1000 mL are infused in 1440 minutes, how many milliliters will be infused in 1 minute?

$$\frac{1000 \text{ mL}}{1440 \text{ min}} = \frac{X \text{ mL}}{1 \text{ min}}$$

$$X = 0.69 \text{ mL}$$

b. If 60 drops are contained in 1 mL, how many drops would be contained in 0.69 mL?

$$\frac{60 \text{ drops}}{1 \text{ mL}} = \frac{X \text{ drops}}{0.69 \text{ mL}}$$

$$X = 41.4 \text{ or } 41 \text{ drops}$$

answer: rate of flow = 26 drops per minute

Example 3:

If a physician prescribes 5 units of insulin to be added to a liter IV solution of D5W and administered to a patient over an 8-hour period, how many drops per min should be administered using an IV set that delivers 10 drops per mL?

By formula method:

Number of drops per minute (or gtt/min) =

$$\frac{1000 \times 10}{8 \times 60}$$

answer: = 20.83 or 21 drops/min

By the method of proportion:

a. If 1000 mL are infused in 480 minutes, how many milliliters will be infused in 1 minute?

$$\frac{1000 \text{ mL}}{480 \text{ min}} = \frac{X \text{ mL}}{1 \text{ min}}$$

$$X = 2.08 \text{ mL}$$

b. If 10 drops are contained in 1 mL, how many drops would be contained in 2.08 mL?

$$\frac{10 \text{ drops}}{1 \text{ mL}} = \frac{X \text{ drops}}{2.08 \text{ mL}}$$

$$X = 21 \text{ drops}$$

answer: rate of flow = 21 drops per minute

Practice Problems

(1) Calculate the IV flow rate for 500 mL D5W to run for 8 hours. The drop factor is 60 gtt/mL.

(2) Calculate the IV flow rate for 200 cc of 0.9% NaCl IV over 2 hours. The drop factor is 20 gtt/mL.

(3) Calculate the IV flow rate for a liter of normal saline to be infused in 6 hours. The infusion set is calibrated for a drop factor of 15 gtt/mL.

(4) A physician's hospital medication is 400 mL D5W to run for 8 hours. If the drop factor is 60 gtt/mL, what should be the flow rate?

(5) A physician ordered 2000 mL D5W IV to run for 24 hours. If the infusion set is calibrated to 15 drops per milliliter, calculate the IV flow rate in gtt/min?

(6) A 1000-mL bag of intravenous solution contains 2.5 million units of ampicillin. How many units of the drug will have been infused after 6 hours with the flow rate of 1.2 mL/minute?

(7) Calculate the flow rate for an IV drug infusion to run for one hour at the rate of 125 mL per hour. The drop factor is 10 gtt/mL.

(8) A patient is to receive 2 µg/kg/min of nitroglycerin from a solution containing 100 mg of the drug in 500 mL of D5W. If the patient weighs 154 lb and infusion set delivers 60 drops per mL, (a) how many mg of nitroglycerin would be delivered per hour and (b) how many drops per min would be delivered?

(9) The drug alfentanil hydrochloride is administered by infusion at the rate of 2.2 µg/kg/min for inducing anesthesia. If a total of 0.55 mg of the drug is to be administered to a 175-lb patient, how long should be the duration of the infusion?

(10) A physician order is for two 500 mL IV units of whole blood to be infused in four hours. If the infusion set is calibrated to 15 drops per milliliter, calculate the IV flow rate in gtt/min?

INSULIN DOSAGE

Insulin, a hormone produced by the pancreas, is essential for the metabolism of glucose, proteins, and fats. Insulins are classified on the basis of the *duration of action* as rapid-, intermediate-, or long-acting; and on the basis of source or *species,* such as human or animal (beef, pork, and mixtures of beef and pork). Table 10.1 summarizes insulin preparations currently available in the United States.

TABLE 10.1. *Insulin Products in the United States.*

Product (Manufacturer)	Strength (Units/mL)	Source
Rapid-Acting Insulins		
Standard		
Regular, Iletin I (Lilly)	40, 100	Beef/pork mixture
Regular (Squibb-Novo)	100	Pork
Semilente, Iletin I (Lilly)	40, 100	Beef/pork mixture
Semilente (Squibb-Novo)	100	Beef
Purified		
Regular, Iletin II (Lilly)	100	Beef or pork
Regular Iletin II, concentrated (Lilly)	500	Pork
Regular, purified (Squibb-Novo)	100	Pork
Velosulin (Nordisk)	100	Pork
Semilente, purified (Squibb-Novo)	100	Pork
Human		
Humulin R (Lilly)	100	Human, biosynthetic
Humulin BR (Lilly)	100	Human, biosynthetic
Novolin R (Squibb-Novo)	100	Human, semisynthetic
Velosulin, human (Nordisk)	100	Human, semisynthetic

TABLE 10.1. (continued).

Product (Manufacturer)	Strength (Units/mL)	Source
Intermediate-Acting Insulins		
Standard		
NPH Iletin I (Lilly)	40, 100	Beef/pork mixture
Lente, Iletin I (Lilly)	40, 100	Beef/pork mixture
NPH (Squibb-Novo)	100	Beef
Lente (Squibb-Novo)	100	Beef
Purified		
NPH Iletin II (Lilly)	100	Pork or beef
Lente, Iletin II (Lilly)	100	Pork of beef
NPH, purified (Squibb-Novo)	100	Pork
Lente, purified (Squibb-Novo)	100	Pork
Insulatard NPH (Nordisk)	100	Pork
Human		
Humulin N (Lilly)	100	Human, biosynthetic
Humulin L (Lilly)	100	Human, biosynthetic
Novolin N (Squibb-Novo)	100	Human, semisynthetic
Novolin L (Squibb-Novo)	100	Human, semisynthetic
Insulatard NPH, human (Nordisk)	100	Human, semisynthetic

(continued)

197

TABLE 10.1. *(continued).*

Product (Manufacturer)	Strength (Units/mL)	Source
Mixtures		
Purified		
Mixtard; 70% NPH: 30 regular premix (Nordisk)	100	Pork
Human		
Novolin 70/30; 70% NPH: 30% regular premix (Squibb-Novo)	100	Human, semisynthetic
Mixtard, human; 70% NPH: 30% regular premix (Nordisk)	100	Human, semisynthetic
Long-Acting Insulins		
Standard		
Ultralente, Iletin I (Lilly)	100	Beef/pork mixture
PZI, Iletin I (Lilly)	40, 100	Beef/pork mixture
Ultralente (Squibb-Novo)	100	Beef
Purified		
PZI, Iletin II (Lilly)	100	Pork or beef
Ultraleate, purified (Squibb-Novo)	100	Beef
Human		
Humulin U (Lilly)	100	Human, biosynthetic

TABLE 10.2.   Types of Insulin Syringes.

A.	*The Standard U-100 Syringe.* It is marked for every 2 units up to 100 units. To measure 70 units with this syringe, withdraw U-100 insulin to the 70 unit mark.
B.	*The 1-cc U-100 Insulin Syringe.* It is marked for every 1 unit up to 100 units. It makes it possible to measure odd numbers, such as 65 units.
C.	*The 50-unit Lo-Dose U-100 Insulin Syringe.* It is marked up to 50. It makes it easier to read and measure low doses of insulin.
D.	*The 30-unit Lo-Dose Insulin Syringe.* It is marked in units up to 30, and most accurately measures small amounts of insulin, such as for children.

The strength of insulin products (see Table 10.1) is expressed in *units of activity* per milliliter. The units of activity, which are derived from biological assay methods, reflect a drug's potency. The doses of insulin are also expressed in units of activity. Insulin should always be measured in insulin syringes, which are available in different designs. Each insulin syringe is calibrated according to the strength of insulin with which it is to be used. The insulin syringe makes it possible to obtain a correct dosage without any mathematical computations or conversions. The smallest capacity insulin syringe possible should be used to most accurately measure insulin dosages. Table 10.2 lists four basic types of insulin syringes.

Example 1:

A patient is required to take 10 units of U-40 isophane insulin suspension and 18 units of U-100 protamine zinc insulin. What volume, in milliliters, of each type will provide the desired dosage?

Sources:

U-40 insulin contains 40 units/mL
U-100 insulin contains 100 units/mL

$$\frac{40 \text{ units}}{1 \text{ mL}} = \frac{10 \text{ units}}{X \text{ mL}}$$

$$X = 0.25 \text{ mL of U-40}$$

$$\frac{100 \text{ units}}{\text{mL}} = \frac{18 \text{ units}}{X \text{ mL}}$$

answer: $X = 0.18$ mL of U-100

Example 2:

A physician orders 1 unit of insulin injection subcutaneously for every 10 mg% of blood sugar over 175 mg% with blood sugar levels and injections performed twice daily in the morning and evening. The patient's blood sugar was 210 mg% in the morning and 320 mg% in the evening. How many total units of insulin injection should be administered?

$$210 \text{ mg}\% - 175 \text{ mg}\% = 35 \text{ mg}\%$$

$$\frac{1 \text{ unit}}{10 \text{ mg}\%} = \frac{X \text{ units}}{35 \text{ mg}\%}$$

$$X = 3.5 \text{ units}$$

$$320 \text{ mg}\% - 175 \text{ mg}\% = 145 \text{ mg}\%$$

$$\frac{1 \text{ unit}}{10 \text{ mg}\%} = \frac{X \text{ units}}{145 \text{ mg}\%}$$

$$X = 14.5 \text{ units}$$

answer: 3.5 units + 14.5 units = 18 units

Example 3:

A medication order in the hospital setting calls for isophane insulin suspension to be administered to a 152-lb patient on the basis of 1 unit per kg per 24 hours. How many units of isophane insulin suspension should be administered daily?

$$152 \text{ lb} = 152/2.2 = 69 \text{ kg}$$

If 1 unit is given per kg of body weight, how many units are needed for 69 kg?

$$\frac{1 \text{ unit}}{1 \text{ kg}} = \frac{X \text{ units}}{69 \text{ kg}}$$

answer: $X = 69$ units

In an emergency situation when an insulin syringe is not available, one may use a tuberculin syringe. The volume of fluid to be withdrawn, *X*, into the tuberculin syringe to administer the prescribed dosage may be calculated by the method of proportion as follows:

$$\frac{\text{Dose on hand}}{\text{Volume of dose on hand}} = \frac{\text{Desired dose}}{X}$$

For example, if 70 U of insulin needs to be administered and no insulin syringe is available, a proportion may be set to calculate the quantity (*X*) to be administered as follows:

$$\frac{100\ U}{1\ cc} = \frac{70\ U}{X}$$

$$X = 70/100 = 0.7\ cc$$

HEPARIN DOSAGE

Heparin is an anticoagulant that prevents the formation of blood clots. Like insulin, it is also measured in *units of activity*. IV heparin may be administered by standard gravity flow or electronic infusion devices. The normal adult heparinizing dosage is 20,000–40,000 units per 24 hours. In general, IV heparin is ordered in units per hour. Heparin may also be ordered by the physician to infuse at a predetermined flow rate in mL per hour.

The heparin dosages may be calculated by the method of proportion. This is explained in the following examples.

Example 1:

A heparin dose of 120 units/kg of body weight has been recommended for a patient undergoing certain type of surgery. How many mL of an injection containing 5000 heparin units/mL should be administered to a 220-lb patient?

$$\frac{120\ units}{2.2\ lb} = \frac{X\ units}{220\ lb}$$

$$X = 12,000\ units$$

$$\frac{5000\ units}{1\ mL} = \frac{12,000\ units}{X}$$

answer: *X* = 2.4 mL

Example 2:

A patient is to receive an IV drip of the following:

Sodium heparin   20,000 units
Sodium chloride injection (0.45%)   500 mL

a. How many milliliters per hour must be administered to achieve a rate of 1200 units of sodium heparin per hour?

b. If the IV set delivers 15 drops/mL, how many drops per minute should be administered?

a.
$$\frac{20,000 \text{ units}}{500 \text{ mL}} = \frac{1200 \text{ units}}{X}$$

answer: $X = 30$ mL per hour

b. Number of drops per minute (or gtt/min)

$$R = \frac{V \times D}{T}$$

$$= \frac{30 \times 15}{60}$$

answer: $= 7.5$ drops/min

Example 3:

For children, heparin sodium is administered by intermittent IV infusion in a range of 60 to 80 units/kg of body weight every four hour. For a 57-lb child, calculate the range, in mL, of a heparin sodium injection containing 5000 units/mL to be administered daily.

$$57 \text{ lb}/2.2 = 25.9 \text{ kg}$$

$$(60 - 80) \times 24/4 = (360 - 480)$$

$$(360 - 480) \times 25.9 \text{ kg} = (9324 - 12,432)$$

$$\frac{5000 \text{ units}}{9324 \text{ units}} = \frac{1 \text{ mL}}{X \text{ mL}}$$

$$X = 1.86 \text{ mL}$$

$$\frac{5000 \text{ units}}{12,432 \text{ units}} = \frac{1 \text{ mL}}{X \text{ mL}}$$

$$X = 2.49 \text{ mL}$$

answer: the range is 1.86 to 2.49 mL

CALCULATIONS INVOLVING RECONSTITUTION OF DRY POWDERS

Certain medications including penicillins and other antibiotics are unstable when stored in solution form and are therefore packaged in powder form. The dry powders must be reconstituted with a sterile diluent such as sterile water for injection or sterile sodium chloride (normal saline) solution. Instructions supplied with the vial state the volume of diluent which should be added. The resulting volume of the reconstituted drug and the approximate average concentration per milliliter are provided in the label or the package information sheet (package insert).

The powdered drug may or may not contribute to the final volume of the reconstituted solution in addition to the amount of diluent added. If the dry powder adds to the final volume of the reconstituted solution, the increase in volume obtained by the drug must be taken into account when calculating the amount of solvent to be used in preparing a solution of specified strength.

Some typical problems associated with reconstitution of dry powders are discussed in the following examples.

Example 1:

A pharmacist receives a medication order for 300,000 units of penicillin G potassium to be added to 500 mL of D5W. A vial of penicillin G potassium 1,000,000 U is on hand, and the directions on the 1,000,000 unit package state "Add diluent 4.6 mL (for a) concentration of solution 200,000 units/mL." How many milliliters of the reconstituted solution must be withdrawn and added to the D5W?

$$\frac{200,000}{1 \text{ mL}} = \frac{300,000}{X}$$

$$X = \frac{300,000}{200,000}$$

answer: = 1.5 mL

Example 2:

℞

Polymixin B sulfate	2,500 units/mL
Sterile Water for Injection	15 mL

Sig. Use as directed.

The source of polymixin B sulfate is a vial containing 50,000 units of the dry powder. The directions on the vial state "Add diluent 9.4 mL (for a) concentration of solution 5000 units per mL." Using water for injection as the diluent, explain how you would obtain the drug needed in compounding the prescription.

Total polymixin B sulfate needed = 2500 × 15 = 37,500 units

$$\frac{5000 \text{ units}}{1 \text{ mL}} = \frac{37,500 \text{ units}}{X}$$

$$X = 7.5 \text{ mL}$$

answer: take 7.5 mL of the reconstituted solution and add water for injection q.s. to 15 mL

Example 3:

A medication order calls for 400 mg of Kefzol® (cefazolin sodium) to be administered IM to a patient every 12 hours. Vials containing 250 mg, 500 mg, and 1 g of cefazolin sodium are available. According to the manufacturer's directions, dilutions may be made as follows:

Vial Size	Solvent to Be Added	Final Volume
250 mg	2 mL	2 mL
500 mg	2 mL	2.2 mL
1 g	2.5 mL	3 mL

Explain how the prescribed amount of cefazolin sodium could be obtained.

From 250 mg vial:

$$\frac{250 \text{ mg}}{2 \text{ mL}} = \frac{400 \text{ mg}}{X}$$

answer: $X = 3.2$ mL

From 500 mg vial:

$$\frac{500 \text{ mg}}{2.2 \text{ mL}} = \frac{400 \text{ mg}}{X \text{ mL}}$$

answer: $X = 1.76$ mL

From 1 g vial:

$$\frac{1000 \text{ mg}}{3 \text{ mL}} = \frac{400 \text{ mg}}{X}$$

answer: $X = 1.2$ mL

Practice Problems

(1) How many mL of Regular U-100 insulin injection should be used to obtain 60 units?

(2) If a 10-mL vial of insulin contains 200 units of insulin per milliliter, and a patient is required to receive 20 units twice daily, how many days will the product last the patient?

(3) Calculate the number of units per milliliter if a 4 mL vial of heparin containing 10,000 units/mL is injected into 1000 mL of normal saline solution.

(4) A patient receives 30 mL of heparin every hour. If there are 40 units in each milliliter, how many units does the patient receive in 24 hours?

(5) An antibiotic for oral suspension, following reconstitution of the dry powder, contains in each 5 mL, 250 mg of the drug in package sizes to prepare 100 mL, 150 mL, or 200 mL of suspension. Which package size should be dispensed for a 20-kg child prescribed to take 50 mg/kg/day total, q.i.d. in divided doses, for a period of 10 days?

(6) A vial contains 1 g of Ancef® (cefazolin sodium). Express the concentrations of cefazolin sodium, in milligrams per milliliter, following reconstitution with sterile water for injection to the following volumes:

a. 2.15 mL

b. 4.2 mL

c. 10 mL

(7) A pharmacist receives a medication order for 275,000 units of penicillin G potassium to be added to 500 mL of D5W. The directions on the 1,000,000 unit package state that if 1.6 mL of solvent are added, the

reconstituted solution will measure 2.2 mL. How many milliliters of the reconstituted solution must be withdrawn and added to the D5W?

(8) A pharmacist receives a medication order for 400,000 units of buffered penicillin G potassium to be added to 500 mL of D5W. A vial of buffered penicillin G potassium 1,000,000 U is on hand, and the directions on the package state "Add diluent 9.2 mL (for a) concentration of solution 100,000 units/mL." How many milliliters of the reconstituted solution must be withdrawn and added to the D5W?

(9) An intravenous infusion for a child weighing 55 lb is to contain 17.5 mg of vancomycin HCl per kg of body weight in 200 mL of NaCl injection. Using a 7.5 mL vial containing 500 mg of dry vancomycin HCl powder, explain how you would obtain the amount needed in preparing the infusion.

(10) A physician orders 1.75 g of an antibiotic to be placed in 1000 mL of normal saline solution (NSS). Using a reconstituted injection which contains 250 mg of the antibiotic per 1 mL, how many mL should be added to the NSS in filling the medication order?

MILLIEQUIVALENTS AND MILLIOSMOLES

Milliequivalents

For a detailed discussion on milliequivalent calculations, please refer to Chapter 5. Some milliequivalent calculations relevant to injectable medications are presented in this section.

The relationship between mEq and mg expressions of the quantity of a substance is as follows:

$$\text{Number of mEq} = \frac{\text{Weight of the substance in mg}}{\text{Milliequivalent weight}}$$

Note: When a quantity of binary compound (e.g., KCl or $CaCl_2 \cdot 2H_2O$) is in a volume of solution, each radical will have exactly the same concentration when expressed in milliequivalents, but the solution will not contain the same weight of each radical. To compute the equivalent weight concentration of a salt hydrate in solution, the milligram weight of the water molecules must be included in the expressed milligram concentration of the salt.

Example 1:

2.5 mEq of Ca^{++} are ordered. Find the amount (in mg) of calcium dihydrate needed. The concentration expressed on the additive container in terms of mg of $CaCl_2 \cdot 2H_2O$ (equivalent weight = 147/2 = 73.5).

The amount (in mg) of calcium dihydrate needed

answer: = 2.5 × 73.5 = 183.75 mg

Note: If calculations were made on the basis of the anhydrous form (equivalent weight of $CaCl_2$ = 115/5 = 55.5), an error would have been made, unless the labelled concentration was also in terms of the anhydrous form.

Example 2:

A physician order for an intravenous infusion for a patient weighing 110 lb calls for a 0.25 mEq of potassium chloride per kilogram of bodyweight to be added to 500 mL of D5W. How many milliliters of a sterile solution containing 50 mEq of potassium chloride per 10 mL should be used in preparing the infusion?

$$\frac{0.25 \text{ mEq}}{2.2 \text{ lb}} = \frac{X}{110 \text{ lb}}$$

$$X = 12.5 \text{ mEq}$$

$$\frac{50 \text{ mEq}}{10 \text{ mL}} = \frac{12.5 \text{ mEq}}{X}$$

answer: X = 2.5 mL

Example 3:

A potassium phosphate solution contains 0.75 g of potassium acid phosphate and 3.5 g of potassium dibasic phosphate in 10 mL. Five milliliters of this solution are added to a liter of D5W. How many milliequivalents of potassium phosphate will be represented in the final D5W solution?

Molecular weight of potassium acid phosphate (KH_2PO_4) = 136

Equivalent weight of potassium acid phosphate = 136 g

Molecular weight of potassium dibasic phosphate (K_2HPO_4) = 174

Equivalent weight of potassium dibasic phosphate = 87 g

$$\text{mEq wt of potassium dihydrogen phosphate} = 136$$

$$\text{mEq wt of potassium monohydrogen phosphate} = 87$$

Number of mEq of potassium phosphate in 10 mL of potassium dihydrogen phosphate can be calculated from:

$$\text{Number of mEq} \times \text{mEq wt} = \text{wt (in mg)}$$

$$\text{Number of mEq} \times 136 = 750 \text{ mg}$$

$$\text{Number of mEq} = 750/136 = 5.51$$

Similarly, the number of milliequivalents of potassium phosphate in 10 mL of potassium monohydrogen phosphate can be calculated as follows:

$$\text{Number of mEq} = 3500/87 = 40.23$$

Total number of milliequivalents of potassium phosphate in 10 mL

$$= 5.51 + 40.23 = 45.74$$

If 10 mL contain 45.74 mEq, 5 mL contain:

$$= 45.74/2 = 22.87$$

answer: 22.87 mEq

Milliosmoles

Electrolytes regulate body water volumes by establishing osmotic pressure which is proportional to the total number of particles in solution. The osmotic pressure of a solution is expressed in units of milliosmoles (mOsm). Osmolar concentrations reflects the number of particles (molecules as well as ions) of total solutes per volume of solution, which in turn determines the osmotic pressure of the solution.

A solute in a given solvent may remain unionized (nonelectrolyte) or may ionize (electrolyte). For nonelectrolytes, 1 millimole (mmol; i.e., one formula weight in mg) represents 1 mOsm. For electrolytes, osmolarity depends on the total number of particles in solution which in turn depends on the degree of dissociation of a solute. For example, 1 mmol of completely dissociated KCl represents 2 mOsm of total particles (i.e., $K^+ + Cl^-$). Similarly, 1 mmol of $CaCl_2$ represents 3 mOsm of total particles (i.e., $Ca^{++} + Cl^- + Cl^-$).

Osmolar concentration (mOsm/L) for each solute in a given product can be calculated using one of the following equations:

For a nonelectrolyte:

$$mOsm/L = \frac{g \text{ of solute/L}}{\text{Gram-molecular weight of solute}} \times 1000$$

For an electrolyte:

$$mOsm/L = \frac{g \text{ of solute/L} \times \text{Number of ions formed}}{\text{Gram-molecular weight of solute}} \times 1000$$

The official injections requiring osmolarity labeling by the USP are listed in Table 10.3. The milliosmolar value of the separate ions of an electrolyte may be obtained by dividing the concentration of the ions in milligrams per liter (mg/L) by the ions' atomic weight. The milliosmolar value of the *whole* electrolyte in solution equals the sum of the milliosmolar values of all the ions in solution.

Note: Each substance dissolved in a solution contributes to its total osmotic pressure.

Example 1:

How many milliosmoles are represented in a liter of NSS (i.e., 0.9% NaCl solution)?

Molecular weight of NaCl = 58.5

0.9% NaCl = 0.9 g/100 mL and 9 g/1000 mL

Number of ions formed = 2 (i.e., Na^+ and Cl^-)

$$mOsm/L = \frac{9 \times 2}{58.5} \times 1000$$

answer: = 307.69 or 308 mOsm/L

Example 2:

How many milliosmoles per liter are represented by a solution that contains 50% anhydrous dextrose in water for injection?

TABLE 10.3.   Official Injections Requiring Osmolarity Labeling by the USP.

Alcohol in dextrose injection
Ammonium chloride injection
Arginine hydrochloride injection
Calcium chloride injection
Calcium gluceptate injection
Calcium gluconate injection
Calcium levulinate injection
Dextrose injection
Dextrose and sodium chloride injection
Fructose injection
Fructose and sodium chloride injection
Magnesium sulfate injection
Mannitol injection
Mannitol in sodium chloride injection
Potassium acetate injection
Potassium chloride injection
Potassium chloride in dextrose injection
Potassium chloride in dextrose and sodium
    chloride injection
Potassium chloride in sodium chloride
    injection
Potassium phosphate injection
Ringer's injection
Lactated ringer's injection
Sodium acetate injection
Sodium bicarbonate injection
Sodium chloride injection
Sodium lactate injection
Sodium phosphate injection

Source: USP XXIII and NF XVIII, 1995.

Molecular weight of anhydrous dextrose = 180

50% solution contains 500 g per liter

$$\text{mOsm/L} = \frac{500 \times 1}{180} \times 1000$$

answer: = 2778 mOsm/L

Note: 1 mmol of anhydrous dextrose = 180 mg

Interconversion between Osmolality and Osmolarity

The interconversion between *molal* and *molar* expressions can be done if the density of solution at 25°C is known. The density should be that of the solution at the freezing point. The grams of solute per milliliter should also be measured at 25°C. The relation can be expressed as:

$$mOsm/L = mOsm/kg \times (density - grams\ of\ solute/mL)$$

Example 3:

What is the *osmolarity* of 0.9% w/v NaCl injection with a reported *osmolality* of 287 mOsm/kg and a density of 1.0046?

$$mOsm/L = 287 \times (1.0046 - 0.009)$$

answer: 285.74 or 286 mOsm/L

Note: For concentrated solutions, the calculated values of mOsm/L may not be accurate because of factors such as solvation and interionic forces which influence the osmotic pressure. Thus, results from the above calculations should be referred to as theoretical or approximate osmolarities. However, since most intravenous infusions are dilute solutions, results obtained from the above calculations are accurate enough to be clinically meaningful.

Practice Problems

Refer to Table 5.1 (in Chapter 5) as needed.

(1) An IV solution contains 40 mEq of potassium chloride in 1000 mL of solution. How many milligrams of potassium chloride are contained in 600 mL of this solution?

(2) 5.0 mEq of potassium ion is to be added to a solution of 5% dextrose injection for IV infusion. The K^+ is to be obtained from a vial of KCl containing 20 mEq of KCl in 25 mL of solution. How many milliliters of KCl solution should be added to the infusion?

(3) A 25 mL vial of NaCl solution was diluted to a liter with sterile water for injection. The concentration (w/v) of the NaCl in the finished product was 0.9%. What was the concentration in terms of mEq/mL, of the original solution?

(4) A medication order for an intravenous infusion for a patient weighing 143 lbs calls for a 0.25 mEq of ammonium chloride per kilogram of body weight to be added to 500 mL of 5% dextrose injection. How many

milliliters of a sterile solution containing 100 mEq of ammonium chloride per 25 mL should be used in preparing the infusion?

(5) A potassium phosphate solution contains 2.75 g of potassium acid phosphate (MW = 136) and 5.75 g of potassium dibasic phosphate (MW = 174) in 25 mL. If 5 mL of this solution are added to a liter of D5W, how many milliequivalents of potassium phosphate will be represented in the infusion?

(6) A liter of a 0.5% intravenous infusion of potassium chloride is to be administered over a period of four hours. How many milliequivalents of potassium are represented in the infusion?

(7) A medication order for an intravenous infusion for a patient weighing 110 lbs calls for a 0.3 mEq of ammonium chloride per kilogram of body weight to be added to 500 mL of 5% dextrose injection. How many milliliters of a sterile solution containing 100 mEq of ammonium chloride per 20 mL should be used in preparing the infusion?

(8) How many milliosmoles are represented in a liter of 10% dextrose (MW = 180) solution?

(9) What is the osmolarity of a liter solution containing 0.45% sodium chloride (MW = 58.5) and 5% dextrose (MW = 180)?

(10) What is the osmolarity of a 1.75% w/v solution of a chemical with a reported osmolality of 462 mOsm/kg and a density of 1.0025?

CHAPTER 11

Calculations Involving Nutrition

A nutritional deficit often exists in hospitalized patients. There are many conditions and diseases for which nutritional support is recommended by enteral or parenteral routes of administration. Provision of nutrients by vein, in amounts sufficient to maintain or achieve anabolism, is referred to as total parenteral nutrition (TPN).

Nutritional status of an individual can be assessed either by subjective global assessment or by prognostic nutritional index (PNI). Subjective global assessment takes into account weight changes, diet history, functional status, type and length of symptoms affecting nutritional status, and metabolic demands of the current disease process. PNI is based on a variety of markers of nutritional status including serum levels of albumin and transferrin, anthropometric measurements including body fat, lean body mass, stature, and various skinfold thickness measurements.

The present chapter deals with calculations associated with calories, nitrogen, protein-calorie percentage, parenteral hyperalimentation, and resting energy expenditure (REE) calculations including REE assessments for geriatric and pediatric populations.

CALCULATIONS OF CALORIES

Nutritional energy values are usually measured in kilocalories (kcal; or simply calories). One kilocalorie represents the amount of heat required to raise the temperature of 1 kg of water by 1°C at room temperature. In the metric system, the energy value is expressed in joules (J), with 1 kcal being equal to 4.184 kilojoules (kJ).

Glucose (dextrose) is the most commonly used energy substrate for TPN,

TABLE 11.1.   Caloric Density of
Nutritional Substrates.

Nutritional Substrate	Caloric Density (kcal/g)
Glucose, anhydrous	3.85
Glucose, monohydrate	3.40
Proteins	4.10
Fat emulsions	9.0
Alcohol	7.0

and may serve as the only nonprotein source of calories during TPN. The calories are also supplied by proteins and fats. The caloric density (kcal/g) of different nutritional substrates are listed in Table 11.1.

The calories represented by large volume parenterals and TPN products may be calculated in three steps as follows:

- Step 1: Find the weight in grams of each nutritional substrate in a specified volume of solution or liquid preparation using the following expression:

Grams of nutritional substrate =

Volume in mL × Percent expressed as decimal

- Step 2: Find the calories represented by each nutritional substrate by multiplying the weight in grams with caloric density.
- Step 3: Add up the calories represented by all the nutritional substrates in the preparation.

Example 1:

How many calories are contained in 3 L of D5W?

D5W is 5% dextrose in water

5% when expressed as decimal = 0.05

Step 1: 3000 mL × 0.05 = 150 g

Step 2: answer: 150 g × 3.4 kcal/g = 510 kcal

Alternatively, the calories represented by large volume parenterals and TPN products may also be calculated by the method of proportion as follows:

D5W = dextrose 5% in water

If 100 mL contain 5 g, 3000 mL contain:

$$\frac{100 \text{ mL}}{5 \text{ g}} = \frac{3000 \text{ mL}}{X \text{ g}}$$

$$X = 150 \text{ g}$$

answer: 150 g × 3.4 kcal = 510 kcal

Example 2:

How many calories are represented by a liter solution containing 20% dextrose, 12.5% proteins, and 5% fats?

Step 1: 1000 × 0.2 = 200 g dextrose
1000 × 0.125 = 125 g proteins
1000 × 0.05 = 50 g fats

Step 2: 200 × 3.4 = 680
125 × 4.1 = 512.5
50 × 9 = 450

Step 3: answer: 680 + 512.5 + 450 = 1642.5 kcal

Example 3:

How many calories are represented by a liter solution containing 12.5% dextrose, 7.5% proteins, and 4.5% fats?

Step 1: 1000 × 0.125 = 125 g dextrose
1000 × 0.075 = 75 g proteins
1000 × 0.045 = 45 g fats

Step 2: 125 × 3.4 = 425
75 × 4.1 = 307.5
45 × 9 = 405

Step 3: answer: 425 + 307.5 + 405 = 1137.5 kcal

Calculations Involving Nitrogen, Calorie:Nitrogen Ratio, and Protein-Calorie Percentage of TPN Solutions

Nitrogen is an essential component of every tissue and organ system. For protein synthesis (anabolism) to occur, the diet must contain adequate nitrogen, usually in the form of protein. The daily requirement for an adult is approximately 0.8 to 1.5 g of protein/kg of body weight. Thus, a 70-kg adult may require between 56 and 105 g of protein every 24 hours in order to prevent negative nitrogen balance. One gram of nitrogen is contained in each 6.25 g of protein or amino acids (i.e., 16% of the total weight). A 70-kg adult will require between 9 and 17 g of nitrogen per 24 hours (i.e., 56/6.25 and 105/6.25).

Grams of nitrogen available from protein sources is calculated as follows:

$$\text{Grams of nitrogen} = \frac{\text{Grams of protein in solution}}{6.25}$$

Example 1:

Calculate grams of nitrogen in 500 mL 8.5% amino acid solution.

8.5% = 8.5 g of amino acids/100 mL

500 mL would contain = 8.5 × 5 = 42.5 g of protein

grams of nitrogen = 42.5/6.25

answer: = 6.8 g

Calorie: Nitrogen Ratio

The ratio of administered calories to grams of nitrogen should promote optimum nitrogen utilization for the synthesis of protein. The calorie to nitrogen ratio (Cal:N) is determined by dividing the total non-nitrogen (non-protein) calories available with grams of nitrogen being provided. The optimal ratio is somewhere between 100 and 200 nonprotein calories per gram of nitrogen, with 135 to 175 being considered best for unstressed patients and slightly lower ratio for severely stressed patients.

Note: Do not take into account the calories from protein sources in computing calorie:nitrogen ratio.

Example 2:

Calculate calorie:nitrogen ratio of a TPN solution consisting of 500 mL of 50% dextrose and 500 mL of 8.5% amino acid solution.

nonprotein calories = 50 × 5 × 3.4 = 850 kcal

grams of amino acids (protein) = 8.5 × 5 = 42.5 g

grams of nitrogen = 42.5 ÷ 6.25 = 6.8 g

Ratio of non-nitrogen calories to grams of nitrogen

= 850 kcal ÷ 6.8 of N

answer: = 125:1

Protein-Calorie Percentage

The protein-calorie percentage of a TPN solution may be calculated as follows:

$$\text{Protein-calorie } \% = \frac{\text{Total \# of calories from protein sources}}{\text{Total \# of calories from all sources}} \times 100$$

Example 3:

Calculate protein-calorie percentage of a liter of 25% dextrose containing 4.25% amino acids.

250 g of dextrose = 250 × 3.4 kcal/g = 850 kcal

42.5 g of amino acids = 42.5 × 4.1 kcal/g = 174.25 kcal

Total calories/liter = 850 + 174.25 = 1024.25 kcal

Protein-calorie percentage of the solution

$$= \frac{174.25}{1024.25} \times 100$$

answer: = 17%

PARENTERAL HYPERALIMENTATION

The administration of large volumes of parenteral fluids containing essential nutrients sufficient to achieve active tissue synthesis and growth is referred to as *parenteral hyperalimentation.* Parenteral hyperalimentation also allows to achieve positive nitrogen balance, weight gain (where necessary), and accelerated wound healing in adults. The preparation of these parenteral admixtures usually involves the addition of a wide variety of additives including electrolytes, vitamins, trace minerals, antibiotics, and other drug combinations to large-volume solutions such as dilute infusions and nutrient fluids for intravenous therapy. Additives may also include heparin and insulin. The quantity of each of the additives required for the medication order is to be obtained from the available component sources. The volume of the additive containing desired quantity of the additive may be calculated by the method of proportion. The following examples illustrate the typical hyperalimentation calculations.

Example 1:

A medication order for a TPN solution includes additives as indicated in the following formula:

TPN Solution Formula	Component Source
Magnesium sulfate 10 mEq	20 mL vial of 10% solution
Potassium acetate 18 mEq	20 mL vial containing 40 mEq
Insulin 10 units	Vial of insulin U-100

To be added to:

  500 mL of 50% dextrose injection
  500 mL 5% protein hydrolysate injection

Using the sources listed, calculate the amount of each component required in filling the medication order.

Magnesium sulfate:

20 mL of 10% solution contains $20/100 \times 10 = 2$ g

$$\text{\# of mEq} \times \text{mEq wt} = \text{wt}$$

$$\text{\# of mEq} \times 60 \text{ mg} = 2000 \text{ mg}$$

$$\text{\# of mEq} = 2000/60 = 33.33 \text{ mEq}$$

$$\frac{33.33}{20 \text{ mL}} = \frac{10 \text{ mEq}}{X}$$

answer: $X = 6$ mL

Potassium acetate:

$$\frac{40 \text{ mEq}}{20 \text{ mL}} = \frac{18 \text{ mEq}}{X}$$

answer: $X = 9$ mL

Insulin:

$$\frac{100 \text{ units}}{1 \text{ mL}} = \frac{10 \text{ units}}{X}$$

answer: $X = 0.1$ mL

Example 2:

A physician order for a TPN solution includes the following additives:

TPN Solution Formula	Component Source
Sodium chloride 30 mEq	20 mL vial of 25% solution
Calcium gluconate 2.5 mEq	10 mL vial containing 12 mEq
Heparin 1000 units	5-mL vial containing 500 U/mL
Insulin 15 units	Vial of insulin U-100

To be added to:

500 mL of 50% dextrose injection
500 mL of 8.5% amino acids injection

Using the sources listed, calculate the amount of each component required in filling the medication order.

Sodium chloride:

20 mL of 25% solution contains $25/100 \times 20 = 5$ g

# of mEq × mEq wt = wt

# of mEq × 58.5 mg = 5000 mg

mEq = 5000/58.5 = 85.47 mEq

$$\frac{85.47}{20 \text{ mL}} = \frac{30 \text{ mEq}}{X}$$

answer: $X = 7.02$ mL

Calcium gluconate:

$$\frac{12 \text{ mEq}}{10 \text{ mL}} = \frac{2.5 \text{ mEq}}{X}$$

answer: $X = 2.08$ mL

Heparin:

$$\frac{500 \text{ units}}{1 \text{ mL}} = \frac{1000 \text{ units}}{X}$$

answer: $X = 2.0$ mL

Insulin:

$$\frac{100 \text{ units}}{1 \text{ mL}} = \frac{15 \text{ units}}{X}$$

answer: $X = 0.15$ mL

Example 3:

A hyperalimentation order for a patient includes 30 mg of amphotericin B, 50 units of heparin, 25 mEq of potassium acetate, and 1.5 mg of folic acid to be administered intravenously in 1000 mL of D5W over an 8 hour period. In filling the medication order, the following sources are available:

- a vial containing 50 mg of amphotericin B in 10 mL
- a syringe containing 10 units of heparin per mL
- a 20 mL vial of 40 mEq of potassium acetate
- an ampul containing 5 mg of folic acid per mL

How many mL of each additive should be used in filling the medication order?

Amphotericin B:

$$\frac{50 \text{ mg}}{10 \text{ mL}} = \frac{30 \text{ mg}}{X}$$

answer: $X = 6$ mL

Heparin:

$$\frac{10 \text{ units}}{1 \text{ mL}} = \frac{50 \text{ units}}{X}$$

answer: $X = 5$ mL

Potassium acetate:

$$\frac{40 \text{ mEq}}{20 \text{ mL}} = \frac{25 \text{ mEq}}{X}$$

answer: $X = 12.5$ mL

Folic acid:

$$\frac{5 \text{ mg}}{1 \text{ mL}} = \frac{1.5 \text{ mg}}{X}$$

answer: $X = 0.3$ mL

Practice Problems

(1) How many calories are contained in 2.5 L of 5% dextrose?

(2) How many calories are represented by a liter solution containing 15% dextrose, 10% proteins, and 8% fats?

(3) A TPN solution consists of 0.75 L of 10% dextrose and 0.25 L of 4.25% amino acid solution. What is the ratio of non-nitrogen calories to grams of nitrogen (Cal:N) for this TPN formula?

(4) A TPN solution contains 0.5 L of 25% dextrose and 0.5 L of 8.5% amino acid solution. What is the non-nitrogen calories to grams of nitrogen ratio (Cal:N) for this TPN formula?

(5) Calculate protein-calorie percentage of a liter of 10% dextrose containing 8.5% amino acids.

(6) A liter of TPN solution is obtained by combining 500 mL of 10% dextrose and 500 mL of 7.5% amino acids. What is the protein-calorie percentage of the solution?

(7) A TPN solution consists of 500 mL of 25% dextrose and 500 mL of 10% amino acid solution. Calculate:

   a. The total number of calories present in the preparation
   b. Grams of nitrogen in the preparation
   c. The ratio of nonprotein calories-to-grams of nitrogen (Cal:N)
   d. The protein-calorie percentage of the solution

(8) A patient is to receive 1 L of the following admixture every eight hours:

   Fre-Amine (10%)   500 mL
   D-50-W   500 mL

   To each liter add:

   • 20 mEq of sodium chloride (Source: NSS solution)
   • 2 mL of magnesium sulfate (Source: 50% solution of magnesium sulfate MW = 120)

   Calculate:

   a. The total number of glucose calories the patient receives per day
   b. The number of mEq of Mg^{++} the patient receives per day
   c. Grams of protein and nitrogen the patient receives per day
   d. Calorie-to-nitrogen ratio (Cal:N)

(9) A patient is to receive 1 L of the following admixture every eight hours:

   50% Dextrose in water   500 mL
   8.5% Fre-Amine   500 mL

   Calculate:

   a. Glucose calories/day

b. Grams of protein received/day
c. Grams of nitrogen received/day
d. Calorie-to-nitrogen ratio (Cal:N)

(10) Using the sources listed below, calculate the amount of each component required in filling the medication order:

TPN Solution Formula	Component Source
Potassium chloride 40 mEq	20 mL vial of 25% solution
Calcium chloride 8.6 mEq	10 mL vial containing 30 mEq
Sodium chloride 30 mEq	20 mL vial of 20% solution
Insulin 12 units	Vial of insulin U-100

To be added to:

Dextrose 40%	500 mL
Amino acid solution 8.5%	500 mL

RESTING ENERGY EXPENDITURE (REE) CALCULATIONS

In order to maintain normal physiological functions, the body needs a continuous supply of energy from food. In hospital settings, particularly in patients requiring total parenteral nutrition, the nutrition requirements are usually assessed on the basis of resting energy expenditure (REE). Many factors affect individual nutritional and energy requirements. These factors include age, height, weight, gender, and physical activity and health status.

The resting energy expenditure (REE), in kilocalories (kcal), may be calculated on the basis of the age (years), weight (kg), height (cm), and sex of the patient (Table 11.2). This is an empirical approach that requires frequent assessment of progress and may necessitate reestablishment of therapeutic goal based upon patient weight gain, laboratory indices, and other objective parameters. These empirical formulae are known as Harris-Benedict equations.

Note: The resting energy expenditure (REE) is also referred to as basal energy expenditure and abbreviated as BEE.

The energy requirement in terms of anabolic goal may be calculated on the basis of REE or body weight:

> **Anabolic Goal**
> *(calories/day)*
> *Based on REE:*
> = REE × 1.75
> *Based on body weight:*
> = 45 kcal × body weight in kg

TABLE 11.2.   Formulae for Resting Energy
Expenditure (REE) Calculations.

For men
  REE (kcal/24 hr)
    = 66.5 + (13.75 × weight in kg)
    + (5.00 × height in cm)
    − (6.76 × age in yrs)

For women
  REE (kcal/24 hr)
    = 655 + (9.56 × weight in kg)
    + (1.85 × height in cm)
    − (4.68 × age in yrs)

Example 1:

Patient profile:

  Sex: Male
  Age: 45 years
  Height: 175 cm
  Weight: 85 kg

Based on the above information, calculate:

a. REE in calories/day
b. Anabolic goal (kcal/day) of the patient based on REE
c. Anabolic goal (kcal/day) of the patient based on his body weight

a. REE (kcal/day)

$$= 66.5 + (13.75 × 85) + (5.00 × 175) − (6.76 × 45)$$

answer: = 1806 kcal/day

b. Anabolic goal based on REE

$$= 1.75 × 1806 = 3161$$

answer: 3161 kcal/day

c. Anabolic goal based on body weight

$$= 45 × 85 = 3825$$

answer: 3825 kcal/day

Example 2:

Patient profile:

Sex:	Female
Age:	26 years
Height:	158 cm
Weight:	48 kg

Based on the above information, calculate:

a. REE in calories/day
b. Anabolic goal (kcal/day) of the patient based on REE
c. Anabolic goal (kcal/day) of the patient based on his body weight

a. REE (kcal/24 hr)

$$= 655 + (9.56 \times 48) + (1.85 \times 158) - (4.68 \times 26)$$

answer: = 1285 kcal/day

b. Anabolic goal based on REE

$$= 1.75 \times 1285 = 2249 \text{ kcal/day}$$

answer: 2249 kcal/day

c. Anabolic goal based on body weight = 45 × 48

$$= 45 \times 48 = 2160$$

answer: 2160 kcal/day

Example 3:

Patient profile:

Sex:	Male
Age:	47 years
Height:	75 inches
Weight:	145.2 pounds

Based on the above information, calculate:

a. REE in calories/day
b. Anabolic goal (kcal/day) of the patient based on REE
c. Anabolic goal (kcal/day) of the patient based on his body weight

a. 145.2 lb = 145.2/2.2 = 66 kg
   75 inches = 75 × 2.54 = 190.5 cm

REE (kcal/day)

$$= 66.5 + (13.75 \times 66) + (5.00 \times 190.5) - (6.76 \times 47)$$

answer: = 1609 kcal/day

b. Anabolic goal based on REE

$$= 1.75 \times 1609 = 2816$$

answer: 2816 kcal/day

c. Anabolic goal based on body weight

$$= 45 \times 66 = 2970$$

answer: 2970 kcal/day

Practice Problems

(1) What is the REE Requirement, in terms of kcal/day, for the patient with the following information?

Patient profile:

Sex:	Female
Age:	35 years
Height:	159 cm
Weight:	70 kg

(2) For the following patient, calculate the REE requirement, in terms of kcal/day.

Patient profile:

Sex:	Male
Age:	57 years
Height:	54 inches
Weight:	108 lb

(3) Calculate the REE requirement, in terms of kcal/hour, for a patient with the following profile.

Patient profile:

Sex:	Female
Age:	42 years
Height:	172 cm
Weight:	154 lb

(4) What is the REE requirement, in terms of kcal/day, for the following patient?

Patient profile:

Sex:	Male
Age:	37 years
Height:	159 cm
Weight:	128 lb

(5) A patient profile is as follows:

Sex:	Male
Age:	47 years
Height:	168 cm
Weight:	132 lb

Calculate:

a. REE in kcal/day
b. The anabolic goal of the patient based on the REE
c. The anabolic goal of the patient based on the body weight
d. How many mL of 50% dextrose solution would be required to provide the calories needed for REE of the patient?

(6) A patient profile is as follows:

Sex:	Female
Age:	32 years
Height:	154 cm
Weight:	110 lb

Calculate:

a. REE in kcal/day
b. The anabolic goal of the patient based on the REE
c. The anabolic goal of the patient based on the body weight
d. How many liters of D5W would be required to provide the calories needed for REE of the patient?

(7) A patient profile is as follows:

Sex: Female
Age: 55 years
Height: 186 cm
Weight: 165 lb

Calculate:

a. REE in kcal/day
b. The anabolic goal of the patient based on the REE
c. The anabolic goal of the patient based on the body weight

(8) Based on the following information, calculate the age of the patient in years.

Sex: Female
Height: 158 cm
Weight: 48 kg
REE: 1285 kcal/day

(9) What is the body weight of the following patient in pounds?

Sex: Male
Height: 168 cm
Age: 47 years
REE: 1285 kcal/day

(10) A patient has the following profile:

Sex: Male
Age: 45 years
Height: 175 cm
Weight: 85 kg

Calculate:

a. REE in calories/day
b. Anabolic goal based on his body weight.

GERIATRIC NUTRITION

There is a decrease in basal metabolic rate with a decline in lean body mass and less physical activity. The caloric requirement may, therefore, be reduced accordingly in the elderly. The use of Harris-Benedict equations to determine REE in the elderly has been questioned in recent times. The following equations have been developed for individuals over age 60:

For men

REE (kcal/24 hr)

$$= (8.8 \times \text{weight in kg}) + (1128 \times \text{height in m}) - 1071$$

For women

REE (kcal/24 hr)

$$= (9.2 \times \text{weight in kg}) + (637 \times \text{height in m}) - 302$$

Example 1:

Patient Profile:

Sex:	Male
Age:	65 years
Height:	175 cm
Weight:	65 kg

Calculate the REE requirement in terms of kcal/day for this patient.

$$\text{REE (kcal/day)} = (8.8 \times 65) + (1128 \times 1.75) - 1071$$

$$= 572 + 1974 - 1071 = 1475$$

answer: 1475 kcal/day

Example 2:

Patient Profile:

Sex:	Male
Age:	68 years
Height:	145 cm
Weight:	48 kg

Calculate the REE requirement in terms of kcal/day for this patient.

$$\text{REE (kcal/day)} = (9.2 \times 48) + (637 \times 1.45) - 302$$

$$= 441.6 + 923.65 - 302 = 1063.25$$

answer: 1063 kcal/day

Note: Increases in energy requirements above the REE are estimated to be 1.2–1.5 times the calculated REE in active healthy elderly.

PEDIATRIC NUTRITION

Body composition varies with age. The pediatric population has unique physiologic needs that make nutritional requirements distinctly different than adults. In children, caloric requirements per kilogram are higher because of their higher basal metabolic rate (BMR). BMR is approximately 50–55 kcal/kg/day in infancy and declines to about 20–25 kcal/kg/day during adolescence.

For children less than three years old, a modified version of the Harris-Benedict equation has been developed by Caldwell-Kennedy:

$$\text{REE (kcal/day)} = 22 + (31 \times \text{wt in kg}) + (1.2 \times \text{height in cm})$$

Example 3:

Calculate the REE (kcal/day) for a 18-month-old child who is 70 centimeters tall and weighs 16 kg.

$$\text{REE (kcal/day)} = 22 + (31 \times 16) + (1.2 \times 70) = 602$$

answer: 602 kcal/day

Practice Problems

(1) A patient profile is as follows:

Sex:	Male
Age:	74 years
Height:	168 cm
Weight:	118 lbs

What is the REE in kcal/day for this patient?

(2) What is the REE (kcal/day) of a 72-year-old female patient who is 162 cm tall and weighs 106 pounds?

(3) What is the REE requirement, in terms of kcal/day, for the following patient?

Patient profile:

Sex:	Male
Age:	71 years
Height:	159 cm
Weight:	122 lbs

(4) What is the REE requirement, in terms of kcal/day, for the following patient?

Patient profile:

Sex:	Female
Age:	76 years
Height:	148 cm
Weight:	121 lbs

(5) What is the REE requirement, in terms of kcal/day, for the following patient?

Patient profile:

Sex:	Male
Age:	71 years
Height:	1.72 m
Weight:	58 kg

(6) What is the REE requirement, in terms of kcal/day, for the following patient?

Patient profile:

Sex:	Female
Age:	76 years
Height:	1.46 m
Weight:	132 lbs

(7) What is the REE (kcal/day) for a two-year-old child who is 82 centimeters tall and weighs 12 kg?

(8) What is the REE (kcal/day) for a 15-month-old child who is 28 inches tall and weighs 28.6 pounds?

(9) What is the REE (kcal/day) for a 24-month-old child who is 85 centimeters tall and weighs 23 kg?

(10) What is the REE (kcal/day) for a 2.5-year-old child who is 88 centimeters tall and weighs 55.6 pounds?

CHAPTER 12

Calculation of Doses and Dose Adjustments

The dose of a drug is the amount at the time of administration to obtain a desired therapeutic response, and the dosage regimen refers to the schedule of dosing. Generally, the manufacturer provides a range of doses for a given drug. Since several factors affect the dose of a drug, the exact amount of a drug to be administered is decided by the health care professionals. Some of the factors affecting the dose of a drug include the type of dosage form, route of drug administration, individual patient's tolerance of the drug, genetic predisposition, concurrent administration of other drugs, patient's age, body weight, gender, length of illness, general physical health, liver and kidney function in the patient, and the rate of absorption, distribution, metabolism and excretion of drugs in the patient. The dose of a given drug is specific to the patient. Thus, a fixed dose of a drug might be an overdose in some patients, whereas the same dose might be considered an under-dose in another group of patients. The inter- and intrasubject variations to the effects of drugs can be avoided by tailoring a dose (or a dosage regimen) to a given patient through the use of clinical pharmacokinetics. Thus, clinical pharmacokinetics may be defined as the applied science in which the pharmacokinetic principles are utilized for tailoring the dose and dosage regimen for an individual patient. The knowledge of clinical pharmacokinetics is essential in providing an optimum drug concentration at the receptor site to obtain the desired therapeutic response, and minimize the drug's adverse or toxic effects.

For an optimal therapeutic response, the clinical pharmacist must select a suitable drug and determine an appropriate dose with the available strengths and a convenient dosing interval. To meet this responsibility, the serum or plasma drug concentrations have to be analyzed, pharmacokinetic parameters have to be evaluated, the drug dose has to be adjusted, and the dosing interval has to be determined.

PLASMA CONCENTRATION VERSUS TIME PROFILE

Figure 12.1 shows the plasma concentration versus time profile of an orally administered hypothetical drug. When the drug concentration in plasma equals the minimum effective concentration (MEC), therapeutic response is initiated. When the concentration exceeds the minimum toxic concentration (MTC), the drug causes toxic responses. Therefore, for ideal therapeutic response, the plasma concentration of drugs should be between the MEC and MTC. This region is called the *therapeutic window.* In Figure 12.1 the MEC is 1.5 ng/mL, and the MTC is 3.5 ng/mL. The therapeutic window is between 1.5 and 3.5 ng/mL.

When a drug is administered, it gets absorbed into the blood, distributed to different sites in the body, metabolized, and finally excreted. As shown in Figure 12.1, initially the plasma concentration increases with time because the rate of absorption is greater than the rate of elimination. When a plateau is reached at the top, the rate of absorption equals the rate of elimination, and finally the concentration goes down because the rate of elimination is greater than the rate of absorption. The time at which the plasma concentration equals the MEC is called the *onset of action,* the length of time for which the drug remains above the MEC is known as the *duration of action,* and the height

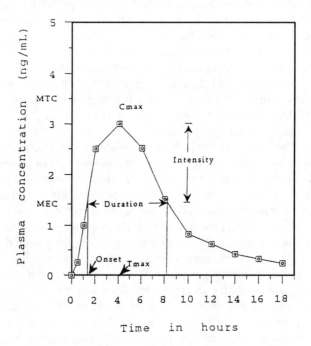

FIGURE 12.1. Plasma concentration versus time profile.

of plasma concentration between the MEC and the maximum plasma concentration is the *intensity of action*. In Figure 12.1, the onset of action is 1.4 hours, the duration of action is 6.7 hours (calculated as 8.1–1.4 hours), and the intensity of action is 1.5 ng/mL (calculated as 3–1.5 ng/mL).

SOME PHARMACOKINETIC PARAMETERS

For understanding the effect of certain drugs, relating the effects of similar drugs, designing dosage regimens, modifying dose for patient specific conditions, and monitoring toxicity, a few pharmacokinetic parameters are very useful. These parameters include area under the plasma level versus time curve (AUC), maximum plasma concentration (C_{max}), time for maximum concentration (T_{max}), elimination half-life of the drug ($t_{1/2}$), elimination rate constant (K_{el}), and the volume of distribution (V_d).

Area Under the Curve (AUC)

Area under the curve, AUC, provides an idea about the extent of drug absorption. It is an essential component of bioavailability studies where the rate and extent of drug absorption are measured. The greater the AUC, the more is the drug absorbed. Although, one cannot determine how much of the drug is absorbed by AUC, the relative performance of different drugs can be evaluated. For example, if the AUC of Drug A is 100 ng·hr/mL and that of a drug B is 200 ng·hr/mL, drug A is one-half as well absorbed as drug B. The AUC is very commonly calculated by the *Trapezoidal Rule* where the blood level curve with time is plotted and trapezoids are constructed at each time point. This is shown in Figure 12.2.

As depicted in the figure, the first and the last segments are triangles. However, in most cases the last segment is a trapezium. The areas of all trapezoids and triangles are calculated and added up to get the AUC. The area of trapezoids is calculated as "$\frac{1}{2} \times w \times$ sum of parallel sides" and the area of triangles is calculated as "$(w \times h)/2$." In these formulae, w represents the width or the class interval for the trapezoids or the triangles, parallel sides are the two heights at the two time points, and h represents the height of the triangle side. These calculations are explained in Example 1 of problems pertaining to pharmacokinetic parameters. The AUC calculation shown in this book is usually from zero to the last time point. The AUC calculations from zero to infinity are beyond the scope of this text.

Maximum Plasma Concentration (C_{max})

Maximum plasma concentration, C_{max}, is a measure of both the rate and extent of drug absorption. It is also an essential component of the bioavailability

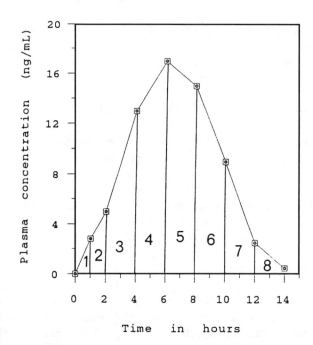

FIGURE 12.2. Plasma concentration versus time profile for area under the curve calculations.

studies. The C_{max} will increase if the drug is more rapidly absorbed. Usually, the C_{max} is read directly from the plasma concentration versus time profile. For example, in Figure 12.2, C_{max} is 17 ng/mL.

Time for Maximum Concentration (T_{max})

The Time for Maximum Concentration, T_{max}, is the third important component of bioavailability studies. It is a measure of the rate of drug absorption. A lower T_{max} represents a faster absorption and a higher T_{max} represents a slower absorption. Similar to C_{max}, the T_{max} is read directly from the plasma concentration versus time profile. The T_{max} in Figure 12.2 is 6 hours.

When the rate and extent of absorption of two drugs are different, they are not considered as equivalent products. When the rate and extent of absorption of two products are equal, they are considered equivalent. In some special cases where rate of absorption is different but the extent is same, the products are considered equivalent.

Elimination Half-Life ($t_{1/2}$)

Elimination half-life, $t_{1/2}$, is the time period in which the plasma concentration becomes one-half of its value. For example, if the plasma concentration is 2 ng/mL at 8:00 A.M. and 1 ng/mL at 11:00 A.M., the $t_{1/2}$ of the drug is 3 hours. It can also be calculated by the equation, $t_{1/2} = 0.693/K_{el}$. The $t_{1/2}$ value is constant for a given therapeutic agent. As a few examples, the $t_{1/2}$ of nitroglycerin, indomethacin, and amitriptyline are 20 min, 2 hours, and 40 hours, respectively.

Elimination Rate Constant (K_{el})

Elimination Rate Constant, (K_{el}), is a crucial pharmacokinetic parameter which measures the rate of elimination of drugs from the body. K_{el} is specific for a given drug, and has the units of time^{-1}. When the K_{el} is greater, the drug is eliminated rapidly. It is calculated from the slope of the terminal portion of the log plasma concentration versus time profile. From the terminal portion of the plasma concentration versus time profile, K_{el} is calculated as,

$$K_{el} = \frac{\ln Y_1 - \ln Y_2}{t_2 - t_1}$$

It can also be calculated from the $t_{1/2}$ as,

$$K_{el} = 0.693/t_{1/2}$$

Volume of Distribution (V_d)

The volume of distribution, V_d, represents a hypothetical volume which relates the amount of drug in the body to the plasma concentration by the equation.

$$V_d = A_b/C$$

where A_b is the amount of drug in the body which also equals the amount of administered drug, and C is the concentration of drug in the plasma. The volume of distribution is defined as an apparent volume in which the drug in the entire body would be contained if it were in the concentration as that found in the plasma. For example, if a 100 mg dose is administered, and the plasma concentration extrapolated to zero time point is 1 mcg/mL, the volume of distribution is 100,000 mcg/1 mcg/mL = 100 L. It is clear from this example that when 100 mg of the drug is administered, only 1 mcg/mL appear in the plasma. Normally the plasma volume of an individual is 3 L. Therefore, plasma accounts for only (1 mcg/mL) × 3000 mL = 3000 mcg or 3 mg. Rest of the drug may be in other areas such as liver, fats, spleen, etc. Therefore, the V_d provides an estimate of the drug which does not appear in the plasma.

In some cases, a given drug may be highly bound to proteins. In such cases, the V_d is very high. The drug quinacrine has a V_d of 50,000 L where as the V_d of tolbutamide is less than 10 L.

Problems Pertaining to Pharmacokinetic Parameters

Example 1:

Assume that the Figure 12.2 was obtained after administration of a marketed antidiabetic drug. Calculate the AUC, C_{max}, T_{max}, K_{el} and $t^1/_2$.

As shown in Figure 12.2, the AUC is divided into eight segments. Segments 1 and 8 are triangles and rest of the segments are trapezoids. The AUC is calculated for all the segments individually. The total AUC is then calculated by adding up the AUC values of all the individual segments. The calculations are shown as follows:

Segment 1: $(w \times h)/2 = (1 \times 2.8)/2 = 1.4$ ng·hr/mL

Segment 2: $\frac{1}{2} \times w \times$ sum of parallel sides $= \frac{1}{2} \times 1 \times (2.8 + 5) = 3.9$ ng·hr/mL

Segment 3: $\frac{1}{2} \times w \times$ sum of parallel sides $= \frac{1}{2} \times 2 \times (5 + 13) = 18$ ng·hr/mL

Segment 4: $\frac{1}{2} \times w \times$ sum of parallel sides $= \frac{1}{2} \times 2 \times (13 + 17) = 30$ ng·hr/mL

Segment 5: $\frac{1}{2} \times w \times$ sum of parallel sides $= \frac{1}{2} \times 2 \times (17 + 15) = 32$ ng·hr/mL

Segment 6: $\frac{1}{2} \times w \times$ sum of parallel sides $= \frac{1}{2} \times 2 \times (15 + 9) = 24$ ng·hr/mL

Segment 7: $\frac{1}{2} \times w \times$ sum of parallel sides $= \frac{1}{2} \times 2 \times (9 + 2.5) = 11.5$ ng·hr/mL

Segment 8: $(w \times h)/2 = (2 \times 2.5)/2 = 2.5$ ng·hr/mL

Therefore, AUC $= 1.4 + 3.9 + 18 + 30 + 32 + 24 + 11.5$

$+ 2.5 = 123.3$ ng·hr/mL

$$C_{max} = 17 \text{ ng/mL}$$

$$T_{max} = 6 \text{ hours}$$

$$K_{el} = (\ln Y_1 - \ln Y_2)/(t_2 - t_1) = (\ln 9 - \ln 2.5)/(12 - 10)$$

$$= 0.64 \text{ hours}^{-1}$$

$$t^1/_2 = 0.693/0.64 \text{ hours} = 1.08 \text{ hours}$$

answer: AUC $= 123.3$ ng·hr/mL; $C_{max} = 17$ ng/mL; $T_{max} = 6$ hr; $K_{el} = 0.64$ hr^{-1} and $t_{1/2} = 1.08$ hr

Note: The $t_{1/2}$ can also be calculated as the time required for the concentration to become one-half of the initial concentration at the elimination stage. In

Figure 12.2, if the initial concentration is 9 ng/mL, the time required for the concentration to become 4.5 ng/mL is 11.1 − 10 = 1.1 hours. Therefore, the $t_{1/2}$ is 1.1 hours. Once the $t_{1/2}$ is known, K_{el} can be easily calculated as K_{el} = $0.693/t_{1/2}$ = 0.693/1.1 = 0.63 hour^{-1}.

Example 2:

After the administration of a generic antidiabetic drug, the following plasma levels were observed at the given time points. Calculate the AUC, C_{max}, T_{max}, $t_{1/2}$ and the K_{el}.

Plasma Conc (mcg/mL)	0	1	3	4	2	1	0.5	0.1
Time in Hours	0	0.5	1	2	4	6	8	10

As shown in Figure 12.3, the AUC is divided into seven segments. Segments 1 and 7 are triangles and rest of the segments are trapezoids. The AUC is calculated for all the segments individually. The total AUC is then calculated by adding up the AUC values of all the individual segments. The calculations are shown as follows:

Segment 1: $(w \times h)/2$ = (0.5 × 1)/2 = 0.25 mcg·hr/mL

Segment 2: 1/2 × w × sum of parallel sides = 1/2 × 0.5 × (1 + 3) = 1 mcg·hr/mL

Segment 3: 1/2 × w × sum of parallel sides = 1/2 × 1 × (3 + 4) = 3.5 mcg·hr/mL

Segment 4: 1/2 × w × sum of parallel sides = 1/2 × 2 × (4 + 2) = 6 mcg·hr/mL

Segment 5: 1/2 × w × sum of parallel sides = 1/2 × 2 × (2 + 1) = 3 mcg·hr/mL

Segment 6: 1/2 × w × sum of parallel sides = 1/2 × 2 × (1 + 0.5) = 1.5 mcg·hr/mL

Segment 7[3]: $(w \times h)/2$ = (2 × 0.5)/2 = 0.5 mcg·hr/mL

Therefore, AUC = 0.25 + 1 + 3.5 + 6 + 3 + 1.5 + 0.5

= 15.75 mcg·hr/mL

C_{max} = 4 mcg/mL

T_{max} = 2 hours

K_{el} = (ln Y_1 − ln Y_2)/(t_2 − t_1) = (ln 1 − ln 0.5)/(8 − 6)

= 0.347 hours^{-1}

$t_{1/2}$ = 0.693/0.347 hours = 2 hours

answer: AUC = 15.75 mcg·hr/mL; C_{max} = 4 mcg/mL; T_{max} = 2 hr, K_{el} = 0.347 hr and $t_{1/2}$ = 2 hr

---

[3]This segment can also be calculated as the area of a trapezium as [1/2 × 2 × (0.5 + 0.1)] = 0.6 mcg·hr/mL.

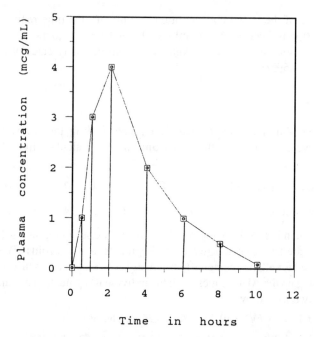

FIGURE 12.3. Plasma concentration versus time profile for area under the curve calculations.

Example 3:

A drug has an elimination half-life of 4 hours. After the administration of a 250 mg dose, plasma concentration at zero time point[4] was found to be 5.65 mcg/mL. What is the volume of distribution of the drug?

$$V_d = D_0/C_0$$

$$D_0 = 250 \text{ mg} = 250{,}000 \text{ mcg}$$

$$= 250{,}000 \text{ mcg}/5.65 \text{ mcg/mL} = 44{,}248 \text{ mL or } 44.3 \text{ L}$$

answer: 44.3 L

Practice Problems

(1) For the problem in Example 2, assume that the data at 1 and 2 hours

---

[4]The plasma concentration at zero time point is calculated by the formula, $\ln C = \ln C_0 - K_{el} \times t$, where C is the plasma concentration at time t and C_0 is the plasma concentration at zero time point. The $K_{si} = 0.693/t_{1/2}$.

was lost due to the instrumental breakdown or a technician's carelessness. What would be the percent error associated with the AUC calculation?

(2) In a pharmacokinetic study, the following data was obtained with a novel antidiabetic drug. Find the AUC of this drug.

Time (hr)	0	0.5	1	2	3	4	6	8	12
Plasma Cone (ng/mL)	0	3.8	5.8	7.1	6.9	6.2	4.8	3.5	1.9

(3) For the following data, find the AUC from the initial time up to six hours.

Time (hr)	0	0.5	1	2	3	4	6	8	12
Plasma Conc (ng/mL)	0	2.8	6.6	8.5	9.5	9.4	8.7	6.6	3.8

(4) The plasma levels listed below are obtained from a patient population and represent averages. Plot the plasma level versus time profile. Determine the elimination rate constant, half-life, C_{max} and the T_{max} of this drug.

Time (hr)	0.25	0.5	1	2	3	4	6	8	12
C_p (ng/mL)	66.2	268	398	422	420	328	180	105	38.4

(5) After the administration of a syrup and tablet dosage form of a drug, the following data was obtained. What is the AUC of the liquid relative to the solid dosage form?

	Plasma Concentration (mcg/mL)	
Time (hr)	Syrup	Tablet
0	0	0
0.5	10	6
1	30	25
2	22	20
4	12	13
6	6	8
8	0.75	1

(6) If the minimum effective concentration is 3 mg/mL, what is the onset, intensity, and duration of action of the administered drug for which the following plasma concentration versus time data is available?

Time (hr)	1	2	4	6	8	10	12	14
C_p(mg/mL)	2.6	3.6	3.5	2.9	2.3	1.7	1.3	1.0

(7) The plasma concentration of a drug immediately following a 50-mg intravenous bolus dose of the drug was found to be 0.84 mcg/mL. What is the apparent volume of distribution of the drug?

(8) If the apparent volume of distribution of a drug is 30 L and the plasma concentration extrapolated to zero time point (C_0) is 0.15 mcg/mL, what is the dose of the drug?

(9) The following data was obtained after the administration of a single 500-mg dose of a drug by slow intravenous infusion. Calculate the AUC, elimination rate constant, and the biological half-life of the drug.

Time (hr)	0	0.5	1	2	4	6	8	10	12
C_p(mg/mL)	0	4.9	7.6	9	9.5	7.4	5.8	4.5	3.6

(10) The average blood concentration of erythromycin observed in a group of twelve adult males following oral administration of 500 mg of erythromycin in a tablet are given below:

Time (hr)	0	0.75	1.5	3	4.5	6	8	10	12	14
C_p(mcg/mL)	0	0.33	1.3	1.44	1.44	0.61	0.27	0.13	0.06	0.03

Calculate the AUC, C_{max}, T_{max}, K_{el} and $t_{1/2}$

FRACTION OF DRUG ABSORBED AND THE DOSING INTERVAL

The fraction of drug absorbed, F, represents the ratio of AUC of drug from a dosage form to the AUC of the same drug from a readily available preparation such as an intravenous injection where the drug is administered directly in the blood stream. This may be expressed as follows:

$$F = \text{AUC of the drug/AUC of the drug by IV injection}$$

If the AUC of an orally administered drug is 8.86 mcg·hr/mL and the AUC of the drug administered by an IV injection is 11.2 mcg·hr/mL, the fraction of drug absorbed is 8.86/11.2 = 0.79.

The F value is also known as "Bioavailability Factor" or "Absolute Bioavailability." It is very useful in the calculation of dosing interval which is described below.

In the plasma concentration versus time profile, after the administration of a dose of a given drug, the drug concentration goes down when the rate of elimination is greater than the rate of absorption. As the drug concentration decreases, it becomes necessary to administer a second dose to maintain the concentration of drug between the MEC and MTC. The duration of time between the administration of two doses is called the dosing interval (τ) which can be calculated from the formula given below:

$$\tau = \frac{F \times D_0}{C_{ave} \times V_d \times K_{el}}$$

where

C_{ave} = average concentration of drug in the blood per L
F = fraction of drug absorbed
D_0 = dose administered
V_d = volume of distribution in liters
K_{el} = elimination rate constant

Example 1:

If the fraction of the drug absorbed is 0.8, dose of the drug is 100 mg, volume of distribution is 25 L, average drug concentration in the blood is 4 mcg/mL, and the elimination rate constant is 0.2 hour^{-1}, when should the second dose be taken if the first dose was taken at 2:00 P.M.?

$$\tau = \frac{F \times D_0}{C_{ave} \times V_d \times K_{el}}$$

$$\tau = \frac{0.8 \times 100}{4 \times 25 \times 0.2}$$

$$\tau = 4 \text{ hours}$$

answer: Since the first dose was taken at 2:00 P.M., the second dose should be taken at 6:00 P.M.

Example 2:

For the problem in Example 1, if the average blood concentration is 10 mcg/mL, what would be the dose of the drug?

$$4 = \frac{0.8 \times D_0}{10 \times 25 \times 0.2}$$

$$D_0 = 10 \times 25 \times 0.2 \times 4/0.8 = 250 \text{ mg}$$

answer: dose of drug $(D_0) = 250$ mg

Example 3:

A therapeutic agent was found to have an F value of 0.75, volume of distribution of 3 L/kg, and an average blood concentration of 2.75 ng/mL.

What would be the dosing interval if the dose of the drug is 0.27 mg, K_{el} value is 0.0315 hr^{-1}, and the weight of the patient is 143 lb?

Convert the weight of patient from pounds to kilograms.

$$143 \text{ lb}/2.2 = 65 \text{ kg}$$

The volume of distribution for the therapeutic agent would be (3 L/kg) × 65 kg = 195 L.

The dosing interval can then be calculated by the formula,

$$\tau = \frac{F \times D_0}{C_{ave} \times V_d \times K_{el}}$$

$$\tau = \frac{0.75 \times 270}{2.75 \times 195 \times 0.0315}$$

$$\tau = 11.99 \text{ or } 12 \text{ hours}$$

answer: dosing interval equals 12 hours

Note: Since the average blood concentration was provided in ng/mL, or mcg/L dose of the drug was taken as 270 mcg instead of 0.27 mg.

Practice Problems

(1) If the fraction of the dose absorbed is 0.6 and the AUC obtained after an IV injection is 24 mcg·hr/mL, what would be the most likely AUC of an oral dose of the same drug?

(2) What would be the dosing interval of a drug which has a volume of distribution of 5 L? When a dose of 250 mg is given, 100 mg[5] of the

---

[5]F value can also be determined as drug absorbed/dose administered. Therefore, F value in the present case is 100 mg/250 mg = 0.4.

drug is absorbed and the average plasma concentration is 2 mcg/mL. The plasma half-life is 3 hours.

(3) If the fraction of the dose absorbed is 0.8 and the AUC obtained after an IV injection is 24 mcg·hr/mL, what would be the most likely AUC of an oral dose of the same drug?

(4) What would be the dosing interval of a drug that has a volume of distribution of 5 L? When a dose of 250 mg is given, 200 mg of the drug is absorbed and the average plasma concentration is 4 mcg/mL. The plasma half-life is 3 hours.

(5) To obtain an average plasma concentration of 25 ng/mL with a dosing interval of 8 hours, what should be the dose of the drug when the fraction of drug absorbed is 0.8? It is known that the drug has a volume of distribution of 75 L and has an elimination rate constant of 0.173 hour^{-1}.

(6) What is the average plasma concentration when a 500 mg drug is adminis-. tered with an interval of 6 hours and has a volume of distribution of 50 L? It is known that the fraction of dose absorbed is 0.8 and the plasma half-life is 2 hours.

(7) If the fraction of drug absorbed is 0.9, dose is 25 mg, dosing interval is 6 hours, volume of distribution is 20 L and the average plasma concentration is 25 mcg/mL, what is the plasma half-life of the drug?

(8) To obtain an average plasma concentration of 25 ng/mL with a dosing interval of 8 hours, what should be the dose of the drug when the fraction of drug absorbed is 0.6? It is known that the drug has a volume of distribution of 75 L and has an elimination rate constant of 0.173 hour^{-1}.

(9) A therapeutic agent was found to have an F value of 0.8, volume of distribution of 3 L/kg, average blood concentration is 2.75 ng/mL, what would be the dosing interval if the dose of the drug is 0.2 mg, K_{el} value is 0.0315 hr^{-1} and the weight of the patient is 143 lb?

(10) What would be the dosing interval of a drug which has a volume of distribution of 50 L? When a dose of 250 mg is given, the 200 mg of the drug is absorbed and the average plasma concentration is 4 mcg/mL. The plasma half-life is 3 hours.

CLEARANCE

Clearance refers to the elimination of drug from the body. It is defined as the volume of blood which is completely cleared of drug per unit time. The drug can be eliminated via excretion through kidneys, and/or metabolism in liver, or through other routes such as saliva, milk, sweat, etc. The clearance associated with the kidney is called the renal clearance (Cl_R), and the clearance associated with other routes including metabolism is known as non-renal clearance (Cl_{NR}). The total clearance (Cl_T) equals the renal and non-renal clearance. Some basic formulae to determine clearance are provided as follows:

$$Cl_T = Cl_R + Cl_{NR}$$

$$Cl_T = \text{Drug elimination/plasma concentration}$$

$$Cl_T = V_d \times K_{el} = V_d \times 0.693/t_{1/2}$$

Example 1:

When a preparation of phenytoin was administered to a patient, the volume of distribution was found to be 70 liters, and the half-life of elimination was 1.5 hours. What is the total clearance of phenytoin?

$$Cl_T = V_d \text{ liters} \times 0.693/1.5 \text{ hours}$$

$$= 70 \times 0.693/1.5 = 32.34$$

answer: 32.34 L/hour

Example 2:

Gentamicin is shown to have a V_d of 0.25 L per kg of the body weight. If the weight of the patient is 132 lb, and the elimination rate constant is 0.33 hour^{-1}, what is the total clearance of gentamicin?

Convert the body weight to kg

$$132/2.2 = 60 \text{ kg}$$

Therefore, the V_d value is $(0.25 \text{ L}/1 \text{ kg}) \times 60 \text{ kg} = 15 \text{ L}$

$$Cl_T = V_d \times K_{el}$$

$$= 15 \text{ L} \times 0.33 \text{ hour}^{-1} = 4.95$$

answer: 4.95 L/hour

Example 3:

In Example 2, if the renal clearance is 4 L/hour, what is the non-renal clearance?

$$Cl_T = Cl_R + Cl_{NR}$$

$$4.95 = 4 \text{ L/hour} + Cl_{NR}$$

$$Cl_{NR} = 4.95 - 4 = 0.95 \text{ L/hour}$$

answer: 0.95 L/hr

Creatinine Clearance (Cl$_{CR}$)

Creatinine is a metabolic breakdown product of muscle and usually has a constant value in an individual. Its value ranges from 0.6 mg/100 mL of serum to 1.2 mg/100 mL of serum. Creatinine is almost exclusively eliminated by the kidneys. Therefore, if the level of creatinine increases in the serum, it is likely that the capability of kidneys to eliminate the drugs is reduced. As a general rule, if the serum creatinine level (C_{cr}) is doubled, the kidney function is one-half. If the C_{cr} is quadrupled, the renal (kidney) function is one-fourth or 25%.

The creatinine clearance, Cl$_{CR}$, is calculated by using the following formulae:

$$Cl_{CR} = \frac{C_U \times V}{C_{cr}}$$

where

C_U = concentration of creatinine in the urine (mg/dL)
V = urine volume in mL/min (collected usually for 24 hours)
C_{cr} = serum creatinine concentration (mg/dL)

For a further understanding of this formula, refer to Example 1.

$$Cl_{CR} \text{ in males} = \frac{(140 - Y) \times (W)}{72 \times C_{cr}}$$

where

Y = age in years
W = body weight in kilograms
C_{cr} = serum creatinine concentration in mg/100 mL
  (sometimes it is written as mg/dL or mg%)

$$\text{Cl}_{CR} \text{ in females} = 0.85 \times \frac{(140 - Y) \times (W)}{72 \times C_{cr}}$$

Example 1:

The serum creatinine concentration of a human volunteer was found to be 1.2 mg/dL. Over a 24-hour period, 1.6 L of urine was collected and the concentration of creatinine in urine was found to be 98 mg/dL. What is the creatinine clearance of the volunteer?

Write down the information provided and use the appropriate formula.

Creatinine concentration in urine (C_U) = 98 mg/dL

Creatinine concentration in serum = 1.2 mg/dL

Volume of urine = 1600 mL

Volume of urine in mL per min

(V) = 1600/(24 hours × 60 min) = 1600/1440 = 1.11 mL/min

$$\text{Cl}_{CR} = \frac{C_U \times V}{C_{cr}}$$

$$= \frac{98 \times 1.11}{1.2}$$

answer: 90.65 mL/min

Example 2:

The serum creatinine concentration of a 60 year old male weighing 150 pounds was found to be 1 mg/dL. What is his creatinine clearance?

$$\text{Cl}_{CR} \text{ in males} = \frac{(140 - Y) \times (W)}{72 \times C_{cr}}$$

$$= \frac{(140 - 60) \times (150/2.2)}{72 \times I}$$

$$\text{Cl}_{CR} = 75.76 \text{ mL/min}$$

answer: 75.76 mL/min

Example 3:

For a 25-year-old female weighing 140 lb, the serum creatinine concentration was found to be 1.4 mg/dL. What is her creatinine clearance?

$$Cl_{CR} \text{ in females} = 0.85 \times \frac{(140 - Y) \times (W)}{72 \times C_{cr}}$$

$$Cl_{CR} \text{ of the 25-year-old} = 0.85 \times \frac{(140 - 25) \times (140/2.2)}{72 \times 1.4}$$

$$Cl_{CR} \text{ of the 25-year-old} = 61.7 \text{ mL/min}$$

answer: 61.7 mL/min

Practice Problems

(1) When a preparation of ibuprofen was administered to a patient, the volume of distribution was found to be 5 L, and the half-life of elimination was 2 hours. What is the total clearance of ibuprofen?

(2) When a preparation of indomethacin was administered to a patient, the volume of distribution was found to be 65 L, and the half-life of elimination was 2 hours. What is the total clearance of indomethacin?

(3) Amantadine is shown to have a V_d of 3.7 L per kilogram of the body weight. If the weight of the patient is 146 lb, and the elimination rate constant is 0.046 hour^{-1}, what is the total clearance of amantadine?

(4) In practice problem 2, if the renal clearance of the drug is found to be 18 L per hour, what would be the non-renal clearance of the drug?

(5) In practice problem number 3, if the non-renal clearance is 1.43 L per hour, what is its renal clearance?

(6) The serum creatinine concentration of a human volunteer was found to be 1.2 mg%. Over a 24-hour period, 2 L of urine was collected and the concentration of creatinine in urine was found to be 110 mg%. What is the creatinine clearance of the volunteer?

(7) The serum creatinine concentration of a 44-year-old male weighing 132 lb was found to be 1 mg/dL. What is his creatinine clearance?

(8) For a 35-year-old female weighing 160 pounds, the serum creatinine concentration was found to be 1.1 mg/dL. What is her creatinine clearance?

(9) The serum creatinine concentration of a 66-year-old male weighing 232 lb was found to be 860 mcg/dL. What is his creatinine clearance?

(10) For a 42-year-old female weighing 186 lb, the serum creatinine concentration was found to be 960 mcg/dL. What is her creatinine clearance?

LOADING AND MAINTENANCE DOSES

A knowledge of steady state concentration is required to understand the calculations associated with loading and maintenance doses. Majority of the drug substances are required in multiple doses. In multiple dosing, a drug is administered repetitively with a constant dosing interval such that a steady-state of drug concentration in the blood is achieved and maintained. As shown in Figure 12.4, when the drug concentration declines, another dose is administered to maintain the blood concentration in the therapeutic window. Again, when the drug declines after the second dose, a third dose is given to bring up the level of drug and maintain it in the therapeutic range. After about the fifth or sixth dose (sixth in Figure 12.4), the C_{max} and C_{min} become constant for each successive dose. The C_{max} after the sixth and the seventh dose is 14.4 ng/mL, and the C_{min} with the same doses is constant with a value of 7 ng/mL. This pattern of uniform fluctuations is called the *Steady-State Concentration.*

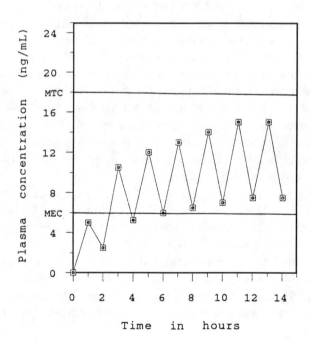

FIGURE 12.4. Plasma concentration versus time profile showing steady-state concentrations following multiple dosing.

At steady-state, the rate of drug absorption is equal to the rate of drug elimination. The C_{max} at steady-state is represented as $C_{max\ ss}$ and the C_{min} at steady-state is $C_{min\ ss}$. The average concentration between the $C_{max\ ss}$ and the $C_{min\ ss}$ is represented by $C_{ave\ ss}$. In Figure 12.4, $C_{max\ ss}$, $C_{min\ ss}$, and the $C_{ave\ ss}$ are 14.4, 7, and 10.7 ng/mL, respectively. The observation of steady-state phenomenon proves that if a proper dose and dosing interval is maintained, the plasma or blood concentration of the drug does not go on increasing forever. For a rational drug therapy, the dose and dosing interval should be maintained such that $C_{max\ ss}$ and the $C_{min\ ss}$ lie within the therapeutic window.

In a multiple dosing regimen involving oral medication, the following equations are useful to find the steady-state parameters:

$$C_{max\ ss} = \frac{D_0/V_d}{1 - e^{-K_{el}\tau}} = \frac{C_0}{1 - e^{-K_{el}\tau}}$$

$$C_{min\ ss} = C_{max\ ss} \times e^{-K_{el}\tau}$$

$$C_{ave\ ss} = \frac{F \times D_0}{K_{el} \times V_d \times \tau} = \frac{C_0}{K_{el} \times \tau}$$

In the above equations, D_0 represents the dose administered, V_d is the volume of distribution, K_{el} is the elimination rate constant, τ is the dosing interval, and C_0 is the plasma concentration at zero time point. It is assumed that the drug is absorbed completely ($F = 1$).

In the case of drug administration by an intravenous infusion, the average steady state concentration (C_{ss}) is obtained by the equation,

$$C_{ss} = R/(V_d \times K_{el})$$

where R represents the rate of intravenous drug infusion.

Loading Dose (D_L)

Since the steady state conditions are achieved after five or six doses because of accumulation of initial doses, it is likely that the first of those doses have a C_{max} which is below the MEC. The second dose may have a C_{max} just equal to or slightly greater than the MEC. In such situations, usually a loading dose is provided which is generally twice the regular or the maintenance dose. This is especially true when the dosing interval of the regimen is equal to the elimination half-life of the drug. The *Loading Dose* helps to achieve the steady state level quickly and also the therapeutic response begins immediately because the plasma levels exceed MEC quickly. The example of loading dose is provided by the 2 *stat* tablets needed for Zithromax® capsules. The loading dose is calculated as,

$$D_L = D_M/(1 - e^{-K_{el}\tau})$$

In the above equation, D_M is the maintenance dose.
  Loading dose is also given by the equation,

$$D_L = C_{ss} \times V_d$$

Maintenance Dose (D_M)

The maintenance dose may be defined as the size of the dose required to maintain the therapeutic range according to the dosage regimen. The maintenance dose needed to replace the amount lost over the dosing interval is the difference between the loading dose and the amount remaining at the end of the interval. It is calculated as,

$$D_M = D_L(1 - e^{-K_{el}\tau})$$

Example 1:

When a 100-mg drug is administered, C_0 was found to be 10 mcg/mL and half-life of the drug was found to be 4 hours. If the drug was administered q4h, what would be the steady-state concentrations?

First write down the information provided

$$D_0 = 100 \text{ mg; } C_0 = 10 \text{ mcg/mL; } t_{1/2} = 4 \text{ hours; } \tau = 4 \text{ hours}$$

$$t_{1/2} = 0.693/K_{el} \text{ or } K_{el} = 0.693/4 = 0.173 \text{ hour}^{-1}$$

$$C_{max\,ss} = \frac{C_0}{1 - e^{-K_{el}\tau}} = \frac{10}{1 - e^{-0.173 \times 4}}$$

answer: 20.023 mcg/mL

$$C_{min\,ss} = C_{max\,ss} \times e^{-K_{el}\tau}$$

$$= 20.023 \text{ mcg/mL} \times e^{-0.173 \times 4} = 10.02$$

answer: 10.02 mcg/mL

Example 2:

What would be the loading dose of an antibiotic drug with a maintenance dose of 300 mg, half-life of 9 hours and a dosing interval also of 9 hours?

$$D_M = 300 \text{ mg}, \ t_{1/2} = 9 \text{ hours}, \ \tau = 9 \text{ hours},$$

$$K_{el} = 0.693/9 = 0.077 \text{ hour}^{-1}$$

$$D_L = D_M/(1 - e^{-K_{el}\tau})$$

$$= 300 \text{ mg}/(1 - e^{-0.077 \times 9}) = {}^{300}/_{0.5} = 600 \text{ mg}$$

answer: 600 mg

Example 3:

In Example 2, if the clinical pharmacist decides to administer 300 mg q8h, what should be the size of the loading dose?

$$\tau = 8 \text{ hours instead of nine hours in Example 2}$$

$$D_L = D_M/(1 - e^{-K_{el}\tau})$$

$$= 300 \text{ mg}/(1 - e^{-0.077 \times 8})$$

$$= 300/0.46 = 652$$

answer: 652 mg

Practice Problems

(1) Calculate the steady-state concentrations of C_{max}, C_{min}, and C_{ave} after the administration of 500 mg of drug every six hours. C_0 of the drug was found to be 25 ng/mL, and the half-life was found to be 2 hours.

(2) What would be the average plasma concentration of drug at steady-state if it is known that the plasma concentration at zero time point is 48 mcg/mL when 50 mg of the dose is given every 12 hours, and the elimination rate constant of the drug is 0.173 hour^{-1}?

(3) After the administration of a 150-mg dose, the plasma concentrations of an antifungal drug were recorded as given below. If the drug was administered every 4 hours, what would be the steady-state concentrations?

Time (hr)	1	2	4	8	12	16	20	24	28
C_p (mcg/mL)	2.9	3.3	2.9	2	1.5	1.0	0.7	0.5	0.4

Find the plasma concentration at zero time point (C_0) by the equation given below:

$$\ln C = \ln C_0 - K_{el} \times t$$

(4) In the practice problem 3, if the dosing interval is changed to 6 hours, what would be the three steady-state concentrations ($C_{max\ ss}$, $C_{min\ ss}$, and $C_{ave\ ss}$)?

(5) What would be the loading dose of an antibiotic drug with a 300 mg of maintenance dose, half-life and dosing interval of 6 hours each?

(6) In practice problem 5, if the dosing interval is changed to 8 hours, what should be the loading dose?

(7) In a clinical situation, if it is known that the loading dose is one gram for a drug administered every 12 hours, what should be the maintenance dose? The plasma half-life of the drug has been reported to be 4 hours.

(8) The maintenance dose of Biaxin® is 250 mg q12h. Its average elimination half-life reported is 5 hours. If it is desired to achieve the steady-state levels sooner, how much loading dose should be recommended?

(9) The maintenance dose of Cleocin® is 150 mg q6h. Its average elimination half-life reported is three hours. If it is desired to achieve the steady state levels sooner, how much loading dose should be recommended?

(10) Lasix®, a loop diuretic drug, is known to be used with a loading dose of 40 mg qd. If it is desired to maintain a once daily dose, how much maintenance dose would you recommend if its half-life is one hour?

DOSE ADJUSTMENTS IN RENAL FAILURE

For drugs that are excreted primarily by the kidneys, extreme care is needed with respect to the dose of drug and its dosing interval in the case of kidney damage (or renal impairment). The renal impairment causes increased drug levels due to reduced excretion. This greater blood concentration of drug relative to the normal state may cause toxicity if the dose of dosing interval or both are not altered. Many drugs including penicillin, aminoglycoside antibiotics, vancomycin, glyburide, digoxin, nadolol, and cimetidine are primarily excreted by the kidneys. Drugs that are highly dependent upon the renal function for elimination are listed in Table 12.1. For these drugs, individualized dosing based on kidney function is recommended. Therefore, in the case of renal damage, their doses and the dosage regimens have to be altered. The following is some useful information with appropriate examples:

$$\tau = \frac{F \times D_0}{C_{ave} \times V_d \times K_{el}}$$

From the above equation, it can be seen that,

TABLE 12.1. *Drugs that Require Dosing Based on Kidney Function.*

Acarbose	Cefonicid	Edrophonium chloride
Acebutolol	Cefotaxime	Eflornithine hydrochloride
Acetaminophen	Cefoxitin	Enalapril
Acetazolamide	Cefpodoxime	Encainide
Acetohexamide	Cefprozil	Enoxacin
Acrivastine	Ceftazidime	Enoxaparin sodium
Acyclovir	Ceftibuten	Epoetin alfa
Albuterol	Ceftizoxime	Erythromycin
Alendronate sodium	Cefuroxime	Ethacrynic acid
Allopurinol	Cephalexin	Ethambutol
Amantadine	Cephalothin	Ethchlorvynol
Amikacin	Cephapirin	Ethionamide
Amiloride	Cephradine	Ethosuximide
Aminocaproic acid	Cetrizime	Etidronate disodium
Aminoglutethimide	Chloral hydrate	Etoposide
Aminosalycilate sodium	Chloroquine	Famatidine
Amoxicillin	Chlorpropamide	Famciclovir
Amoxicillin clavulanic acid	Chlorthalidone	Fentanyl citrate
Amphotericin B	Choline salicylate	Flecainide
Ampicillin	Cimetidine	Fluconazole
Ampicillin sulbactum	Cinoxacin	Flucytosine
Amrinone	Ciprofloxacin	Fludarabine phosphate
Atenolol	Cisplatin	Fluoxetine
Auranofin	Clarithromycin	Foscarnet
Azathioprine	Clofibrate	Fosinapril
Azlocillin	Clonidine	Furosemide
Aztreonam	Clordiazepoxide	Gabapentin
Bacampicillin	Codeine	Gallium nitrate
Baclofen	Colchicine	Gancyclovir
Bactrim	Cotrimoxazole	Gentamycin
Benzazepril	Cyclophosphomide	Glimepiride
Betaxolol	Cycloserine	Glipizide
Bismuth	Cytarabine	Glyburide
Bleomycin	Dacarbazine	Granisetron
Bretylium	Dapsone	Guanadrel
Bupropion	Daunorubicin	Guanethidine
Butorphanol	Deferoxamine	Hydralazine
Captopril	Demeclocycline	Hydrochlorthiazide
Carbamazepine	Dezocine	Hydroxyurea
Carbenicillin	Didanosine	Idarubicin
Carboplatin	Diflunisal	Imipenam
Carteolol	Digitoxin	Immunoglobulin
Cefaclor	Digoxin	Insulin
Cefadroxil	Diltiazem	Isoniazid
Cefamandole	Diphenhydramine	Isosfamide
Cefazolin	Disopyramide	Isosorbide dinitrate
Cefepime	Doxacurium	Itraconazole
Cefimetazole	Doxorubicin	Kanamycin
Cefixime	Dyphylline	Ketorolac

TABLE 12.1.   Drugs that Require Dosing Based on Kidney Function
(continued)

Levoflaxacin	Nizatidine	Rimantadine
Lincomycin	Nodolol	Rimapril
Lisinopril	Norfloxacin	Risperidone
Lithium	Ofloxacin	Salicylate
Lomefloxacin	Oxacillin	Simvastin
Lomustine	Oxytetracycline	Sotalol
Loracarbef	Pancuronium	Sparfloxacin
Magnesium salts	Paroxetine	Spironolactone
Mecamylamine hydrochoride	Pemoline	Stavudine
Mefenamic acid	Penicillin V potassium	Streptomycin
Melphanan	Penicillin G potassium	Streptozocin
Meperidine	Pentamidine	Succimer
Mephobarbital	Pentazocine	Sucralfate
Meprobamate	Pentobarbital	Sulfamethoxazole
Mercaptopurine	Pentostatin	Sulfasalazine
Meropenem	Perindopril erbumine	Sulfinpyrazone
Metformin	Phenazopyridine	Sulfisoxzole
Methadone	Phenobarbital	Tacrolimus
Methanamine	Pindolol	Teicoplanin
Methicillin	Piperacillin tazobactam	Teniposide
Methotrimeprazine	Piperacillin	Terbutaline
Methyldopa	Pipercuronium bromide	Tetracycline
Metoclopramide	Plicamycin	Thiabendazole
Metocurine	Polymixin B sulfate	Thioguanine
Metronidazole	Pralidoxime chloride	Thiopental
Mexiletine	Pramipexole	Thiotepa
Mezlocillin	Primidone	Ticarcillin
Midazolam	Probenecid	Ticarcillin clavulanate
Milrinone	Procainamide	Tobramycin
Minocycline	Procarbazine	Tocainide
Mitomycin	Propoxyphen	Tolazoline
Mivacurium chloride	Propronolol	Tranexamic acid
Moexipril hydrochloride	Propylthiouracil	Triameterene
Moricizine	Pseudoephedrine	Trimethoprim
Morphine	Pyrazinamide	Tubocurarine
Moxalactam	Pyridostigmine	Valacyclovir
Mycophenolate mofetil	Quinacrine	Vancomycin
Naficillin	Quinapril	Venlafaxime
Nalidixic acid	Quinidine	Verapamil
Naratriptan	Quinine	Vidarabine
Neomycin sulfate	Ramipril	Vinorelbine
Neostigmine	Ranitidine	Zalcitabine
Netilimicin	Reserpine	Zidovudin
Nitrofurantoin	Riluzole	

$$C_{ave} \propto \frac{D_0}{\tau \times K_{el}}$$

If the same C_{ave} as a normal individual is desired in a patient with renal impairment, then the following equality should hold:

$$\frac{D_{On}}{\tau_n \times K_{eln}} = \frac{D_{Ori}}{\tau_{ri} \times K_{elri}}$$

In the previous equation, the subscripts "n" and "ri" indicate normal and renally impaired conditions respectively. This equation is very useful in calculating the dose and the dosing interval in individuals with renal impairment. The examples that follow this discussion show that the dosage regimen in renally impaired patients may be corrected either by adjusting the dose and maintaining the same dosing interval, or by adjusting the dosing interval and maintaining the same dose, or by adjusting both the dose and dosing interval simultaneously.

Example 1:

Upon the administration of 0.27 mg of a therapeutic agent to a normal individual, the elimination rate constant was found to be 0.0315 hour^{-1}. The normal dosing regimen included 0.27 mg qid. If the elimination rate constant in renally impaired condition is 80% of the normal elimination rate constant, how can the dose be adjusted maintaining the same dosing interval of six hours?

The information given is as follows:

$$D_{On} = 0.27 \text{ mg}, \tau_n = 6 \text{ hours}, K_{eln} = 0.0315 \text{ hour}^{-1}$$

$$D_{Ori} = ?, \tau_{ri} = 6 \text{ hours}, K_{elri} = 80\% \text{ of } 0.0315 = 0.0252 \text{ hour}^{-1}$$

$$\frac{D_{On}}{\tau_n \times K_{eln}} = \frac{D_{Ori}}{\tau_{ri} \times K_{elri}}$$

$$\frac{0.27 \text{ mg}}{6 \text{ hr} \times 0.0315 \text{ hr}^{-1}} = \frac{X}{6 \text{ hr} \times 0.0252 \text{ hr}^{-1}}$$

X = Dose for the renally impaired condition = 0.216 mg

answer: 0.216 mg

Thus, this example shows that the dose has to be reduced from 0.27 mg to 0.216 mg in order to maintain the same plasma concentration in renally impaired patient.

Example 2:

In the problem in Example 1, if it is decided to administer the same dose of 0.27 mg to the renally impaired patient, what should be the dosing interval?

$$\frac{0.27 \text{ mg}}{6 \text{ hr} \times 0.0315 \text{ hr}^{-1}} = \frac{0.27 \text{ mg}}{X \times 0.0252 \text{ hr}^{-1}}$$

X = Dosing interval for the renally impaired patient = 7.5 hours

answer: 7.5 hr

Thus, this example shows that if it is desired to maintain the same dosage of 0.27 mg, the dosing interval should be changed from 6 to 7.5 hours in a renally impaired patient to maintain the same average plasma concentration. This adjustment is very useful in cases where it is not physically possible to split the dosage form and administer the modified dose.

Example 3:

In the problem in Example 1, if it is decided to administer the drug every eight hours, what should be the amount of dose required?

$$\frac{0.27 \text{ mg}}{6 \text{ hr} \times 0.0315 \text{ hr}^{-1}} = \frac{X \text{ mg}}{8 \times 0.0252 \text{ hr}^{-1}}$$

X = Dose required for renally impaired condition = 0.288 mg

answer: 0.288 mg

This example illustrates a situation in which it is not very convenient to administer drug every 7.5 hours. A dosing interval of 8 hours makes it convenient because of q8h administration. Thus, the dose has to be changed to 0.288 mg.

Another situation in which a dose and the dosing interval are required to be modified in renally impaired conditions is the availability of a particular strength of medication so that an alternate dose can be provided, and the dosing interval can be determined. In the above problem, if a dosage form of 0.3 mg is already available and is convenient for the clinical pharmacist to administer that dose, the dosing interval can be easily calculated as follows:

$$\frac{0.27 \text{ mg}}{6 \text{ hr} \times 0.0315 \text{ hr}^{-1}} = \frac{0.3 \text{ mg}}{X \times 0.0252 \text{ hr}^{-1}}$$

X = Dosing interval for the renally impaired condition and with a dose of 0.3 mg is 8.33 hours

answer: 8.33 hr

Practice Problems

(1) Upon the administration of 250 mg of an antihypertensive drug to a normal individual, the elimination rate constant was found to be 0.17 hour^{-1}. The normal dosing regimen included 0.25 g tid. If the elimination rate constant in renally impaired condition is 0.14 hour^{-1}, how can the dose be adjusted maintaining the same dosing interval?

(2) In the practice problem 1, if it is decided to administer the same dose of 0.25 g to the renally impaired patient, what should be the dosing interval?

(3) In the practice problem 1, if it is decided to administer the drug every 6 hours, what should be amount of dose required?

(4) The elimination rate constants of an antitubercular drug in normal and a renally impaired patient were found to be 0.2 and 0.08 hour^{-1}, respectively. It is usually administered once daily in a dose of 300 mg. How can the dose be adjusted in the renally impaired patient to provide similar plasma levels as in the normal patient by maintaining the same dosing interval of 24 hours?

(5) In practice problem number 4, if it is decided to keep the dose of 300 mg constant, how would you change the dosing interval of drug in the renally impaired patient to provide the same plasma concentration as that of a normal individual?

(6) In practice problem number 4, if it is decided to provide a dose of 150 mg, how would you change the dosing interval of drug in the renally impaired patient to provide the same plasma concentration as that of a normal individual?

(7) A clinical pharmacist has recommended that the dose of a cardiac drug be reduced from 0.25 mg to 0.2 mg in a renally impaired patient. In both the normal and renally impaired patient, the dosing interval was

TABLE 12.2.   Drugs that Require Dosing Based on Liver Function.

Acebutolol	Mephobarbital	Quinidine
Acetaminophen	Meprobamate	Rifampin
Acetohexamide	Methadone	Risperidone
Alprazolam	Methotrexate	Sertraline
Amiodarone	Mexiletine	Sulindac
Amlodipine	Morphine	Testosterone
Buspiron	Nalbuphine	Theophylline
Chloral hydrate	Naproxen	Tiagabine
Chloramphenicol	Nifedipine	Tocainide
Chlordiazepoxide	Nimodipine	Tolazamide
Chlorpromazine	Nortriptylline	Tolbutamide
Cimetidine	Ocycodone	Triazolam
Citalopram	Olanzapine	Trovafloxacin
Cyclosporine	Paramethadiaone	Valproic acid
Diazepam	Paroxetine	Vancomycin
Digitoxin	Pentazocine	Verapamil
Disopyramide	Pentobarbital	Vincristine sulfate
Doxepin	Perphenazine	Warfarin sodium
Doxorubicin	Phenobarbital	Zidovudine
Fluorouracil	Phenylbutazone	
Fluoxetime	Phenytoin	
Glipizide	Pimozide	
Glyburide	Pindolol	
Grepafloxacin	Piroxicam	
Ibuprofen	Propafenone	
Isoniazid	Propoxyphene	
Ketoconazole	Pyrazinamide	
Meperidine	Quazepam	

six hours. If the elimination rate constant of the drug in normal individual was 0.18 hour^{-1}, what would be the elimination rate constant in the renally impaired patient?

(8) A clinical pharmacist has recommended that the dose of a diuretic be reduced from 250 mg to 225 mg in a renally impaired patient. In both the normal and renally impaired patients, the dosing interval was six hours. If the elimination rate constant of the drug in normal individual was 0.18 hour^{-1}, what would be the elimination rate constant value in the renally impaired patient?

(9) In problem number 7, if it is decided to use the same dose of 0.25 mg of the cardiac drug in the renally impaired patient, what should be the dosing interval?

(10) In problem number 8, if it is decided to use a 300-mg tablet which is already available in the market, what should be the dosing interval of the diuretic drug?

DOSE ADJUSTMENTS IN HEPATIC FAILURE

A vast majority of the drugs are metabolized by the liver. Selected drugs that require individualized dosing based on liver function are listed in Table 12.2. The drug elimination process is comprised of drug metabolism and drug excretion. Therefore, if the liver is damaged, it is very likely that the drug may get accumulated and cause toxicity. Therefore, the dose or dosing interval may required to be changed for a rational drug therapy. However, unlike the renal damage, there is no specific method of adjusting the dosing regimen in the cases of liver impairment. The dosage regimen in each patient is required to be titrated to his/her clinical response.

CHAPTER 13

Pediatric and Geriatric Dosing

The adjustment of dose and dosing regimen for children and the elderly needs a special consideration because of several differences as compared to an adult individual. The differences may be due to many factors which include changes in pharmacokinetic parameters, age, body weight, surface area, and genetic predisposition. The present chapter provides some basic explanation about their differences and the dosage calculations because of these differences.

As explained in Chapter 12, the dose and dosing interval of drugs depend to a large extent on the rate of their absorption, distribution, metabolism and excretion. An important determinant of drug distribution is the volume of distribution, and the determinant for drug metabolism and excretion is elimination half-life. It is an established fact that the volume of distribution and elimination half-lives of drugs in newborn and adults have considerable differences. For example, the volume of distribution of diazepam in newborns was found to be 1.6 L/kg and in adults, it was 2.4 L/kg. The elimination half-life of the same drug was found to be in the range of 25 to 100 hours in newborns, and 15 to 25 hours in adults. As another example, the cephalosporin drug ceftriaxone, was shown to have an average clearance of 7.7 mL/min in children with an average age of 3.5 years. The clearance value of the same drug was shown to have an average value of 17 mL/min when the average age of the population was 33.5 years. Similarly, the pharmacokinetic parameters of children were found to be different from adults for drugs which include morphine, theophylline, caffeine, indomethacin, and tolbutamide. Because the enzyme system for metabolism of drugs is not well developed in children, generally it can be expected that the elimination half-life of drugs is greater. Therefore the t^1_2 of diazepam, meperidine, and indomethacin is greater in children as compared to adults. However, certain drugs such as clindamycin, valproic acid, and theophylline have shown to metabolize and excrete faster

263

in children as compared to adults. All these examples clearly demonstrate the need to change the dose and dosing interval for newborns and children.

The dosing regimen of the elderly also needs special consideration because of several differences with a young adult. As an example of a major difference, the change in body composition of elderly is substantially different from a young adult. The percent fat tissues of total body weight have an average value of 36% in elderly men and 48% in elderly women. The composition of percent fat tissue of total body weight in young adults was found to be 18% in men and 33% in women. The muscle mass of the elderly is also different as compared to young adults. Other examples include changes in renal function, cardiac output, hepatic clearance, and metabolizing enzymes.

DOSAGE CALCULATIONS BASED ON AGE

Age of a patient is one of the most important considerations for drug dosage modifications. As explained in the previous section, some of the important pharmacokinetic parameters change with age. In general, the drug elimination (which is comprised of drug metabolism and excretion) is less functional in newborns, and improves with age as they grow into healthy adult individuals. Finally, as they grow further to an age of 65 years or above, the elimination declines. A few general equations for the dosage calculations based on age are provided below. However, the use of these equations is rapidly declining. It is important to remember that age is not the only valid criterion for dose modifications. Therefore, after adjusting the dose with one of the formulae given below, it is important to monitor the response in the patient for some more time. The guidelines provided by the manufacturers as *usual pediatric dose* in the drug inserts and pharmaceutical literature are valuable for drug dosage calculations in children.

Young's Equation (preferably from one to twelve years of age):

$$\text{Dose of child} = \frac{\text{Age in years}}{\text{Age in years} + 12} \times \text{Adult dose}$$

Cowling's Equation:

$$\text{Dose of child} = \frac{\text{Age in years at next birthday}}{24} \times \text{Adult dose}$$

Fried's Equation (preferably from birth to one year of age):

$$\text{Dose of child} = \frac{\text{Age in months}}{150} \times \text{Adult dose}$$

Note: It should be remembered that in many situations, the information given for dosage conversion from adult to children is not direct. The dose prescribed on a prescription or a medication order may be for an adult while the patient profile may reveal that the age of the patient is a few months or a few years and the patient is a child.

Example 1:

Calculate the dose of Valium® of a thirteen-month-old child by the Young's method if the adult dose is 10 mg. Valium® is available as a 5 mg/5 mL oral solution. How would you administer this medication to the child?

$$\text{Dose of child} = \frac{\text{Age in years}}{\text{Age in years} + 12} \times \text{Adult dose}$$

$$\text{Dose of child} = \frac{(13/12)}{(13/12) + 12} \times 10 \text{ mg}$$

$$\text{Dose of child} = 0.83 \text{ mg}$$

$$5 \text{ mg/5 mL} = 0.83 \text{ mg in } 0.83 \text{ mL}$$

answer: Therefore a medicinal dropper will be calibrated to determine the number of drops which would constitute 0.83 mL and the drug will be administered.

Example 2:

Henry Huxtable, M.D.
61-40 Flushing Avenue
Monroe, LA 71208
Phone No. 555-1234

Name : Savannah Bell   **Age**: 2 mo.
Address: 96 Havana Blvd., LA.71209   **Date**: 4/22/96

R℞

    EES 200
              2 Fl. oz.

    Sig: tsp qid

REFILL _____

DAW _____

              HHuxtable
         DEA # AD 7973142

It can be seen in the above prescription that age of the child is just two months, and one teaspoonful (containing 200 mg/5 mL) three times daily appears to be high. Therefore the dose has to be lowered. The usual adult dose of erythromycin is 400 mg every six hours. In the present problem, Fried's Equation will be used as follows:

$$\text{Dose of child} = \frac{\text{Age in months}}{150} \times \text{Adult dose}$$

$$\text{Dose of child} = \frac{2 \text{ months}}{150} \times 400 = 5.33 \text{ mg}$$

answer: 5.33 mg every six hours

The above medication is required to be calibrated to provide the number of drops which would provide 5.33 mg of the drug. The required number of drops should be given four times daily. The dose change should be made after consulting the physician.

Example 3:

Product information on Lorabid® shows that its usual adult dose is 200–400 mg q12h. What would be the range of this medication for a patient born on February 9, 1993. How would you administer the drug from one of the available Lorabid® medications? Assume that the prescription was written on May 1996.

The patient is a child and would be four years old on the following birthday. Therefore Cowling's Equation will be used as follows:

$$\text{Dose of child} = \frac{\text{Age in years at next birthday}}{24} \times \text{Adult dose}$$

$$\text{Dose of child} = \frac{4 \text{ years}}{24} \times 200$$

Dose of child = 33.33 mg for the lower drug range

answer: range of drug for the patient = 33.33 mg to 66.67 mg

The drug Lorabid® is available as 100 mg/5 mL suspension besides other strengths.

$$100 \text{ mg/5 cc} = 33.33 \text{ mg}/X$$

answer: The volume of Lorabid® 100 mg/5 mL required would be 1.67 to 3.34 cc

Practice Problems

(1) How many milliliters of meclizine hydrochloride (50 mg/mL) should be provided to a patient who is six years old? The average dose of meclizine for an adult is 50 mg.

(2) The usual dose of Minocin® is 50 mg qid. If it is to be prescribed for a child born on May 20, 1990, how would you determine the amount of medication to be administered based upon Minocin® 50 mg/5 mL liquid suspension? The prescription was dated May 1, 1996.

(3) Pepcid® liquid suspension is available in a strength of 40 mg/mL. The normal maintenance dose in an adult patient is 20 mg qhs. How many milliliters of this medication would you administer to an eight-year-old patient at bedtime?

(4) How would you dispense the following medication if it is known that the average adult dose of prednisone is 10 mg three times daily?

Henry Huxtable, M.D.
61-40 Flushing Avenue
Monroe, LA 71208
Phone No. 555-1234

Name : Baby Imran   Age: 10 mo.
Address: 96 Shady Blvd., LA.71209   Date: 3/20/96

R

Prednisone Liquid 5 mg / 5 mL
2 Fl. oz.

Sig: 2tsp tid

REFILL _____

DAW _____

HHuxtable
DEA # AD 7973142

---

(5) Prochlorperazine is prescribed for a child whose date of birth is 05/21/93. If the usual adult dose is 5 mg, how many milligrams would be administered to the child? The prescription is dated 01/01/96.

(6) For certain infections, the usual adult dose of Ceclor® is 500 mg q8h. For an eighteen-month-old child how many milliliters of 125 mg/5 mL Ceclor® suspension should be recommended?

(7) Cleocin® 150 mg is prescribed for a child who is four years old. If the usual adult dose is 150 mg q8h, how many milliliters of Cleocin® 75 mg/5 mL suspension will be required for 10 days?

(8) How many milliliters of Reglan® injection (5 mg/mL) should be given to a patient who is eight months old? The usual dose of metoclopramide hydrochloride is 10 mg.

(9) The usual dose of Tylenol® is 500 mg qid, prn fever. If Tylenol® is to be prescribed for a two-month-old baby, how many milliliters of Tylenol® drops (80 mg/mL) should be given as a single dose to this patient?

(10) For a patient born on March 12, 1992, what is the quantity of Vantin® liquid suspension (100 mg/5 mL) needed if the medication is required for 14 days? The adult dose for Vantin® is 200 mg bid, and the prescription is written on August 30, 1996.

DOSAGE CALCULATIONS BASED ON BODY WEIGHT

Dose adjustments based on weight are common in children and also in obese patients. From the previous discussion, it is known that the dosing regimen may have to be altered if the volume of distribution changes. The volume of distribution is a function of the total body water and the extracellular fluids which in turn are related to the body weight. Therefore, the volume of distribution may change with the change in body weight. In the case of an obese patient, the proportion of body fat is greater and the ratio of body water and lean body weight to total body weight is smaller. The percent of body fat and lean body weight can be estimated by the equations,

$$\% \text{ Fat} = 90 - 2 \text{ (Height in inches}$$
$$- \text{ Girth in inches at umbilical level at exhalation)}$$

$$\text{Lean body weight (males)} = 50 + 2.3 \text{ kg per inch over } 5'$$

$$\text{Lean body weight (females)} = 45.5 + 2.3 \text{ kg per inch over } 5'$$

When the percent fat is greater, the extracellular fluid is less. Therefore, there is less distribution of polar drugs. As a result, the plasma concentration of polar drugs will be higher and there may be a need to lower the dose of such drugs. In the case of nonpolar or lipid soluble drugs, their distribution in cellular tissues will be more and there may be a need to increase the dose of such drugs. For this reason, extreme care is needed for changes in the dosing regimen of obese patients. Often, the dosing regimens based simply on milligrams of drug per kilogram of body weight without due consideration of percent fats may lead to erroneous results. However, the dose adjustment in children based on body weight are fairly common. The product information and package inserts express the pediatric doses of many drugs on the basis of body weight per kilogram. As an example, the recommended dose of ibuprofen for fever in children is 5 mg/kilogram of body weight. A well-known equation for the dosage calculation based on body weight is the Clarke's Equation. The use of this equation is also declining.

Clarke's Equation:

$$\text{Dose of the child} = \frac{\text{Weight in pounds} \times \text{Adult dose}}{150 \text{ lb (average weight of an adult)}}$$

The milligram per kilogram doses of many drugs are greater for children than the adults. For example, the usual dose of digoxin for children in the age group of two to twelve years is 10 to 15 mcg per kilogram of body weight per day. For adults, the dose of digoxin is 4 to 5 mcg per kilogram per day. These doses have shown to provide an average digoxin plasma concentration of 1 to 1.5 ng/mL. The larger mg/kg doses for children are required because of a higher percentage of total body water and extracellular fluid in children as compared to adults. At birth, newborns have approximately 78% body water. In adults, the total body water decreases to about 60%. Because of the higher total body water and the extracellular fluid content, there is more distribution of digoxin, and less appearance of drug in the plasma.

DOSAGE CALCULATION BASED ON BODY SURFACE AREA

The dose of drugs for children as well as adults may be adjusted based on the body surface area. The normal adult body surface area is 1.73 m². The body surface area may be calculated in many ways. The following equation provides a useful estimate of the surface area when the height (in cm) and weight (in kg) of the patient are known:

$$\text{Surface area in m}^2 = (\text{height} \times \text{weight})^{1/2}/60$$

Body surface area may also be calculated by using a nomogram. Figure 13.1 shows the nomogram for children and Figure 13.2 shows the nomogram for adults. One can find out the body surface area by joining the body weight and height by a straight line, and reading the value at the point where the

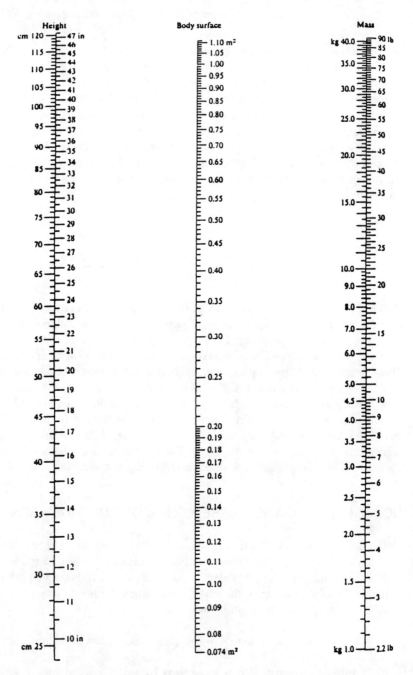

FIGURE 13.1 A nomogram for determination of the body surface area of children. (Source: *Geigy Scientific Tables,* 8th Edition, p. 226.)

270

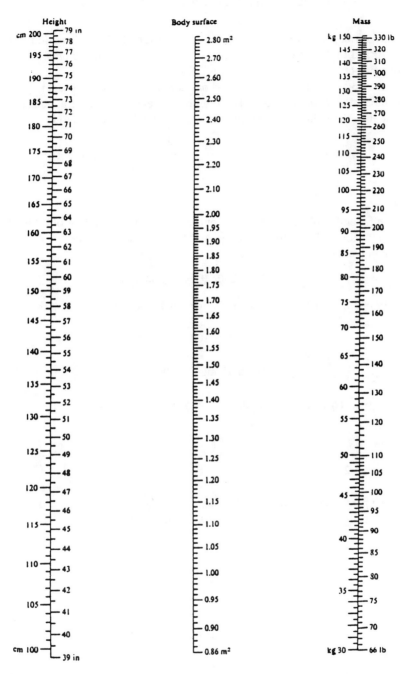

FIGURE 13.2 A nomogram for determination of the body surface area of adults. (Source: *Geigy Scientific Tables,* 8th Edition, p. 227.)

body surface area column is intersected. For example, if the height in inches is 70 and the body weight in pounds is 150, the body surface area in square meters obtained from Figure 13.2 is 1.94.

The dose modifications based on body surface area provide a better approximation of dose than the dose based on body weight. The general equation to calculate the child's dose by the surface area method is as follows:

$$\text{Child's dose} = \frac{\text{Surface area of child (m}^2)}{1.73 \text{ m}^2} \times \text{Adult dose}$$

Example 1:

In juvenile arthritis, Advil® is required to be given in a dose of 30 mg/kg/day. How many milliliters of the Advil® suspension (100 mg/5 mL) should be given to a child weighing 74 lb?

$$74 \text{ lb} = 74/2.2 = 33.64 \text{ kg}$$

In one day, Advil® required is 30 mg per kg or 30/1 kg = X/33.64 kg

$$X = 1009 \text{ mg}$$

$$100 \text{ mg/5 mL} = 1009 \text{ mg}/X$$

Therefore, X = milliliters of Advil® required = 50.5 mL

answer: 50.5 mL

Example 2:

Alupent® has a normal adult dose of 20 mg tid for asthma. How much Alupent® should be given to a child weighing 75 lb by the Clarke's Equation?

$$\text{Dose of the child} = \frac{\text{Weight in pounds} \times \text{Adult dose}}{150 \text{ lb}}$$

$$\text{Dose of the child} = \frac{75 \text{ lb} \times 20 \text{ mg}}{150 \text{ lb}} = 10 \text{ mg}$$

answer: dose of the child = 10 mg

Example 3:

The height of a child is 120 cm and the weight is 130 lb. The usual adult dose of Elavil® (Amitriptyline HCl) is 75 mg/day. What would be the dose for the child based on body surface area?

When height and weight of a child are known, surface area may be calculated by using the formula:

$$\text{Surface area in m}^2 = (\text{height} \times \text{weight})^{1/2}/60$$

$$130 \text{ lb} = 130/2.2 = 59.1 \text{ kg}$$

$$\text{Surface area in m}^2 = (120 \times 59.1)^{1/2}/60$$

$$= 1.40 \text{ m}^2$$

$$\text{Child's dose} = \frac{\text{Surface area of child (m}^2)}{1.73 \text{ m}^2} \times \text{Adult dose in mg/day}$$

$$\text{Child's dose} = \frac{1.4 \text{ (m}^2)}{1.73 \text{ m}^2} \times 75 \text{ mg/day}$$

answer: Child's dose = 60.7 mg

Practice Problems

(1) Keflex® has a normal adult dose of 250 mg, q6h. If this medication is required for 14 days for a child weighing 46 lb, how many fluidounces of Keflex® 125 mg/5 mL should be dispensed?

(2) The usual maintenance dose of Klonopin® for children is 0.1 mg/kg/day in three divided doses. For a child weighing 66 lb how many Klonopin® 1 mg tablets should be dispensed if the medication is required for 10 days?

(3) For a 67 inches tall person weighing 138 lb, what is the estimated percent fat? The girth of the person in inches is 32.

(4) The height of a child is 98 cm and the weight is 80 lb. The usual adult dose of Mycostatin® is 500,000 units five times daily for 14 days. How many fluid ounces of Mycostatin® oral suspension (100,000 units/mL) should be dispensed for the child when the surface area estimation is performed by using the nomogram?

(5) What should be the size of a dose of Nalfon® for an arthritic patient with a body surface area of 0.87 square meters? The usual adult dose of Nalfon® is 600 mg tid for arthritis.

(6) Benadryl® may be given in a daily dose of 150 mg per square meter. If a child weighs 72 lb and stands 48 inches tall, how many milligrams of Benadryl® should be given per day?

(7) By using Clarke's Equation determine the dose of Tegretol® for a child weighing 62 lb. The usual adult dose of Tegretol® is 100 mg bid.

(8) What is the average intravenous dose of Adriamycin® (doxorubicin) for

a child who weighs 50 kg and has a height of 156 cm? The average intravenous dose of doxorubicin for a child is 30 mg/m^2.

(9) The height of a child is 110 cm and the weight is 35 kg. The usual adult dose of Zovirax® is 20 mg/kg/day. What would be the dose of Zovirax® for the child when the surface area estimation is performed by using the nomogram?

(10) The average adult dose of Demerol® is 100 mg q3h. For a child weighing 28 kg, what should be the recommended dose?

DOSAGE REGIMEN IN PATIENTS USING AMINOGLYCOSIDES

Aminoglycosides are antibacterial agents used for the treatment of infections, primarily caused by gram-negative bacteria. Plague, tuberculosis, meningitis, and urinary tract infections are some of the indications for aminoglycosides. The most common aminoglycosides include streptomycin, kanamycin, gentamycin, tobramycin, and neomycin. These antibiotics cause severe renal damage and ototoxicity in many patients. Renal excretion is the major route of elimination for the aminoglycosides. Therefore, it is important that the dosing regimen of these drugs be closely monitored. The half-life of tobramycin, gentamycin, and amikacin in normal patients is about 2.5 hours but it increases considerably with renal impairment. This necessitates a lowering of dosage. Infants less than 7 days and the elderly also need a reduction in dosage.

The steady-state maximum plasma concentration, $C_{max\ ss}$, of gentamycin and tobramycin are 6 to 10 mcg/mL. The $C_{max\ ss}$ of amikacin is 25 to 30 mcg/mL. The $C_{min\ ss}$ of both gentamycin and tobramycin is 0.5 to 1.5 mcg/mL, while that of amikacin is 5 to 8 mcg/mL. In order for these drugs to be effective, it is important to closely monitor their therapeutic concentrations. An important observation of these antibiotics is that with prolonged therapy, the $C_{min\ ss}$ values increase. This increase is due to the renal impairment. In the case where $C_{min\ ss}$ is less than the desired $C_{min\ ss}$, the dose may be insufficient.

Table 13.1 presents suggested changes in dose or dosing interval based on blood (serum) concentrations of the aminoglycoside antibiotics. One should consider the table as an approximate guide to the suggested change in the dose or dosing regimen. However, for a closer titration of the dose, the following information is very useful.

New Dose to Adjust the Steady-State Concentration

When it is desired to change the $C_{min\ ss}$ of an aminoglycoside, it can be done by either changing the dose or the dosing interval of the drug. In the present case, it is being assumed that the dosing interval is same and only dose is

TABLE 13.1. Suggested Changes in Dose or Dosing Interval Based on Measured Serum Aminoglycoside Concentration.*

Measured $C_{max\ ss}$ Compared to Desired Values		Suggested Change in Dosage Regimen	
$C_{max\ ss}$	$C_{min\ ss}$	Dose	Dosing Interval
Desired	Desired	No change	No change
Higher	Higher	Decrease/no change	Increase
Lower	Higher	Increase	Increase
Lower	Lower	Increase/no change	Decrease
Higher	Lower	Decrease	Decrease
Higher	Desired	Decrease	No change
Lower	Desired	Increase	No change
Desired	Higher	No change/increase	Increase
Desired	Lower	No change/decrease	Decrease

* Source: Adapted from Cipolle et al., Gentamycin/Tobramycin. Therapeutic use and serum concentration monitoring. In *Individualizing Drug Therapy. Practical Applications of Drug Monitoring. Vol. 1.* Edited by W. J. Taylor and A. L. Finn. New York, Gross, Towsend, Frank. 1980, pp. 113–147.

modified. The following equation may be used when the plasma concentration of the drug is directly proportional to the dose of the drug (linear kinetics).

$$C_{min\ ss}/C_{min\ ssn} = \text{Dose of the drug } (D_0)/\text{New dose of the drug } (D_{0n})$$

After determining the new dose, the new plasma concentration at zero time (C_{0n}) can be calculated by the equation,

$$C_0/C_{0n} = \text{Dose } (D_0)/\text{New dose } (D_{0n})$$

Because of the increase in dose for an increase in $C_{min\ ss}$, the $C_{max\ ss}$ also changes as it is a function of C_0 which changes to C_{0n}. The new $C_{max\ ssn}$ can be calculated by the equation,

$$C_{max\ ssn} = C_{0n}/(1 - e^{-K_{el}\tau})$$

The manufacturer's suggested regimen is very useful for determining the dose of aminoglycosides. As an example, for vancomycin hydrochloride injection, the product information is available for the usual adult dose, the average adult dose with reduced renal functions, the dosing information for children, and the dosing information for neonates. Aminoglycosides are mainly distributed in the extracellular fluid volume. Therefore the dose of aminoglycosides in children is generally higher than that of adults.

Example 1:

The steady-state serum concentrations of a patient taking gentamycin were found to be 10 mcg/mL ($C_{max\ ss}$) and 2.5 mcg/mL ($C_{min\ ss}$). The patient was taking the usual dose of 3 mg/kg/day of gentamycin. Would you recommend a change in dosing schedule? If so, how?

It is known from the text above that the $C_{max\ ss}$ and $C_{min\ ss}$ of gentamycin are 6 to 10 mcg/mL and 0.5 to 1.5 mcg/mL. Therefore, the steady-state concentrations in the given problem indicate that the $C_{max\ ss}$ level is still normal while the $C_{min\ ss}$ level is higher. The table presented reveals that a change in dosage regimen is suggested. The dose of gentamycin need not be changed or slightly increased, while the dosing interval should be increased.

Example 2:

Upon the administration of 1 gram of an aminoglycoside every 12 hours, the $C_{min\ ss}$ was found to be 8 mcg/mL. The plasma concentration at time zero was 63 mcg/mL and elimination rate constant was 0.14 hour^{-1}. If it is desired to increase the $C_{min\ ss}$ to 10 mcg/mL, what should be the dose of the drug, and the new $C_{max\ ss}$? Assume that the drug follows linear kinetics.

$$C_{min\ ss}/C_{min\ ssn} = \text{Dose of the drug } (D_0)/\text{New dose of the drug } (D_{0n})$$

$$8\ mcg/mL/10\ mcg/mL = 1000\ mg/D_{0n}$$

$$D_{0n} = 1250\ mg$$

After determining the new dose, the plasma concentration at zero time (C_{0n}) can be calculated by the equation,

$$C_0/C_{0n} = \text{Dose } (D_0)/\text{New dose } (D_{0n})$$

$$63\ mcg/mL/C_{0n} = 1000\ mg/1250\ mg$$

$$C_{0n} = 78.75\ mcg/mL$$

Because of the increase in dose from 1000 mg to 1250 mg for an increase in $C_{min\ ss}$ from 8 mcg/mL to 10 mcg/mL, the $C_{max\ ss}$ also changes. The new $C_{max\ ssn}$ can be calculated by the equation,

$$C_{max\ ssn} = C_{0n}/(1 - e^{-K_{el}\tau})$$

$$78.75/(1 - e^{-0.14 \times 12})$$

$$C_{\text{max ssn}} = 97.22 \text{ mcg/mL}$$

answer: The desired $C_{\text{min ssn}}$ of 10 mcg/mL can be obtained when the dose is changed from 1000 mg to 1250 mg. C_{0n} and the $C_{\text{max ssn}}$ values are 78.75 and 97.22 mcg/mL, respectively.

Example 3:

When a single 250 mg bolus dose of an antibiotic is given, the C_0 was found to be 25 mcg/mL and the elimination half-life was 5 hours. What would be the dose required to achieve a new minimum steady-state concentration of 12 mcg/mL with a dosing interval of 6 hours? Also what would be the new maximum steady-state concentration? Assume that the drug follows first-order kinetics.

$$C_{\text{min ss}} = (C_0 \times e^{-K_{\text{elT}}})/(1 - e^{-K_{\text{elT}}})$$

$$= (25 \times e^{-0.139 \times 6})/(1 - e^{-0.139 \times 6})$$

$$= (25 \times 0.434)/(1 - 0.434)$$

$$= 19.16 \text{ mcg/mL}$$

$$C_{\text{min ss}}/C_{\text{min ssn}} = \text{Dose of the drug } (D_0)/\text{New dose of the drug } (D_{0n})$$

$$19.16 \text{ mcg/mL}/12 \text{ mcg/mL} = 250 \text{ mg}/D_{0n}$$

$$D_{0n} = 156.58 \text{ or } 157 \text{ mg}$$

After determining the new dose, the plasma concentration at zero time (C_0) can be calculated by the equation,

$$C_0/C_{0n} = \text{Dose } (D_0)/\text{New dose } (D_{0n})$$

$$25 \text{ mcg/mL}/C_{0n} = 250 \text{ mg}/157 \text{ mg}$$

$$C_{0n} = 15.7 \text{ mcg/mL}$$

Because of the decrease in dose from 250 mg to 157 mg for a decrease in $C_{\text{min ss}}$ from 19.16 mcg/mL to 12 mcg/mL, the $C_{\text{max ss}}$ also changes. The new $C_{\text{max ssn}}$ can be calculated by the equation,

$$C_{\text{max ssn}} = C_{0n}/(1 - e^{-K_{\text{el}}\tau})$$

$$C_{\text{max ssn}} = 15.7/(1 - e^{-0.139 \times 6})$$

$$C_{\text{max ssn}} = 27.75 \text{ mcg/mL}$$

answer: By changing the dosing regimen from 250 mg to 157 mg every 6 hours, the minimum steady-state concentration has changed from 19.16 mcg/mL to the desired level of 12 mcg/mL. Also, the new maximum steady-state concentration is 27.75 mcg/mL

Practice Problems

(1) The steady-state maximum concentration ($C_{\text{max ss}}$) after the administration of amikacin was 38 mcg/mL, and the steady-state minimum serum concentration was 10 mcg/mL. If the dosing regimen has to be changed, how should it be done?

(2) The product information on gentamycin shows that the recommended dose of gentamycin sulfate is 1–2 mg/kg for adults, 6 to 7.5 mg/kg/day for children, and 5 mg/kg/day for patients in the age group of one or less. How much gentamycin should be given to a five-day-old child weighing 12 lb?

(3) With references to the product information in problem #2, how much drug should be given to a seven-year-old child weighing 46 lb?

(4) Neomycin sulfate is given in a dose of 292 mg/m² orally for infants as well as children for preoperative bowel sterilization. If it is given every four hours for three days, how many tablets of the available strength (350 mg/tablet) should be dispensed to a child with a body surface area of 1.2 m²?

(5) For adult patients, neomycin sulfate is given in a dose of 10.3 mg/kg every four hours for three days. How many tablets (350 mg/tablet) should be dispensed for a patient weighing 150 lb?

(6) When a single 25-mg bolus dose of an antibiotic is given, the C_0 was found to be 2.5 mcg/mL and the elimination half-life was 2.5 hours. What would be the dose required to achieve a new minimum steady-state concentration of 0.45 mcg/mL with a dosing interval of 6 hours? Also what would be the new maximum steady-state concentration? Assume that the antibiotic follows linear kinetics?

(7) Upon the administration of 0.5 g of an aminoglycoside every 12 hours, the $C_{\text{min ss}}$ was found to be 8 mcg/mL, the plasma concentration at time zero was 36 mcg/mL, and elimination half-life was 5 hour⁻¹. If it is desired to increase the $C_{\text{min ss}}$ to 10 mcg/mL, what should be the dose of the drug, and the new $C_{\text{max ss}}$? Assume that the drug follows linear kinetics.

(8) The steady-state serum concentrations of a patient taking gentamycin were found to be 4 mcg/mL ($C_{max\,ss}$) and 0.5 mcg/mL ($C_{min\,ss}$). The patient was taking the usual dose of 3 mg/kg/day of gentamycin. Would you recommend a change in dosing schedule? If so, how?

(9) Intravenous bolus dose of a 500-mg dose of an antibiotic every six hours in a patient produces minimum steady-state concentration of 10 mcg/mL. If the desired minimum steady-state concentration in this patient is 16 mcg/mL, calculate the size of dose needed to change this concentration. Assume that the drug follows linear kinetics.

(10) A single bolus dose administration of 50 mg of a drug showed the following pharmacokinetic parameters: $C_0 = 2.5$ mg/mL, and $t_{1/2} = 5.5$ hours. If the desired minimum steady-state concentration is 2 mg/mL, calculate the dose that should be administered every six hours, and the expected maximum steady-state concentration with the new dose.

CRITICAL CARE

In a critical care situation, the patient is seriously ill and is under constant monitoring for vital signs in an in-patient setting. The clinical conditions requiring critical care include serious heart conditions, septic shocks, and severe asthma. The drug dose and the rate of administration are frequently altered in accordance with clinical monitoring of the vital signs. A simple mistake in the amount of drug administered or the rate at which the drug is administered could be fatal for the patient. The amount of drug to be mixed with the specified vehicle is determined to make an intravenous preparation. Following the preparation, the liquid is administered at designated infusion rate to provide a certain amount of medication in a given period of time. As indicated in Chapter 10, the infusion sets are designed to deliver 10 to 60 drops per milliliter. The set which delivers 60 drops per milliliter is the "microdrop" (also known as microdrip). The sets which deliver less drops, i.e., 10–20 drops per milliliter are known as "macrodrop" sets. Generally, the number of drops per milliliter are provided on the sets. It is preferable to use macrodrop sets when the infusion volume rate is higher (e.g., 100 mL/hr) and microdrop sets when the infusion rate is lower than 100 mL/hr.

The calculations involved in critical care include determination of solution strengths, flow rates in terms of drops per minute or hour, and flow rates in volume per unit time. Since the administration of medications requires dose adjustments under a clinical monitoring, it is very important to calculate a "titration factor" which is the amount of medication in units of weight per drop. Most of these calculations are presented in Chapter 10, but the present section will highlight the calculations which involve the titration factor. The titration factor will help the health care professional to rapidly determine the amount or the exact concentration of the infusion when the rate of intravenous flow is increased or decreased for the patient. The following example will show the calculations involved with dose titration.

Example 1:

Explain how one would titrate dopamine starting from 4 mcg/kg/min to maintain a mean systolic pressure between 100–120 mmHg. The patient weighs 165 lb and the IV preparation is dopamine 200 mg in 125 mL of D5W.

The titration factor will be mcg/drop in the present problem because the dose is to be titrated from 4 mcg/kg/min. To find the titration factor, the flow rate in micrograms per minute and the number of drops per minute should be known.

$$\text{Titration factor} = \frac{\text{mcg/min}}{\text{drops/min}} = \text{mcg/drop}$$

To calculate micrograms of dopamine per minute,

$$165 \text{ lb} = 75 \text{ kg}$$

$$4 \text{ mcg/kg/min} = 4 \times 75 \text{ mcg/min for the 75 kg patient}$$

$$= 300 \text{ mcg/min}$$

To find the drops per minute, amount in milliliters per hour is required,

$$200 \text{ mg or } 200,000 \text{ mcg/125 mL} = X \text{ mcg/1 mL}$$

$$X = 1600 \text{ mcg/mL}$$

$$\text{Drops/min} = \frac{300 \text{ mcg/min}}{1600 \text{ mcg/mL}}$$

$$= 0.1875 \text{ mL/min which equals}$$

$$0.1875 \times 60 = 11.25 \text{ mL/hour}$$

Note: Whenever microdrop IV set is used, mL/hour = drops/min

$$11.25 \text{ mL/hour} = 11.25 \text{ drops/min}$$

$$\text{Titration factor} = \frac{\text{mcg/min}}{\text{drops/min}} = \text{mcg/drop}$$

$$\frac{300 \text{ mcg/min}}{11.25 \text{ drops/min}} = 26.67$$

answer: 26.67 mcg/drop

Determination of Amount Infused by the Titration Factor

In the above problem, when the infusion rate increases by two drops, the amount infused per minute is,

$$26.67 \text{ mcg/drop} \times 2 = 53.34 \text{ mcg}$$

i.e., 300 + 53.34 mcg/min = 353.34 mcg/min

When the infusion rate increases by two drops, its value in volume per hour is

$$2 \text{ drops} + 11.25 \text{ drops/min} = 13.25 \text{ drops/min}$$

By the microdrop rule, 13.25 drops/min = 13.25 ml/hr

When the infusion rate decreases by 3 drops, the amount in micrograms per minute is,

$$26.67 \text{ mcg/drop} \times 3 = 80 \text{ mcg/min}$$

i.e., 300 − 80 mcg = 220 mcg/min

When the infusion rate decreases by 3 drops, the infusion rate in volume per hour is,

$$11.25 \text{ drops} - 3 \text{ drops} = 8.25 \text{ drops/min}$$

By the microdrop rule, 8.25 drops/min = 8.25 mL/hr

Example 2:

An infusion of 50 mg of nitroprusside in 250 mL of D5W is to be provided to a patient weighing 132 pounds. What is the titration factor of this infusion between 0.5 to 1.5 mcg/kg/min to maintain mean blood pressure at 100 mmHg.

$$50{,}000 \text{ mcg}/250 \text{ mL} = 200 \text{ mcg/mL}$$

$$132 \text{ lb} = 60 \text{ kg}$$

$$0.5 \text{ mcg/kg/min} = 0.5 \times 60 = 30 \text{ mcg/min (lower limit)}$$

$$1.5 \text{ mcg/kg/min} = 1.5 \times 60 = 90 \text{ mcg/min (higher limit)}$$

$$\frac{30 \text{ mcg/min}}{200 \text{ mcg/mL}} = 0.15 \text{ mL/min or } 0.15 \times 60 = 9 \text{ mL/hour}$$

$$\frac{90 \text{ mcg/min}}{200 \text{ mcg/mL}} = 0.45 \text{ mL/min or } 0.45 \times 60 = 27 \text{ mL/hour}$$

$$9 \text{ mL/hr} = 9 \text{ drops/min by the microdrop rule, and}$$

$$27 \text{ mL/hour} = 27 \text{ drops/min by the same rule}$$

$$\text{Titration factor} = \frac{\text{mcg/min}}{\text{drops/min}} = \text{mcg/drop}$$

$$\frac{30 \text{ mcg/min}}{9 \text{ drops/min}} = 3.33 \text{ mcg/drop}$$

or

$$\text{Titration factor} = \frac{\text{mcg/min}}{\text{drops/min}} = \text{mcg/drop}$$

$$= \frac{90 \text{ mcg/min}}{27 \text{ drops/min}} = 3.33 \text{ mcg/drop}$$

answer: 3.33 mcg/drop

Example 3:

For the problem in Example 2, what would be the concentration per minute and volume per hour when the infusion rate is increased by 4 drops/minute? Similarly what would be the concentration/minute and volume per hour when the infusion rate is decreased by 5 drops?

When the infusion rate is increased by 4 drops/min.

$$4 \times 3.33 \text{ mcg/drop} = 13.32 \text{ mcg}$$

$$13.32 \text{ mcg} + 30 \text{ mcg} = 43.32 \text{ mcg/min}$$

$$4 \text{ drops} + 9 \text{ drops/min} = 13 \text{ drops/min or } 13 \text{ mL/hr}$$

When the infusion rate is decreased by 5 drops/min,

$$5 \times 3.33 = 16.65 \text{ mcg}$$

$$30 - 16.65 = 13.35 \text{ mcg/min}$$

$$9 \text{ drops} - 5 \text{ drops} = 4 \text{ drops/min or } 4 \text{ mL/hr}$$

answer: 43.32 mcg/min, 13 mL/hr; 13.35 mcg/min, 4 mL/hr

Practice Problems

(1) In Example 1, if the infusion rate decreases by 2 drops, what would be the amount infused in micrograms per minute and in volume per hour?

(2) In Example 1, if the infusion rate increases by 3 drops, what would be the amount infused in micrograms per minute and in volume per hour?

(3) Explain how one would titrate dopamine starting from 3 mcg/kg/min to maintain a mean systolic pressure between 100 and 120 mmHg. The patient weighs 136 lb and the IV preparation is dopamine 200 mg in 125 mL of D5W.

(4) In problem 3, what would be the amount infused in micrograms per minute and in volume per hour when the infusion rate increases by one drop?

(5) In problem 3, what would be the infusion rate in micrograms per minute and in volume per hour when the infusion rate decreases by one drop?

(6) In problem 3, what would be the amount infused in micrograms per minute and in volume per hour when the infusion rate increases by 3 drops?

(7) In problem 3, what would be the infusion rate in micrograms per minute and in volume per hour when the infusion rate decreases by 3 drops?

(8) An infusion of 50 mg of nitroprusside in 200 mL of D5W is to be provided to a patient weighing 132 lb. What is the titration factor of this infusion between 0.5 to 1.5 mcg/kg/min to maintain mean blood pressure at 100 mmHg.

(9) In problem 8, what would be the amount infused in micrograms per minute and in volume per hour when the infusion rate increases by 3 drops?

(10) In problem 8, what would be the infusion rate in micrograms per minute and in volume per hour when the infusion rate decreases by 3 drops?

PEDIATRIC CRITICAL CARE

The titration factor calculations are important for critical care in the adults because of dose modifications for individualized therapy. In pediatric patients, the dose calculations based on body weight are fairly reliable. However, extreme precautions are necessary to limit the volume intake of medications. Because of very small body surface areas, any small addition to the volume of medication for increasing the dose might cause a fluid overload in the pediatric patients. Therefore, if additional dose is required, the concentration of the drug in IV medication should be changed rather than increasing the volume. The important considerations in pediatric critical care include calculation and verification of the dilution parameters in medication orders, and the assurance that excessive fluid is not being administered to children in critical situations. In general, wt/mL obtained from dose and administration rate should be at least approximately equal to wt/mL of the dilution.

Example 1:

A medication order for a nine-month-old child weighing 8 kg includes dopamine in a dose of 5 mcg/kg/min. The drug available is dopamine 400 mg/5 mL. The physician ordered 70 mg of dopamine in 200 mL of D5W to be administered at 6.75 mL per hour to this child who is in septic shock. Check for the accuracy of the dilution order.

Drug administration rate = 6.75 mL/hour

Dose for the child = 5 mcg/kg/min = 5 × 8 = 40 mcg/min

Dose per hour = 40 mcg/min × 60 = 2400 mcg/hour

$$\text{Concentration of the solution} = \frac{2400 \text{ mcg/hr}}{6.75 \text{ mL/hr}}$$

Concentration of the solution = 2400/6.75 = 356 mcg/mL

The dilution order is prepared as follows:

$$400 \text{ mg/5 mL} = 70 \text{ mg}/X$$

$$X = 0.875 \text{ mL or } 0.88 \text{ mL}$$

Take 0.88 mL of the available dopamine preparation and add it to 200 mL of D5W.

Accuracy of the dilution order is performed as follows:

$$70 \text{ mg/201 mL} = 0.35 \text{ mg/mL or } 350 \text{ mcg/mL}$$

answer: The concentration of solution determined was 356 mcg/mL. Therefore, the dilution order is fairly accurate.

Example 2:

A medication order provided for a one-year-old child weighing 9 kg includes sodium nitroprusside in a dose of 1.5 mcg/kg/min. The drug available is sodium nitroprusside 25 mg/5 mL. The physician wanted 20 mg of sodium nitroprusside in 200 mL of D5W to be administered at 20 mL per hour to this child who is in shock. Check for the accuracy of the dilution order.

Concentration of the solution in mcg/mL is calculated as follows:

$$1.5 \text{ mcg/kg/min} = 1.5 \times 9 = 13.5 \text{ mcg/min}$$

$$\text{Dose per hour} = 13.5 \times 60 = 810 \text{ mcg per hour}$$

$$\text{Concentration of the solution} = \frac{810 \text{ mcg/hr}}{20 \text{ mL/hr}}$$

Concentration of the solution = 810/20 = 40.5 mcg/mL

The dilution for administration is prepared as follows:

The physician ordered 20 mg/200 mL of the sodium nitroprusside

$$25 \text{ mg/5 mL} = 20 \text{ mg}/X$$

X = 4 mL of the 25 mg/5 mL available solution should be measured accurately and added to 200 mL of D5W.

The concentration of the dilution is 20 mg/(200 + 4) mL = 20 mg/204 mL

$$= 0.098 \text{ mg/mL or } 98 \text{ mcg/mL}$$

answer: The concentration of the solution calculated was 40.5 mcg/mL and the dilution concentration is 98 mcg/mL. Therefore, the dilution order is inaccurate.

Example 3:

For a five-year-old child weighing 25 kg and suffering from tachycardia, a physician prescribed 20 mcg/kg/min lidocaine. The instruction was to add 200 mg of lidocaine in 200 mL of D5W and administer at a rate of 30 mL per hour. The available drug is lidocaine 1 g/25 mL. Check if the dilution factor is accurate.

Concentration of the solution in mcg/mL is calculated as follows:

$$20 \text{ mcg/kg/min} = 20 \times 25 = 500 \text{ mcg/min}$$

$$\text{Dose per hour} = 500 \times 60 = 30,000 \text{ mcg per hour}$$

$$\text{Concentration of the solution} = \frac{30,000 \text{ mcg/hr}}{30 \text{ mL/hr}}$$

Concentration of the solution = 30,000/30 = 1000 mcg/mL

The dilution for administration is prepared as follows:

The physician wants 200 mg of lidocaine in 200 mL

$$1000 \text{ mg/25 mL} = 200 \text{ mg/}X$$

X = 5 mL of the 1 g/25 mL available solution should be measured accurately and added to 200 mL of D5W.

The concentration of the dilution is

$$200 \text{ mg/(200 + 5) mL} = 0.98 \text{ mg/1 mL} = 980 \text{ mcg/mL.}$$

answer: The concentration of the solution calculated was 1000 mcg/mL and the concentration of the dilution is 980 mcg/mL. Therefore, the dilution is fairly accurate.

Practice Problems

(1) For a five-week-old infant weighing 3 kg and suffering from shock, a physician prescribed 2.0 mcg/kg/min of dobutamine. The instruction was to add 6 mg of dobutamine in 25 mL of D5W and administer at a rate of 1 mL per hour. The available drug is dobutamine 0.125 g/10 mL. Check if the dilution factor is accurate.

(2) For the above problem, if the instruction was to add 9.3 mg of dobutamine in 25 mL of D5W, is the dilution factor accurate?

(3) For an eight-year-old child weighing 28 kg and suffering from tachycardia, a physician prescribed 20 mcg/kg/min lidocaine. The instruction was to add 195 mg of lidocaine in 200 mL of D5W and administer at a rate of 35 mL per hour. The available drug is lidocaine 1 g/25 mL. Check if the dilution factor is accurate.

(4) For a six-year-old child weighing 30 kg and suffering from tachycardia, a physician prescribed 20 mcg/kg/min lidocaine. The instruction was to add 200 mg of lidocaine in 200 mL of D5W and administer at a rate of 25 mL per hour. The available drug is lidocaine 1 g/25 mL. Check if the dilution factor is accurate.

(5) For the problem number 4, if the child weighs 20.5 kg, check for the accuracy of the dilution factor.

(6) For a five-year-old child weighing 25 kg and suffering from tachycardia, a physician prescribed 20 mcg/kg/min lidocaine. The instruction was to add 125 mg of lidocaine in 100 mL of D5W and administer at a rate of 25 mL per hour. The available drug is lidocaine 1 g/25 mL. Check if the dilution factor is accurate.

(7) If the patient in problem 6 was a three year old weighing 15 kg, what would be the concentration of the solution and the dilution factor? Check for its accuracy.

(8) For a one-year-old child weighing 5.5 kg and suffering from a serious asthma problem, a physician prescribed 0.85 mg/kg/min of aminophylline. The instruction was to add 50 mg of aminophylline in 500 mL of D5W and administer at a rate of 40 mL per hour. The available drug is aminophylline 2.5% w/v. Check if the dilution factor is accurate.

(9) In the above problem (problem 8), if the child weighs 22 kg and is four years old, what would be the concentration of the solution and the dilution factor? Is the amount to be administered accurate?

(10) For the patient in problem 8, if the prescribed dose is changed to 0.25 mg/kg/min, what should be the concentration of the solution and the dilution factor? Check for the accuracy of the dilution factor.

Calculations Involving Immunizing Agents and Vaccines

As defined by the Food and Drug Administration (FDA), immunizing agents are known as biologics. Immunization is the process of acquiring immunity through the use of biologics. Vaccination refers to active immunization through the administration of a vaccine, a type of biologic. Vaccination is meant to prevent the occurrence of a disease rather than treat it. Since pharmacists are in close contact with their patients, they can provide an effective pharmaceutical care plan by recommending appropriate vaccines to their patients in high-risk conditions. In some states, pharmacists are even allowed to administer vaccination. The recommended immunization schedules from the Center for Disease Control and Prevention (CDC, USA) are given in Tables 14.1 and 14.2.

There are two general types of biologics available for active immunity:

- vaccines
- toxoids

A vaccine consists of a suspension of live (attenuated) or killed (inactivated) microorganisms (in whole or fractions), whereas a toxoid is a detoxified bacterial toxin that has the ability to trigger the production of antitoxin once administered into the body.

Types of Vaccines:

1. Bacterial
2. Viral

BACTERIAL VACCINES

The organisms for these vaccines are grown in suitable media under con-

TABLE 14.1. *Recommended Childhood Immunization Schedule—United States, January–December 1998.*

Vaccines[1] are listed under the routinely recommended ages [rectangle] areas indicate range of acceptable ages for immunization. [oval] areas indicate vaccines to be assessed and given if necessary during the early adolescent visit. Shaded areas indicate vaccines to be assessed and given if necessary during the early adolescent visit.

Age ► Vaccine ▼	Birth	1 mo	2 mos	4 mos	6 mos	12 mos	15 mos	18 mos	4-6 yrs	11-12 yrs	14-16 yrs
Hepatitis B[2,3]	Hep B-1	Hep B-2			Hep B-3					Hep B[3]	
Diphtheria, Tetanus, Pertussis[4]			DTaP or DTP	DTaP or DTP	DTaP or DTP			DTaP or DTP[4]	DTaP or DTP	Td	
H. influenzae type b[5]			Hib	Hib	Hib	Hib					
Polio[6]			Polio[6]	Polio		Polio[6]			Polio		
Measles, Mumps, Rubella[7]							MMR		MMR[7]	MMR[7]	
Varicella[8]							Var			Var	

Approved by the Advisory Committee on Immunization Practices (ACIP), the American Academy of Pediatrics (AAP), and the American Academy of Family Physicians (AAFP).

Further information can be obtained from www.cdc.gov/nip/child.htm.

290

TABLE 14.2. Vaccines and Toxoids Recommended for Adults, by Age Groups. United States.

AGE	VACCINE/TOXOID						
	Influenza	Pneumococcal	Measles	Mumps	Rubella	Varicella	Td[1]
18-24			X	X	X	X	X
25-64			X[2]	X	X[3]	X	X
65	X	X				X	X

[1] Td = Tetanus and diphtheria toxoids, adsorbed (for adult use), which is a combined preparation containing <2 flocculation units of diphtheria toxoid
[2] One dose for all persons born in 1957 or later, two doses for health care workers, college students, and travelers born in 1957 or later.
[3] Those born after 1956.
Adapted from CDC. Further information can be obtained from www.cdc.gov/nip/adultov.htm.

trolled conditions. Examples include cholera, pertussis, plague, typhoid, anthrax, haemophilus b conjugate, and haemophilus b polysaccharide vaccines. The bacterial vaccines are available as suspensions of resuspended cells, filtrate adsorbed on aluminum hydroxide, or as lyophilized powder. The vaccine product may contain a single immunogen (called *monovalent*) or multiple immunogens (called *polyvalent*). Further, the product may be a mixed vaccine with different immunogens for different diseased states or a mixed biologic. MMR (Measles, Mumps, and Rubella) is a mixed vaccine with three immunogens for three different diseased states. A mixed biologic, e.g., diphtheria, tetanus, and pertussis (DTP) is a combination of a vaccine and a toxoid.

Strength of Bacterial Vaccines

The strength of bacterial vaccines may be expressed in one of three different forms, each of which is correlated with the dosage regimen and schedule of specific vaccines on the basis of theoretical computations and clinical trials.

1. The strength may be expressed in the form of colony forming units (e.g., BCG vaccines). This is the number of organisms or colony forming units required for stimulating the immune system to produce adequate antibodies for immunity against the organism.
2. The strength may be in terms of total protective units per milliliter or per dose (e.g., pertussis vaccine). This is the number required to protect the body from a lethal dose of the organism.
3. The strength may be expressed in terms of the total amount (μg) of immunogen present in each milliliter or dose of vaccine (e.g., meningococcal vaccine).

Example 1:

Pertussis vaccine is intended for infants and children 6 weeks through 6 years at 16 protective units (PU) administered over four injections for active immunization. Calculate how many milliliters of injection are required for each administration if the vaccine is supplied at a dose of 60 PU/7.5 mL vial.

Number of PU required for each injection = 16 PU/4 injections = 4 PU

answer: Required volume per injection = 7.5 mL/60 PU × 4 PU = 0.5 mL

Example 2:

Every mL of BCG vaccine contains greater than or equal to 8 million to less than or equal to 26 million colony forming units (CFU) upon reconstitution. Calculate the number of CFUs injected for the usual 0.05 mL intradermal dose recommended for infants under 3 months of age.

$$0.05 \text{ mL} \times 8,000,000 \text{ CFU} = 400,000$$

$$0.05 \text{ mL} \times 26,000,000 \text{ CFU} = 1,300,000$$

answer: Therefore, 400,000 CFU < usual recommended dose < 1,300,000

Example 3:

If the recommended dose for meningococcal vaccine is 1 injection of 0.5 mL at 0.1 mg/mL, how many immunizations can a 10-mL multi-use vial yield?

Strength per injection = 0.1 mg/mL × 0.5 mL = 50 μg

Total strength of the vial = 10 mL × 0.100 mg/mL = 1 mg

answer: Number of immunizations per vial = 1000 μg/50 μg = 20

Practice Problems

(1) An anthrax vaccine contains 0.0025% benzethonium chloride as preservative. When a subcutaneous injection of 0.5 mL is given as a booster dose, how many micrograms of the preservative does the patient get?

(2) The BCG vaccine has an average of 17 million colony forming units

per milliliter. How many units would an infant get when the recommended dose of 0.05 mL is given?

(3) Plague vaccines have strength of 2×10^9 organisms per milliliter. How many organisms are present in a dose of 0.2 milliliter?

(4) Each dose of pneumococcal vaccine contains 25 micrograms of polysaccharide immunogens. How many doses of the vaccine can be obtained with two grams of the polysaccharide immunogens?

(5) Typhoid vaccine contains not more than one million organisms per milliliter based on a potency of 8 units per milliliter. For children less than 10 years old, two injections of 0.25 milliliter are given four weeks apart for vaccination. How many units are given in this vaccination dose of two injections?

(6) Typhoid vaccine contains not more than one million organisms per milliliter based on a potency of 8 units per milliliter. For children less than 10 years old, two injections of 0.25 milliliter are given four weeks apart for vaccination. How many organisms are given in this vaccination dose of two injections?

(7) Typhoid vaccine contains not more than one million organisms per milliliter based on a potency of 8 units per milliliter. For children over 10 years old and adults, the initial dose is 0.5 milliliter. From the available vial of 25 mL, how many children over 10 years old and adults can be vaccinated with the initial dose?

(8) Haemophilus b conjugate vaccine contains 25 micrograms of a purified capsular polysaccharide and 18 micrograms of diphtheria toxoid protein in a single dose of 0.5 mL. How many micrograms of diphtheria toxoid proteins are there in a vial containing 2.5 mL of the vaccine?

(9) Every mL of BCG vaccine contains greater than or equal to 8 million to less than or equal to 26 million colony forming units (CFU) upon reconstitution. Calculate the number of CFUs injected for the usual 0.1-mL intradermal dose.

(10) Pertussis vaccine is intended for infants and children 6 wk through 6 yr at 16 protective units (PU) administered over four injections for active immunization. Calculate how many mL of injection is required for each administration if the vaccine is supplied in a strength of 8 PU/mL.

VIRAL VACCINES

Viral vaccines are cultivated on inanimate media. Some examples include hepatitis b vaccine, influenza virus vaccine, measles virus vaccine, rabies vaccine, rubella vaccine, and yellow fever vaccine. The viral vaccines are available as lyophilized powder for reconstitution, or suspension for injections, or in a liquid drop form for oral use. Similar to bacterial vaccines, viral vaccines are available as monovalent or polyvalent types.

Strengths of Viral Vaccines

Viral vaccines may have their strength expressed as one of five general forms.

1. The strength may be in the form of the quantity of virus estimated to infect half (50%) of the inoculated culture, tissue culture infectious doses ($TCID_{50}$). For example, rubella virus vaccine contains 1,000 $TCID_{50}$, which means each dose contains one thousand times the amount of virus present in one tissue culture infectious dose.
2. Similar to bacterial vaccines, the strength of viral vaccines may be expressed in the total amount (μg) of virus or immunogen present in each mL or dose (e.g., influenza vaccines).
3. The strength of certain viral vaccines is expressed as international units (IU), which are based on animal potency tests (e.g., rabies vaccine).
4. The strength may be expressed as plaque forming units (PFU) as in the case of yellow fever vaccine.
5. The D antigen unit is another form of strength expression of viral vaccines. The D antigen units are determined on the basis of radial immunodiffusion (e.g., poliovirus vaccine).

Example 1:

Each mL of the Measles, Mumps, and Rubella (MMR) virus vaccine contains not less than 2,000 $TCID_{50}$ of the US Reference Measles virus; 10,000 $TCID_{50}$ of the US Reference Mumps virus; and 2,000 $TCID_{50}$ of the US Reference Rubella virus. The first dose (half mL SC) of this vaccine is recommended at the age of 12 to 15 months. What is the dose strength for the Measles virus?

answer: 2,000 $TCID_{50}$ / mL × 0.5 mL dose = 1,000 $TCID_{50}$

Example 2:

In example 1, What is the dose strength for the Mumps virus?

answer: 10,000 $TCID_{50}$ / mL × 0.5 mL dose = 5,000 $TCID_{50}$

Example 3:

What is the dose strength for the Rubella virus?

answer: 2,000 $TCID_{50}$ / mL × 0.5 mL dose = 1,000 $TCID_{50}$

Practice Problems

(1) Thiomersal is a preservative used in hepatitis B vaccine. Its usual concentration is 1:20,000. How many micrograms of the preservative are present in a single pediatric dose of 0.5 milliliter?

(2) The strength of a 0.5 milliliter dose of measles vaccine is 1,000 $TCID_{50}$. The vaccine is available as a single dose, 10- and 50 doses. What is the total strength of vaccines in the 50-dose vial?

(3) Each mL of the Measles, Mumps, and Rubella (MMR) virus vaccine contains not less than 2,000 $TCID_{50}$ of the US Reference Measles virus; 10,000 $TCID_{50}$ of the US Reference Mumps virus; and 2,000 $TCID_{50}$ of the US Reference Rubella virus. The first dose (half mL SC) of this vaccine is recommended at the age of 12 to 15 months. What is the tissue culture infectious dose of measles virus in a 50-milliliter vial?

(4) Each mL of the Measles, Mumps, and Rubella (MMR) virus vaccine contains not less than 2,000 $TCID_{50}$ of the US Reference Measles virus; 10,000 $TCID_{50}$ of the US Reference Mumps virus; and 2,000 $TCID_{50}$ of the US Reference Rubella virus. The first dose (half mL SC) of this vaccine is recommended at the age of 12 to 15 months. What is the tissue culture infectious dose of measles virus in a 50-milliliter vial?

(5) Each mL of the Measles, Mumps, and Rubella (MMR) virus vaccine contains not less than 2,000 $TCID_{50}$ of the US Reference Measles virus; 10,000 $TCID_{50}$ of the US Reference Mumps virus; and 2,000 $TCID_{50}$ of the US Reference Rubella virus. The first dose (half mL SC) of this vaccine is recommended at the age of 12 to 15 months. What is the tissue culture infectious dose of mumps virus in a 25-milliliter vial?

(6) Polio vaccine contains 27 ppm of formaldehyde. How many micrograms of formaldehyde are present in a 0.5-mL booster dose of this vaccine?

(7) Tetanus immune globulin (TIG) is usually given in a dose of 10 mg/kg of body weight. For a child weighing 66 pounds, how much TIG vaccine should be administered?

(8) If a poliovirus vaccine was prepared to contain 40-D antigen units per dose of 0.5 mL, how many antigen units would be present in a bulk vial containing 10 mL?

(9) Each poliovirus vaccine dose of 0.5 mL contains 105.4 to 106.4 infective titers for Type I live attenuated poliovirus. How many infective titers are present in a 50-dose disposable pipette container?

(10) If a poliovirus vaccine was prepared to contain 32-D antigen units per dose of 0.5 mL, how many antigen units would be present in a bulk vial containing 10 mL?

TOXOIDS

Toxoids are immunogens obtained by the detoxification of toxins. The toxins are obtained by the processing of filtrates of bacterial cultures. Similar to bacterial and viral vaccines, the toxoids may also contain single, multiple, or mixed immunogens. The toxoid preparations are cloudy when they are plain and suspensions when they are absorbed on aluminum compounds.

Strength of Toxoids

Toxoids are usually expressed in terms of flocculating units (Lf), which represent the smallest amount of toxin that would flocculate one unit of standard antitoxin (within mixtures of varying amounts of toxin and constant amounts of antitoxin).

Example 1:

If every 0.5 mL of tetanus toxoid (TT) contains 5 Lf units and the complete schedule for TT is 3 IM or SC injections of 0.5 mL administered in 4–8 weeks followed by a fourth dose of 0.5 mL in 6 to 12 months, how many complete immunization courses of TT can be administered from a 7.5 mL dosage form of TT.

Total number of injections required = 4

Total volume injected = 4 × 0.5 mL = 2 mL

7.5 mL / 2.0 mL = 3.75

answer: Therefore, a total of three complete immunization courses can be administered per dosage form

Example 2:

In the example above, how many Lf units are injected for the complete immunization course?

Total volume injected = 0.5 × 4 = 2.0 mL

answer: Total Lf units injected = 2.0 mL × 5 Lf units / 0.5 mL = 20 Lf units

Example 3:

How would your answer change if the potency of TT were 4 Lf units per 0.5 mL?

Total volume injected = 0.5 × 4 = 2.0 mL

answer: Total Lf units injected = 2.0 mL × 4 Lf units / 0.5 mL = 16 Lf units

Practice Problems

(1) Diphtheria toxoid adsorbed on to aluminum hydroxide is available in strength of 30 Lf units per mL. Its usual dose is 2 injections of 0.5 mL 6 to 8 weeks apart, and a third reinforcing dose approximately one year later. From the available dosage form containing 5 milliliters how many complete courses can be provided?

(2) In the example above, how many Lf units are injected for the complete immunization course?

(3) How would your answer change if the potency of TT was 40 Lf units per mL?

(4) Tetanus toxoid is given as two injections of 0.5 mL given 4 to 8 weeks apart, followed by a third dose of 0.5 mL 6 to 12 months later. If a 5-mL vial is available, how many individuals can be vaccinated with the first dose only?

(5) If each milliliter of tetanus contains 10 Lf units, how many units would one patient receive with the complete vaccination? Refer to problem #4 for complete vaccination.

(6) For the complete vaccination of all ten individuals, how many milliliters of tetanus toxoid are required? Refer to problem #4 for complete vaccination.

(7) An ultrafine diphtheria and tetanus toxoid preparation contains 15 Lf units of diphtheria and 10 Lf units of tetanus toxoids per 0.5-mL dose. In a dosage form containing 5 mL, how many Lf units of tetanus are present?

(8) In problem #7, how many Lf units of diphtheria are present?

(9) The tri-immunal preparation from Wyeth-Ayerst contains 6.7 Lf units of diphtheria toxoid, 5 Lf units of tetanus toxoid, and 4 protective units of pertussis vaccine in each dose of 0.5 mL. In a 7.5-mL dosage form of the tri-immunal preparation, how many Lf units of diphtheria toxoid are present?

(10) In the above preparation, how many Lf units of pertussis vaccine are present?

CHAPTER 15

Calculations Involving Radiopharmaceuticals

A radiopharmaceutical is a chemical containing a radioactive isotope for use in humans for the purpose of diagnosis, mitigation, or treatment of a disease. Isotopes may be defined as atoms having the same atomic number, but different masses. Isotopes may be stable and unstable. The unstable isotopes are radioactive.

UNITS OF RADIOACTIVITY

Radioactivity is expressed in units known as *curies*. A *curie* is defined as the disintegration rate of 1 g of radium, which was considered to be 3.7 × 10^{10} (i.e., 37 billion) disintegrations per second (dps) or 2.22 × 10^{12} disintegrations per minute (dpm).

The millicurie (mCi) is one thousandth (i.e., 10^{-3}) of a curie, and the microcurie (μCi) is one millionth (i.e., 10^{-6}) of a curie, and the nanocurie (nCi) is one billionth (i.e., 10^{-9}) of a curie. The *curie* units are summarized in Table 15.1.

The System Internationale (SI) unit for radioactivity is becquerel (Bq), which is defined as one disintegration per second. The SI units and the conversion factors between curie and SI units are listed in Table 15.2.

Radiopharmaceuticals are prescribed according to units of radioactivity. A pharmacist practicing nuclear pharmacy may need to convert radio activity units from curies to SI unit, becquerel and its multiples, and vice versa. The following examples illustrate the interconversion of radioactive units.

TABLE 15.1. Curie Units.

1 curie (Ci)	=	3.7×10^{10} dps
	=	2.22×10^{12} dpm
1 millicurie (mCi)	=	3.7×10^{7} dps
	=	2.22×10^{9} dpm
1 microcurie (μCi)	=	3.7×10^{4} dps
	=	2.22×10^{6} dpm
1 nanocurie (nCi)	=	$3.7 \times 10^{1} = 37$ dps
	=	2.22×10^{3} dpm
1 Ci = 1000 mCi		
= 1,000,000 μCi		
= 1,000,000,000 nCi		

TABLE 15.2. Conversion between Curie and SI Units.

1 becquerel (Bq)	=	1 dps	=	2.7×10^{-11} Ci
1 kilobecquerel (kBq)	=	10^{3} dps	=	2.7×10^{-6} Ci
1 megabecquerel (MBq)	=	10^{6} dps	=	2.7×10^{-4} Ci
1 gigabecquerel (GBq)	=	10^{9} dps	=	2.7×10^{-2} Ci
1 terabecquerel (TBq)	=	10^{12} dps	=	27 Ci
1 Ci	=	3.7×10^{10} Bq	=	37 GBq
1 mCi	=	3.7×10^{7} Bq	=	37 MBq
1 μCi	=	3.7×10^{4} Bq	=	37 kBq
1 nCi	=	3.7×10^{1} Bq	=	37 Bq

Example 1:

The inhalation dose of krypton Kr 81m is the equivalent of 5 mCi. Express this dose in terms of megabecquerels.

$$\frac{1 \text{ mCi}}{37 \text{ MBq}} = \frac{5 \text{ mCi}}{X \text{ MBq}}$$

answer: $X = 37 \times 5 = 185$ MBq

Example 2:

The intravenous dose of indium hydroxide In 113m injection is the equivalent of 0.37 gigabecquerel. Express this dose in terms of mCi.

$$1 \text{ GBq} = 0.027 \text{ Ci} = 27 \text{ mCi}$$

$$\frac{1 \text{ GBq}}{27 \text{ mCi}} = \frac{0.37 \text{ GBq}}{X \text{ mCi}}$$

$$X = 0.37 \times 0.27 = 9.99 \text{ or } 10 \text{ mCi, answer}$$

Example 3:

The usual oral dose of cyanocobalamin Co 60 capsules is equivalent of 0.5 to 1 μCi. Express this dose range in terms of megabecquerels.

$$0.5 \text{ μCi} = 0.0005 \text{ mCi}$$

$$\frac{1 \text{ mCi}}{37 \text{ MBq}} = \frac{0.0005 \text{ mCi}}{X \text{ MBq}}$$

$$X = 0.0005 \times 37 = 0.0185 \text{ MBq}$$

Similarly,

$$1 \text{ μCi} = 0.001 \text{ mCi}$$

$$\frac{1 \text{ mCi}}{37 \text{ MBq}} = \frac{0.001 \text{ mCi}}{X \text{ MBq}}$$

$$X = 0.001 \times 37 = 0.037 \text{ MBq}$$

answer: The dose range of cyanocobalamin Co 60 is 0.0185 to 0.037 MBq

HALF-LIFE OF RADIOPHARMACEUTICALS

Half-life is defined as the time required for a radioisotope to reduce its initial radioactivity (disintegration rate) to one-half (or 50%). The half-life is represented by the symbol, $t^1{}_2$, and it is unique for a given radioisotope. The useful lifetimes of radiopharmaceuticals are usually determined by radioactive decay, which constantly decreases the amount of radioactivity present. The half-life is related to decay constant, λ of a radioisotope (discussed in the subsequent section), as follows:

$$\lambda = 0.693/t_{1/2}$$

or

$$t_{1/2} = 0.693/\lambda$$

The $t^1{}_2$ of a radioisotope is determined by plotting the radioactivity (or disintegration rate) as a function of time on a semi-logarithmic paper. The slope of the resulting straight line is equal to λ. The $t^1{}_2$ of the radioisotope may then be calculated from the above expression.

Example 1:

The disintegration constant of ^{55}Fe is 0.2665 years^{-1}. Calculate the half-life of the radioisotope.

$$\lambda = 0.2665 \text{ years}^{-1}$$

$$t_{1/2} = 0.693/\lambda$$

$$= 0.693/0.2665$$

answer: 2.6 years

Example 2:

The disintegration constant of a radioisotope is 0.07452 hours^{-1}. What is the half-life of that radioisotope?

$$\lambda = 0.07452 \text{ hours}^{-1}$$

$$t_{1/2} = 0.693/\lambda$$

$$= 0.693/0.07452$$

answer: 9.299 or 9.3 hours

Example 3:

The half-life of ^{45}Ca is 165 days. Calculate the disintegration constant of the radioisotope.

$$t_{1/2} = 165 \text{ days}$$

$$\lambda = 0.693/t_{1/2}$$

$$= 0.693/165$$

answer: 0.0042 days^{-1}

MEAN LIFE

Mean life of a radioisotope is the average life of a group of the radioisotopes. The mean life, represented by the symbol, τ, is related to decay constant λ and half-life $t'_{/2}$ as follows:

$$\tau = 1/\lambda$$

or

$$\tau = t_{1/2}/0.693$$

$$\tau = 1.44 \times t_{1/2}$$

Note: In one mean life, the activity of a radioisotope is reduced to 37% of its initial value.

Example 1:

If the half-life of a radioisotope is 13.3 hours, calculate the mean life of the isotope.

$$t_{1/2} = 13.3 \text{ hours}$$

$$\tau = 1.44 \times t_{1/2}$$

$$= 1.44 \times 13.3$$

answer: 19.2 hours

Example 2:

The half-life of radioisotope, ^{131}I, is 8.05 days. Calculate the mean life of that isotope.

$$t_{1/2} = 8.05 \text{ days}$$

$$\tau = 1.44 \times t_{1/2}$$

$$= 1.44 \times 8.05$$

answer: 11.59 or 11.6 days

Example 3:

The mean life of ^{24}Na is 21.6 years. What is the half-life of ^{24}Na?

$$\tau = 21.6 \text{ years}$$

$$t_{1/2} = \tau/1.44$$

$$= 21.6/1.44$$

answer: 15.0 years

Practice Problems

(1) A ^{99m}Tc sample is found to contain activity equivalent to 20 μCi. Express this activity in megabequerels.

(2) The intravenous dose of albumin microspheres containing Tc 99m for lung imaging is equivalent of 4 mCi. Express this dose in terms of megabecquerels.

(3) The usual intravenous dose of pentetate calcium trisodium Yb 169 injection for brain and kidney imaging is the equivalent of 0.037 GBq. Express this dose in terms of millicuries.

(4) In the process of calibrating a radionuclide generator, 18.4 GBq activity was shown for a radioisotope. Express this in millicuries.

(5) For *scintigraphy of the pancreas*, an intravenous dose of selenomethionine Se 75 injection, the equivalent of 250 μCi is needed. Express this quantity in bequerels.

(6) The disintegration constant of ^{24}Na is 0.0462 years^{-1}. Calculate the half-life of the radioisotope.

(7) The disintegration constant of ^{64}Cu is 0.05414 hours^{-1}. Calculate the half-life of the radioisotope.

(8) The half-life of ^{59}Fe is 45 days. Calculate the disintegration constant of the radioisotope.

(9) If the half-life of ^{76}Se is 120.4 days, calculate the mean life of the isotope.

(10) The mean life of ^{67}Ga is 112.32 hours. What is the half-life of the isotope?

RADIOACTIVE DECAY OF RADIOISOTOPES

Radioisotopes are unstable and decay by particle emission, electron capture, or γ-ray emission. The decay is a random process, i.e., one cannot predict which atom from a group of atoms will decay at a specific time. The decay of radioisotopes, therefore, is described in terms of the average number of radioisotopes disintegrating during a period of time. The disintegration rate (or the number of disintegrations per unit time), $-dN/dt$, of a radioisotope at any time is proportional to the total number of undecomposed radioisotopes present at that time. This may be expressed as follows:

$$-dN/dt = \lambda N$$

where

N = number of undecomposed radioisotopes at time t
λ = decay constant

The disintegration rate, $-dN/dt$, may also be termed the radioactivity or simply the activity of a radioisotope, is represented by the symbol, A.

Thus, one can write an expression for A as follows:

$$-dN/dt = A = \lambda N$$

Upon integration, the above equation becomes:

$$N_t = N_0 \times e^{-\lambda t}$$

where N_0 and N_t are the number of undecomposed radioisotopes present at time 0 and t, respectively.

The above exponential decay expression may also be represented in terms of radioactivity or disintegration rate as follows:

$$A_t = A_0 \times e^{-\lambda t}$$

where

A_t = radioactivity remaining after time t
A_0 = initial activity
e = base of the natural logarithm (2.7183)
λ = decay constant

Decay Calculations of Radiopharmaceuticals

Since radiopharmaceuticals are prepared in advance prior to the actual administration, calculations must take into account corrections for loss of radioactivity by radioactive decay. Using the expression, $A_t = A_0 \times e^{-\lambda t}$, one can calculate the radioactivity of an isotope remaining at any time t after the initial assay. This is explained in the following examples.

Example 1:

A radioisotope sample with a half-life of 10 days contains 250 mCi radioactivity. What is the radioactivity of the sample after 23 days?

$$A_0 = 250 \text{ mCi}$$

$$t_{1/2} = 10 \text{ days}$$

$$t = 23 \text{ days}$$

$$\lambda = 0.693/10 = 0.0693 \text{ days}^{-1}$$

$$A_t = A_0 \times e^{-\lambda t}$$

$$= 250 \times e^{-0.0693 \times 23}$$

answer: 50.8 mCi

Example 2:

A sample of ^{131}I has an initial activity of 30 mCi. Calculate the activity at the end of exactly 20 and 30 days. The half-life of ^{131}I is 8.05 days.

$$A_0 = 30 \text{ mCi}$$

$$\lambda = 0.693/t_{1/2}$$

$$= 0.693/8.05$$

$$= 0.0861 \text{ days}^{-1}$$

At the end of 20 days:

$$= A_0 \times e^{-\lambda t}$$

$$= 30 \times e^{-0.0861 \times 20}$$

$$= 30 \times e^{-1.7217}$$

answer: 5.36 mCi

At the end of 30 days:

$$= 30 \times e^{-0.0861 \times 30}$$

$$= 30 \times e^{-2.583}$$

answer: 2.27 mCi

Example 3:

At 8:00 A.M., the ^{99m}Tc radioactivity was found to be 9 mCi. If half-life for ^{99m}Tc is 6 hours, calculate the activity at 5:00 A.M. and 1:00 P.M. on the same day. Express the answers in curies as well as SI units.

Time from 5:00 A.M. to 8:00 A.M. is 3 hours

$$A_t = 9 \text{ mCi (or } 37 \times 9 = 333 \text{ MBq)}$$

$$A_0 = ?$$

$$A_t = A_0 \times e^{-\lambda t}$$

$$9 \text{ mCi} = A_0 \times e^{-0.1155 \times 3}$$

$$A_0 = 9 \times e^{0.3465}$$

$$= 12.7 \text{ mCi at 5:00 A.M.}$$

In MBq units:

$$\frac{1 \text{ mCi}}{37 \text{ MBq}} = \frac{12.7 \text{ mCi}}{X \text{ MBq}}$$

answer: $X = 469.9$ or 470 MBq

Time from 8:00 A.M. to 1:00 P.M. is 5 hours

$$A_t = A_0 \times e^{-\lambda t}$$

$$A_t = 9 \times e^{-0.1155K5}$$

$$A_0 = 9 \times e^{-0.5775}$$

$$= 5.05 \text{ mCi at 1:00 P.M.}$$

In MBq units:

$$\frac{1 \text{ mCi}}{37 \text{ MBq}} = \frac{5.05 \text{ mCi}}{X \text{ MBq}}$$

answer: $X = 186.85$ or 187 MBq

The half-life values of selected radioisotopes are listed in Table 15.3.

PERCENTAGE ACTIVITY

The factor "$e^{-\lambda t}$" in the equation, $A_t = A_0 \times e^{-\lambda t}$ is called the decay factor, where λ is decay constant and t is time. The decay constant, as discussed in the previous section, can be calculated from the relation: $\lambda = 0.693/t_{1/2}$.

The percentage of radioisotope remaining after time, t, is calculated as $100 \times e^{-\lambda t}$.

Example 1:

The half-life of ^{99m}Tc is 6 hours. Calculate the percentage of ^{99m}Tc remaining after 4 hours.

$$\lambda = 0.693/t_{1/2}$$

$$= 0.693/6 = 0.1155 \text{ hours}^{-1}$$

$$\% \text{ remaining} = 100 \times e^{-\lambda t}$$

$$= 100 \times e^{-0.1155 \times 4}$$

$$= 100 \times e^{-0.462}$$

answer: 63.00%

TABLE 15.3. Half-Life Values of Selected
Radioisotopes.*

Radioisotope	Half-Life
^{11}C	20.3 minutes
^{14}C	5730 years
^{22}Na	2.6 years
^{24}Na	15.0 years
^{32}P	14.3 years
^{38}S	88 days
^{42}K	12.4 hours
^{43}K	22.4 hours
^{49}Ca	165 days
^{51}Cr	27.8 days
^{55}Fe	2.6 years
^{59}Fe	45 days
^{57}Co	270 days
^{56}Co	71.3 days
^{60}Co	5.26 years
^{64}Cu	12.8 hours
^{62}Zn	9.3 hours
^{65}Zn	245 days
^{67}Ga	78 hours
^{78}Se	120.4 days
^{81m}Kr	13 seconds
^{85}Kr	10.76 years
^{86}Sr	64 days
^{99m}Tc	6 hours
^{113m}In	100 hours
^{123m}Te	117 days
^{123}I	13.3 hours
^{126}I	60 days
^{131}I	8.05 days
^{127}Xe	36.4 days
^{133}Xe	5.3 days
^{169}Yb	32 days
^{195m}Au	31 seconds
^{196}Au	2.7 days
^{197}Hg	64.8 hours
^{203}Hg	46.9 days

* Source: *Remington's Pharmaceutical Sciences*, 18th Ed., Mack Publishing Co.

Example 2:

The half-life of ^{131}I is 8.05 days. Calculate the percentage of ^{131}I remaining after 12 days.

$$\gamma = 0.693/t_{1/2}$$

$$= 0.693/8.05 = 0.0861 \text{ days}^{-1}$$

$$\% \text{ remaining} = 100 \times e^{-\lambda t}$$

$$= 100 \times e^{-0.0861 \times 12}$$

$$= 100 \times e^{-1.033}$$

answer: 35.6%

Example 3:

The half-life of ^{85}Sr is 64 days. Calculate the percentage of ^{85}Sr remaining after 3 months.

$$\lambda = 0.693/t_{1/2}$$

$$= 0.693/64 = 0.0108 \text{ days}^{-1}$$

$$\% \text{ remaining} = 100 \times e^{-\lambda t}$$

$$= 100 \times e^{-0.0108 \times 90}$$

$$= 100 \times e^{-0.972}$$

answer: 37.83

Note: In hospital setting, the radioactive decay charts for radiopharmaceuticals may be used for quick reference to determine the percentage of radioactivity remaining at a given time. A representative decay chart for ^{131}I is shown in Table 15.4.

DISPENSING OF RADIOPHARMACEUTICALS

Specific Activity and Concentration

Radiopharmaceuticals are prescribed in units of radioactivity, and the actual dispensing of the patient dose involves calculating how much radiopharmaceu-

TABLE 15.4.   Radioactive Decay* of ^{131}I.

Time (days)	Percentage Remaining
1	91.8
2	84.2
3	77.2
4	70.9
5	65.0
6	59.7
7	54.7
8	50.2
9	46.0
10	42.3
11	38.8
12	35.6
13	32.6
14	29.9
15	27.5
16	25.2
17	22.9
18	21.2
19	19.5
20	17.9

* The decay constant, λ is calculated as (0.693/8.05) day^{-1}. The decay factor is $e^{-\lambda t}$. The % remaining is calculated as $100 \times e^{-\lambda t}$.

tical, in terms of volume, is required to provide the prescribed amount of radioactivity at a given time.

SPECIFIC ACTIVITY

Specific activity of a radiopharmaceutical may be defined as the amount of radioactivity per unit mass of a radioisotope or a labeled compound. For example, if 100 mg ^{131}I-labeled albumin contains 150 mCi ^{131}I radioactivity, its specific activity would be 150/100, i.e., 1.5 mCi/mg. Specific activity is usually expressed in units such as Ci/g, mCi/mg, or MBq/mg. It is also expressed in terms of the radioactivity per mole of a labeled compound, e.g., mCi/mole, MBq/mole, mCi/μmole, or MBq/μmole. Specific activity is usually provided on the product label.

ACTIVITY CONCENTRATION

Activity concentration is defined as the amount of radioactivity per unit volume (mCi/mL) of a sample. A 10 mL solution containing 42 mCi radioactivity will have a concentration of 4.2 mCi/mL. The majority of radiopharmaceuticals are liquids, and, therefore, the amount of radioactivity per volume (or activity concentration) must be known for a given time such that the desired amount of radioactivity may be dispensed. If the activity concentration of a radiopharmaceutical is known, the quantity of dose in milliliters may be calculated as follows:

$$\text{Quantity of dose (in mL) to be dispensed} = \frac{\text{Activity required}}{\text{Activity concentration}}$$

Example 1:

A 10 mCi dose is ordered and the radiopharmaceutical activity concentration is presently 16 mCi/mL. What is the quantity to be dispensed to provide the necessary radioactivity?

Activity needed = 10 mCi

Activity concentration = 16 mCi/mL

$$\text{Quantity needed} = \frac{10 \text{ mCi}}{16 \text{ mCi/mL}}$$

answer: 0.63 mL

Example 2:

A dose equivalent to 30 mCi is ordered and the radiopharmaceutical activity concentration is presently 15 mCi/mL. What is the quantity to be dispensed to provide the necessary radioactivity?

$$\text{Quantity needed} = \frac{30 \text{ mCi}}{15 \text{ mCi/mL}}$$

answer: 2.0 mL

Carrier-Free Radiochemicals

Carrier-free radiochemical is a radionuclide that is not contaminated with a stable or radioactive nuclide of the same element. The "no carrier added" (NCA) designation applies to most of the elements to which the term "carrier free" is indicated. The specific activity of a carrier-free radioisotope can be calculated by the following formula:

$$\text{Specific activity (mCi/mg)} = \frac{3.13 \times 10^9}{A \times t_{1/2}}$$

where

A = mass number of the radioisotope

$t_{1/2}$ = half-life in hours of the radioisotope

Example 3:

What is the specific activity of carrier free ^{99m}Tc? The $t_{1/2}$ of ^{99m}Tc is 6 hours.

$$\text{Specific activity (mCi/mg)} = \frac{3.13 \times 10^9}{99 \times 6}$$

answer: 5.27×10^6 mCi/mg

Useful Equations Pertaining to Radiopharmaceuticals

$$\lambda = 0.693/t_{1/2}$$

$$t_{1/2} = 0.693/\lambda$$

$$\tau = 1/\lambda$$

$$\tau = t_{1/2}/0.693$$

$$A_t = A_0 \times e^{-\lambda t}$$

$$\text{Dose (mL)} = \frac{\text{Activity required}}{\text{Activity concentration}}$$

$$\text{Specific activity (mCi/mg)} = \frac{3.13 \times 10^9}{A \times t_{1/2}}$$

Practice Problems

Refer to Table 15.3 as required.

(1) A sample of ^{113m}In has an initial activity of 16 mCi. Calculate the activity at the end of exactly 5 hours.
(2) A radioisotope sample with a half-life of 2.34 years contains 182 mCi radioactivity. What is the radioactivity of the sample after 6.4 years?

(3) A sample of ^{62}Zn has an initial activity of 100 μCi. Calculate the activity at the end of exactly 30 hours.

(4) At 12:00 P.M., the ^{11}C radioactivity was found to be 28 mCi. If half-life for ^{11}C is 20.3 minutes, calculate the activity at 1:30 P.M. and 2:30 P.M. on the same day. Express the answers in curies as well as SI units.

(5) The half-life of ^{51}Cr is 27.8 days. Calculate the percentage of ^{51}Cr remaining after 72 days.

(6) The half-life of ^{85}Sr is 64 days. Calculate the percentage of ^{85}Sr remaining after 200 days.

(7) Calculate the percentage of ^{75}Se remaining after a year (365 days).

(8) Calculate the percentage of ^{195m}Au remaining after 2 minutes.

(9) A 150 MBq dose is ordered and the radiopharmaceutical activity concentration is 225 MBq/mL. What is the quantity to be dispensed to provide the necessary radioactivity.

(10) What is the specific activity of carrier free ^{123}I?

REVIEW SET 1

(1) A bottle of Children's Tylenol® contains 30 teaspoons of liquid. If each dose is 3/4 teaspoon, how many doses are available in this bottle?

(2) If Nebcin® (tobramycin sulfate injection USP) contains 800 mg of tobramycin per 2 mL of solution, how many mL of solution would be needed to deliver 15 mg of tobramycin?

(3) How many milliliters of a 1:100 w/v solution of ferrous sulfate should be used to prepare 1 liter of a 1:600 w/v solution?

(4) If 100 mL of mannitol solution weighs 125 g, what is its specific gravity?

(5) If Lactulose Syrup USP contains 10 g of lactulose in 15 mL of the syrup, how many milliliters would provide the equivalent of 1.33 g of lactulose?

(6) Lanoxin® Elixir contains 50 μg of digoxin/mL. How much additional digoxin should be added to 4 fluid ounces of the elixir so that each teaspoonful will contain 1 mg of digoxin?

(7) What is the percentage strength (v/v) of alcohol in a mixture of 500 mL of 15% v/v alcohol, 150 mL of 20% v/v alcohol, and 350 mL of 30% v/v alcohol?

(8) What is the percentage strength of a solution containing 20 mEq of potassium chloride per 15 mL?

(9) Four anthralin ointment (Anthra-Derm®) preparations are available containing 0.1, 0.25, 0.5, and 1.0% w/w active ingredient. Express these concentrations in terms of mg/g.

(10) In what proportions 2%, 10%, and 12% sulfur ointments must be mixed to prepare 7% sulfur ointment?

(11) How many grams of sodium chloride should be used in compounding the following prescription?

R̸

Atropine Sulfate	2%
Sodium Chloride	q.s.
Sterile Water for Injection ad	60
Make isoton. sol.	

(12) 1% sulfacetamide sodium solution has a freezing point depression of 0.14°C. Calculate the volume of iso-osmotic solution obtained by 1 g of sulfacetamide sodium.

(13) Calculate the hydronium ion concentration of the following solutions (at 25°C) at pH value of:

a. 4.50
b. 8.20
c. 5.40
d. 7.8

(14) A physician ordered: "2000 mL D5W IV run for 24 hours." If the drop factor is 15 gtt/mL, what would be the IV flow rate?

(15) A patient is required to receive 20 units of insulin twice daily. If the patient has a 10-mL vial of insulin on hand that contains 1000 units of insulin per milliliter, how many days will the product last the patient?

(16) An IV solution contains 25 mEq of potassium chloride in 500 mL of solution. How many milligrams of potassium chloride are contained in 325 mL of this solution?

(17) If 100 mL D5W are infused per hour, how many calories will be given in 24 hours?

(18) What is the REE requirement, in terms of kcal/hour for a patient with the following information?

Patient data

Sex:	Female
Age:	30 years
Height:	142 cm
Weight:	70 kg

(19) The usual intravenous dose of thallium TI 201 chloride injection for myocardial ischemia imaging is equivalent of 1.5 mCi. Express this dose in terms of megabecquerels.

(20) Lasix® (furosemide) oral solution contains 10 mg of furosemide per milliliter, how many grams of furosemide would be contained in 5 pt of the solution?

(21) If a vial of gentamycin contains 80 mg of drug in 2 mL, how many micrograms of the drug are present in 0.02 mL?

(22) A doctor ordered morphine sulfate gr 4/9 and the pharmacist has a stock solution of gr 1/8 per mL of morphine sulfate. How many milliliters of the stock solution are required to fill the prescription?

(23) Suprax® suspension contains 100 mg/5 mL of cefixime. If the patient takes one-half teaspoonful of the suspension twice daily for 10 days, how many grams of the drug does the patient consume?

(24) Tylenol with Codeine® elixir contains 12 mg of codeine per 5 mL of the elixir. If a pharmacist dispenses 6 fluidounces of the elixir to a patient, how many grains of codeine does the patient receive?

(25) ℞

Cephalexin 250 mg/5 mL

Sig: ii tsp tid, 7 days

How many f℥ of cephalexin suspension would the patient receive?

(26) What are the errors and omissions of the following prescriptions?

Jack Ramos, M.D.
911 Hollywood Avenue
Detroit, MI-71208
Phone No. 555-1234

Name : John Doe   Age: 70
Address: 96 Havana Blvd., MI-71208   Date: 2/28/96

℞

Keflex 500 mg

Sig: i cap qid, 7 days

REFILL None

DAW

                    JRamos
              DEA # AD 7973142

```
┌─────────────────────────────────────────┐
│            NORTHEAST PHARMACY            │
│             169 Hillside Avenue          │
│        Monroe, LA 71206    555-0342      │
│                                          │
│  ℞ # 123456          Date: 2/28/95       │
│  Ramos, Jack                             │
│  911 Hollywood Ave                       │
│  Take one capsule four times a day for   │
│  seven days                              │
│  Cephalexin Caps 500 mg #40              │
│  Refill 1              J. Doe, M.D.       │
└─────────────────────────────────────────┘
```

(27) What is the minimum amount that can be weighed on a Class A prescription balance with a potential error of not more than 8%?

(28) If it is desired to weigh 50 mg of salicylic acid on a Class A prescription balance with a sensitivity requirement of 6 mg, and potential error of not more than 5%, explain how you would perform the weighing.

(29) How would you measure 0.03 mL of a concentrate which is to be diluted to 60 mL following the measurement? You are provided with a 5-mL piper with marking in units of 1 mL, a measuring cylinder, and a container to dispense the final product.

(30) Atenolol is available in a strength of 50 mg. If a prescription is written for 100 mg daily for three weeks as directed, how many tablets should be dispensed?

(31) How would you fill the following prescription? Show all the calculations, procedure, and the label for the product.

```
┌─────────────────────────────────────────────────┐
│              Henry Huxtable, M.D.                 │
│             61-40 Flushing Avenue                 │
│               Monroe, LA 71208                    │
│              Phone No. 555-1234                    │
├─────────────────────────────────────────────────┤
│  Name : Sonya Burns              Age: 36          │
│  Address: 96 Havana Blvd., FL 31207   Date: 3/18/96 │
│                                                   │
│  ℞                                                │
│                                                   │
│     Hydrochlorothiazide      10 mg                │
│     Triamterene             20 mg                 │
│     Lactose q.s.                                  │
│                                                   │
│     M. ft caps.  DTD # 10                         │
│                                                   │
│     Sig: i cap bid, UD                            │
│                                                   │
│  REFILL  1 x                                      │
│                                                   │
│  DAW                                              │
│                               HHuxtable           │
│                         DEA # AD 7973142          │
└─────────────────────────────────────────────────┘
```

Tablets available: HCTZ 25 mg and Triameterene 25 mg

(32) Show how you will prepare the following prescription.

℞

    Iodine 0.5%
    Boric acid 5 g
    Lactose qs 30 g
    Ft. ℥ -iv

    Sig: AAbid, UD

(33) After the administration of a novel drug, the following plasma levels were observed at the given time points. Calculate the AUC, C_{max}, T_{max}, $t_{1/2}$, and the K_{el}.

Plasma conc (mg/mL)	0	0.1	0.3	0.4	0.2	0.1	0.05	0.01
Time in hours	0	1	2	4	6	8	10	12

(34) If the fraction of the drug absorbed is 0.6, dose of the drug is 50 mg,

volume of distribution is 25 L, average drug concentration in the blood is 4 mcg/mL, and the elimination rate constant is 0.2 hour^{-1}, when would the second dose be taken if the first dose was taken at 6:00 A.M.?

(35) Gentamycin is shown to have a V_d of 0.25 L per kilogram of the body weight. If the weight of the patient is 162 lb, and the elimination rate constant is 0.33 hour^{-1}, what is the total clearance of gentamycin?

(36) Upon the administration of 0.27 mg of a therapeutic agent to a normal individual, the elimination half-life was found to be 2 hour^{-1}. The normal dosing regimen included 0.27 mg qid. If the elimination rate constant in renally impaired condition is 70% of the normal elimination rate constant, how can the dose be adjusted maintaining the same dosing interval of six hours?

(37) In juvenile arthritis, Advil® is required to be given in a dose of 30 mg/kg/day. How many milliliters of the Advil® suspension (100 mg/5 mL) should be given to child weighing 54 lb?

(38) The steady-state serum concentrations of a patient taking gentamycin were found to be 8 mcg/mL ($C_{max\,ss}$) and 2 mcg/mL ($C_{min\,ss}$). The patient was taking a dose of 2.5 mg/kg/day of gentamycin. Would you recommend a change in dosing schedule? If so, how?

(39) Intravenous bolus dose of 500 mg dose of an antibiotic every six hours in a patient produces minimum steady-state concentration of 8 mcg/mL. If the desired minimum steady-state concentration in this patient is 14 mcg/mL, calculate the size of dose needed to change the minimum steady-state concentration. Assume that the drug follows linear kinetics.

(40) A medication order provided for a nine-month-old child weighing 8 kg includes dopamine in a dose of 5 mcg/kg/min. The drug available is dopamine 200 mg/5 mL. The physician wanted 70 mg of dopamine in 200 mL of D5W to be administered at 6 mL per hour to this child who is in septic shock. Check for the accuracy of the dilution order.

REVIEW SET 2

(1) If each Tegretol® (carbamazepine) chewable tablet contains 100 mg of carbamazepine, how many Tegretol® tablets can be made from 1 kg of carbamazepine?

(2) Vistaril® (hydroxyzine pamoate) oral suspension contains 25 mg of hydroxyzine in each 5-mL dose. How many mg of hydroxyzine would be contained in a 120-mL container of the syrup?

(3) How many milliliters of purified water should be added to 50 mL of a 1:10 w/v solution to make a solution such that 20 mL diluted to 100 mL will provide a 1:5000 dilution?

(4) The specific gravity of a solvent is 0.850. What is its specific volume?

(5) A physician ordered: "Benadryl® 50 mg PO h.s. p.r.n." If the available Benadryl® (diphenhydramine HCl) elixir contains 2.5 mg of drug in each milliliter, how many teaspoons will be administered to the patient?

(6) If one fluidounce of a cough syrup contains 20 gr of sodium citrate, how many milligrams of sodium citrate are contained in 5 mL?

(7) If Benadryl® elixir containing 25 mg diphenhydramine hydrochloride per 10 mL is evaporated to 80% of its volume, what is the strength of diphenhydramine hydrochloride in the remaining solution?

(8) How many grams of potassium chloride are required to provide 40 mEq of potassium ion?

(9) What is the percentage (w/w) of coal tar in the finished product when 10 g of coal tar is mixed with 200 g of a 5% coal tar ointment?

(10) How many grams of coal tar should be added to a kilogram of zinc oxide paste to prepare an ointment containing 5% of coal tar?

(11) How much of sodium chloride should be used in compounding the following prescription?

℞

Zinc Sulfate	0.1
Sodium chloride	q.s.
Purified Water ad	50.0
Make isotonic solution.	

(12) If the freezing point depression of a 5% solution of boric acid is 1.55°C, how many grams of boric acid should be used in preparing a liter of an isotonic solution?

(13) What is the pH of solution containing 0.1 mole of ephedrine and 0.01 mole of ephedrine hydrochloride per liter of solution? The pK_b of ephedrine is 4.64.

(14) An IV flow rate is set at 48 gtt/mL. The infusion set has a drop factor of 15 gtt/mL. How many milliliters of IV fluid will be infused in 8 hours?

(15) A physician ordered: "1000 mL D5W IV with 40,000 U heparin to infuse at 40 mL/h." What is the hourly dosage of heparin?

(16) How many milliequivalents of potassium chloride are there in 5 mL ampul containing 1 g of potassium chloride?

(17) A TPN solution contains 0.5 L of 10% dextrose and 0.5 liter of 8.5% amino acid solution. What is the non-nitrogen calories to grams of nitrogen ratio for this TPN formula?

(18) Calculate the REE requirement, in terms of kilocalories/hour for a patient with the following profile.

Patient data

Sex:	Male
Age:	45 years
Height:	158 cm
Weight:	78 kg

(19) In the process of calibrating a radionuclide generator, 22.8 GBq activity was shown for a radioisotope. Express this in millicuries.

(20) A sample of ^{62}Zn has an initial activity of 60 μCi. Calculate the activity at the end of exactly 20 hours.

(21) Pediaprofen® pediatric suspension contains 80 mg of ibuprofen in 5 mL of the suspension. While taking 2.5 mL of this medication, the patient spilled 1 mL of the suspension. How many grams of ibuprofen did the patient receive?

(22) If 2 pt of guaifenesin elixir is present in the inventory, how many ʒ iv prescriptions can be filled?

(23) In the calibration of a medical dropper, 2 mL of a pediatric drop solution was found to give 48 drops. If it is desired to administer 0.3 mL of the medication to a baby, approximately how many drops should be given?

(24) Halcion® tablet contains 0.25 mg of triazolam. How many grains of the drug triazolam would be present in 50 tablets of Halcion®?

(25) ℞

Keflex caps 500 mg

Sig: i cap bid, 7 days

If the pharmacist has only 250 mg capsules in the inventory, how many capsules should be given to the patient?

(26) Write the errors and omissions in the following prescriptions.

```
┌─────────────────────────────────────────┐
│            Pat Moody                      │
│          96 Alonzo Drive                  │
│          Miami, FL-71208                  │
│         Phone No. 555-1234                │
├───────────────────────────────────────────┤
│ Name : Baby Starks          Age: 6 mo.    │
│ Address: 96 Havana Blvd., FL-71208  Date: 2/29/96 │
│                                           │
│  Rx                                       │
│                                           │
│       Vantin 100 mg                       │
│                                           │
│       Sig: ss ℥ bid, 7 days               │
│                                           │
│  REFILL _None_____                     │
│                                           │
│  DAW _____                            │
│                      _PMoody__            │
└───────────────────────────────────────────┘
```

```
┌────────────────────────────────────────┐
│         NORTHEAST PHARMACY               │
│            169 Hillside Avenue           │
│         Monroe, LA 71206   555-0342      │
│                                          │
│  Rx # 123456         Date: 2/29/96       │
│  Starks, Baby                            │
│  96 Havana Blvd.                         │
│  Take one-half tablet twice daily for seven │
│  days                                    │
│  Vancomycin 100 mg tablets               │
│  Refill 1            P. Moody            │
└────────────────────────────────────────┘
```

(27) If the pointer moves two divisions when a 10 mg weight is placed on the right-hand side of a prescription balance, what is its sensitivity requirement?

(28) Explain how you would weigh gr ss of atropine sulfate on a prescription balance with a sensitivity requirement of 6 mg.

(29) Rx

Gentian violet   0.03 g
Purified water qs ad   f℥ iv

Show how you would prepare this prescription using a Class A prescription balance.

(30) If a prescription requires a stat dose of 0.375 mg of Lanoxin (gen) and the pharmacist has digoxin tablets of strength, 0.25 mg, how many digoxin tablets should the patient take?

(31) How would you dispense the following prescription? Show all the calculations involved.

Patrick Mills, M.D.
61-40 Flushing Avenue
New York, NY 12345
Phone No. 555-1234

Name : Samuel Doe   Age: 32
Address: 96 Main St., NY 12345   Date: 3/9/96

R

ASA   0.20 g
Phenobarb.   0.02 g
Lactose   qs

Ft. caps. *M et. Div.* # 15

Sig: i cap q8h

REFILL _None_

DAW _____

                                         PMills
                              Lic # 333444

Tablets available: ASA 5 gr (325 mg) and Phenobarbital 0.5 gr (32 mg).

(32) Show how you will prepare the following prescription.

R

Iodine 1%
Boric acid 5 g
Lactose qs 30 g
Ft.℥ −v

Sig: AAbid, UD

(33) For the following data, find the AUC from the initial time up to 12 hours.

Time (hr)	0	0.5	1	2	3	4	6	8	12
Plasma conc (ng/mL)	0	2.8	6.6	8.5	9.5	9.4	8.7	6.6	3.8

(34) A therapeutic agent was found to have an F value of 0.8, volume of distribution of 2 L/kg, average blood concentration is 1.75 ng/mL, what would be the dosing interval if the dose of the drug is 0.27 mg, K_{el} value is 0.0315 hr^{-1} and the weight of the patient is 132 lb?

(35) When a 50-mg drug is administered, C_0 was found to be 4 ng/mL. The half-life of the drug was found to be 4 hours. If the drug was administered q4h, what would be the steady-state concentrations?

(36) Upon the administration of 500 mg of an antihypertensive drug to a normal individual, the elimination rate constant was found to be 0.17 hour^{-1}. The normal dosing regimen included 0.5 g bid. If the elimination rate constant in renally impaired condition is 0.14 hour^{-1}, how can the dose be adjusted maintaining the same dosing interval?

(37) The height and weight of a child are 110 cm and 35 pounds respectively. The usual adult dose of Elavil® (Amitriptyline HCl) is 75 mg/day. What would be the dose for the child?

(38) When a single 250 mg bolus dose of an antibiotic is given, the C_0 was found to be 20 ng/mL and the elimination half-life was 5 hours. What would be the dose required to achieve a new minimum steady-state concentration of 10 ng/mL with a dosing interval of 6 hours? Also what would be the new maximum steady-state concentration? Assume that the drug follows first-order kinetics.

(39) An infusion of 60 mg of nitroprusside in 250 mL of D5W is to be provided to a patient weighing 165 lb. What is the titration factor of this infusion between 0.5 to 1.5 mcg/kg/min to maintain mean blood pressure at 100 mmHg?

(40) For a three-year-old child weighing 27 kg and suffering from tachycardia, a physician prescribed 20 mcg/kg/min lidocaine. The instruction was to add 200 mg of lidocaine in 200 mL of D5W and administer at a rate of 25 mL per hour. The available drug is lidocaine 1 g/25 mL. Is the dilution factor accurate?

REVIEW SET 3

(1) If each Dalmane® (flurazepam hydrochloride) capsule contains 15 mg of flurazepam hydrochloride, how many grams of flurazepam hydrochloride are contained in 650 capsules?

(2) What is the percentage strength of a solution prepared by dissolving 750 mg of potassium chloride in 20 mL of water?

(3) How many milliliters of water should be added to 20 mL of a 1:10 w/v solution to make a solution such that 10 mL diluted to 100 mL will provide a 1:1000 dilution?

(4) What is the weight of 100 mL of propylene glycol having a specific gravity of 1.24?

(5) A physician prescribes Amoxil (amoxicillin) oral pediatric suspension for a patient to be taken in doses of 1/2 teaspoonful four times a day for seven days. How many milliliters of the suspension should be dispensed to provide the quantity for the prescribed dosage regimen?

(6) A physician ordered: "Lithium citrate 600 mg t.i.d. PO." If 300 mg of lithium citrate are equal to 8 mEq of lithium, how many milliequivalents of lithium will be given to the patient in a day?

(7) If Benadryl® Elixir containing 12.5 mg diphenhydramine hydrochloride in each 5 mL is evaporated to 90% of its volume, what is the strength of diphenhydramine hydrochloride in the remaining solution?

(8) A patient's potassium level in the blood plasma was found to be 26 mg%. Express this concentration in terms of milliequivalents/liters.

(9) What is the percentage (w/w) of hydrocortisone in the finished product when 600 mg of hydrocortisone is mixed with 20 g of Cortril® ointment containing 1% hydrocortisone?

(10) How many grams of coal tar should be added to 600 g of zinc oxide paste to prepare an ointment containing 5% of coal tar?

(11) How many milliliters of a 0.9% solution of sodium chloride are used in compounding the prescription?

℞

Atropine sulfate	0.5
Chlorobutanol	0.25
Sodium Chloride	q.s.
Purified Water ad	50.0
Make isoton. sol.	

Sig. Use as directed.

(12) How many mg of sodium chloride are needed to compound the following prescription?

℞

Ephedrine sulfate	2%
Sodium chloride	q.s.
Isotonic solution	40 mL

Sig. gtt ii each nostril q6h

(13) What is the molar ratio of bicarbonate to carbonic acid at pH 6.4? The pK_a of the carbonic acid is 6.1 at 25°C.

(14) A physician ordered: "2000 mL D5W IV to run for 24 hours." If the infusion set is calibrated to deliver 60 drops per milliliter, calculate the IV flow rate in gtt/min.

(15) A physician ordered: "1 liter D5W IV with heparin 40,000 U to infuse at 0.5 mL/min." What is the hourly heparin dosage?

(16) 600 mL of a 0.25% intravenous infusion of potassium chloride is to be administered over a period of four hours. How many milliequivalents of potassium are represented in the infusion?

(17) An IV solution contains 500 mL of 10% dextrose and 500 mL of 7% amino acids. What is the protein-calorie percentage of the solution?

(18) What is the basal energy expenditure (BEE) in kcal/day for a patient with the following information?

    Sex: Female
    Age: 45 years
    Height: 168 cm
    Weight: 128 lb

(19) A physician ordered: "Carbenicillin 1.5 g IM q.6h." A 5 g Geopen® (carbenicillin) was on hand. If the reconstitution directions on Geopen® state "Add 9.5 mL sterile water to provide 1 g in 2.5 mL," how many milliliters of this reconstituted solution are needed per day?

(20) If each Xanax® tablet contains 0.25 mg of alprazolam, how many Xanax® tablets can be prepared with 5 g of alprazolam?

(21) Fer-In-Sol® drops contain 75 mg of ferrous sulfate in 0.6 mL of the solution. If a pharmacist dispensed 60 mL of the solution, how many grams of ferrous sulfate were dispensed?

(22) If you fill approximately ten prescriptions of f℥-vi Ventolin® syrup per day, how many gallons of the syrup would be used in 15 days?

(23) If a patient needs one teaspoonful of Amoxil® oral liquid three times a day for 7 days, how many fluidounces of medication should the pharmacist dispense?

(24) A prescription requires gr ii of phenolphthalein in f℥ iv of an emulsion. If the patient takes 2 tsp of the emulsion at bedtime, how many milligrams of phenolphthalein does this dose represent?

(25) Write the errors and omissions in the following prescription.

Medication profile and a prescription.

Susan Monroe				
20 Main Street				
Monroe, LA 71201			Allergy:Aspirin	
Date	Dr.	R #	Patient	Drug
3/1/95	Quinn	12340	Susan	Synthroid 0.2 mg #100, 1 daily
5/6/95	Quinn	12350	Susan	Hygroton 2.5 mg #70, 1 qd
7/7/95	Quinn	12369	Susan	Tylenol #3 #30, ii tid, prn

Doc Rogers, M.D.
12 Desiard Street
Monroe, LA-71208
Phone No. 555-1234

Name : Evelyn Monroe_____   **Age:** 58 yrs
Address: 20 Main Street, Monroe   **Date:** 7/9/95

Rx

Fiorinal
       # 20

Sig: ii caps, q4h daily

REFILL 1_____

DAW ✓_____

DRogers
DEA # DR 1234567

(26) Rx

Dr. Zogg's otic drops
    15 cc

Sig: 0.1 cc au tid, prn pain

If a calibrated dropper delivers 40 drops per 2 mL, how many drops should the patient instill in each ear every time?

(27) To achieve 80% accuracy, the amount to be weighed must be how many times greater than the sensitivity requirement of the balance?

(28) Show how you would weigh 0.01 g of aspirin on a Class A prescription balance.

(29) How would you prepare the following prescription?

℞

    KI solution   0.003 mL
    Water qs ad 50 mL

(30) ℞

    Phenobarbital gr ii
                #21 tablets

    Sig: i tablet tid, finish all

A pharmacist had twelve 32-mg tablets of phenobarbital. After notifying the physician, he dispensed those tablets to the patient. How long would the medication last?

(31) How would you dispense the prescription. Show the calculations involved.

Patrick Mills, M.D.
61-40 Flushing Avenue
New York, NY 12345
Phone No. 555-1234

Name : Samuel Doe   **Age:** 32
Address: 96 Main St., NY 12345   **Date:** 3/9/96

℞

    Methyldopa   1.2 g
    Hydralazine 0.1 g
    Lactose qs 3.25 g

    Ft. caps. # 10

    Sig: i cap qid

REFILL _None_

DAW _____

                       PMills
                  Lic # 333444

Available tablets: Methyldopa 250 mg weighing 600 mg each, and Hydralazine tablets 50 mg weighing 200 mg each.

(32) Explain the compounding procedure.

℞

Precipitated calcium carbonate USP	1 g
Sodium bicarbonate USP	0.5 g
Lactose qs	3.0 g

M. Ft. chart DTD #12

(33) If the minimum effective concentration is 3 mg/mL, what is the onset, intensity and duration of action of the administered drug for which the following plasma concentration versus time data is available?

Time (hr)	0.5	1	2	4	6	8	10	124
C_p (mg/mL)	1.6	2.6	2.5	1.9	0.3	0.7	0.3	0.1

(34) If the fraction of the dose absorbed is 0.6 and the AUC obtained after an IV injection is 24 mcg·hr/L, what would be the most likely AUC of an oral dose of the same drug?

(35) What would be the loading dose of an antibiotic drug with a maintenance dose of 100 mg, half-life of 3 hours and a dosing interval also of 3 hours?

(36) The elimination rate constants of an antitubercular drug in normal and a renally impaired patient were found to be 0.2 and 0.08 hour^{-1}. The drug is usually administered twice daily in a dose of 25 mg. How can the dose be adjusted in the renally impaired patient to provide similar plasma levels as in the normal patient by maintaining the same dosing interval of 12 hours?

(37) For a 71 inches tall person weighing 148 lb, what is the estimated % fat? The girth of the person in inches is 34.

(38) The product information on gentamycin shows that the recommended dose of gentamycin sulfate is 1–2 mg/kg/day for adults, 6 to 7.5 mg/kg/day for children, and 5 mg/kg/day for patients in the age group of one or less. How much gentamycin should be given to an eight-month-old child weighing 30 lb?

(39) Explain how one would titrate dopamine starting from 3 mcg/kg/min to maintain a mean systolic pressure between 100–120 mmHg. The patient weighs 165 lb and the IV preparation is dopamine 200 mg in 250 mL of D5W.

(40) For a three-year-old child weighing 27 kg and suffering from tachycardia, a physician prescribed 20 mcg/kg/min lidocaine. The instruction was to

add 200 mg of lidocaine in 200 mL of D5W and administer at a rate of 25 mL per hour. The available drug is lidocaine 1 g/25 mL. Check if the dilution factor is accurate.

REVIEW SET 4

(1) A pharmacist had 20 g of codeine sulfate. If he used it in preparing fifteen capsules each containing 0.025 g, and ten capsules each containing 0.015 g, how many g of codeine sulfate were left after he prepared the capsules?

(2) How many liters of 2% w/v iodine tincture can be made from 78 g of iodine?

(3) How many milliliters of sterile water for injection must be added to a liter of a 50% w/v dextrose injection to reduce the concentration to 10% w/v?

(4) What is the volume of 55 g of a solution with a specific gravity of 1.28?

(5) The pediatric dose of cefadroxil is 30 mg/kg/day. A child is receiving a daily dose of 1 1/2 tsp of a pediatric cefadroxil suspension based on the body weight. If the child's weight is 26.4 lb, how many mg of the drug is child receiving in each dose?

(6) If Keflex® oral suspension contains 3 g of cephalexin in 120 mL, how many milligrams of cephalexin are contained in each teaspoonful dose?

(7) How many milliliters of a 1:500 v/v solution of methyl salicylate in alcohol can be made from 150 mL of 10% v/v solution?

(8) How many grams of potassium chloride should be used in preparing 10 L of a solution containing 40 mEq per liter?

(9) What is the percentage of ichthammol in the finished product when 10 g of 10% ichthammol ointment, 40 g of 5% ichthammol ointment, and 50 g of petrolatum (diluent) are mixed?

(10) A physician ordered: "Librium 25 mg IM q.6h p.r.n." Reconstitution directions state "Add 2 mL special diluent to yield 100 mg per 2 mL." How many milliliters of reconstituted drug solution is required per day?

(11) How many milliliters of a 0.9% sodium chloride solution should be used in compounding the prescription?

℞

Oxymetazoline Hydrochloride	2.5%
Sodium Chloride Solution	q.s.
Purified Water ad	50.0
Make isoton. sol.	

Sig. Use as directed.

(12) How do you adjust the isotonicity of the preparation in problem #11 using 5% boric acid solution as the isotonic agent?

(13) What is the pH value of a solution containing a 5:1 molar ratio of sodium acetate to acetic acid at 25°C? The pK_a of the acetic acid is 4.76.

(14) At 1 A.M., it is found that 160 mL of an IV is running at a flow rate of 33 gtt/min. The drop factor is 60 gtt/mL. At what time will this 160 mL be completed?

(15) An intravenous infusion for a child weighing 42 lb is to contain 15 mg of vancomycin HCl per kg of body weight in 200 mL of NaCl injection. Using a 7.5-mL vial containing 500 mg of dry vancomycin HCl powder, how would you obtain the amount needed in preparing the infusion.

(16) A potassium phosphate solution contains 3.5 g of potassium dihydrogen phosphate (MW = 136) and 6.5 g of potassium monohydrogen phosphate (MW = 174) in 40 mL. If 5 mL of this solution are added to a liter of D5W, how many milliequivalents of potassium phosphate will be represented in the infusion?

(17) A patient is to receive 1 L of the following admixture every six hours.

Fre-Amine (10%)   500 mL
D-50-W   500 mL

Calculate:

a. The total number of glucose calories the patient will receive per day
b. Grams of protein and nitrogen patient receive per day
c. Calorie-to-nitrogen ratio

(18) A patient profile is as follows:

Sex: Male
Age: 74 years
Height: 62 inches
Weight: 78 kg

Calculate:
a. REE in kcal/day
b. The anabolic goal of the patient based on the REE
c. The anabolic goal of the patient based on the body weight

(19) A physician orders Tylenol® 10 mg/kg/dose for a child weighing 12 kg. How many mg of Tylenol® per dose should the child receive?

(20) If each Slow-K® extended-release tablet contains 600 mg of potassium chloride, how many milliequivalents are represented by each Slow-K® tablet?

(21) When an intravenous solution containing 0.2 g of a sulfa drug in 1 L of the solution is administered to a patient at the rate of 100 mL per hour, how many micrograms of the drug will the patient receive in a 10 minute period?

(22) How many apothecary ounces are present in lbs iiss?

(23) A child received 5 f℥ of amoxicillin suspension containing 250 mg/5 mL for one week. If one teaspoonful was taken three times a day, how many grams of amoxicillin did the child take?

(24) Zovirax® tablets, containing the antiviral drug acyclovir, are given in a dose of 80 mg/kg for five days for treating chickenpox. If the patient weighs 120 lb, how many ounce(s) of acyclovir would the patient consume if he has to take the full dose prescribed?

(25) ℞

Aspirin   gr v
Caffeine   gr i
Lactose qs
Ft. cap. DTD # xv

How many grams of aspirin would be needed to fill the above prescription?

(26) What are the errors and omissions in the prescription?

Henry Huxtable, M.D.
61-40 Flushing Avenue
Monroe, LA 71208
Phone No. 555-1234

Name : Pat O'Neal_____   **Age:** 23___
Address: 96 Havana Blvd., FL 31207   **Date:** 2/28/96

℞

Neosynephrine 1.5%
10 mL

Sig: i gtt os tid

REFILL _____

DAW _____
            _HHuxtable__
        DEA # AD 7973142

```
        NORTHEAST PHARMACY
           169 Hillside Avenue
        Monroe, LA 71206   555-0342

    ℞ # 123456          Date: 2/28/96
    O'Neal, Pat
    96 Havana Blvd.
    Instill one drop in each nostril three
    times daily
    Neosynephrine 1.5%
                    H. Huxtable, M.D.
```

(27) If 2 g of sulfur is weighed on a prescription balance with a sensitivity requirement of 4 mg, what would be the potential percent error?

(28) How would you weigh 0.03 g of APAP on a Class A prescription balance?

(29) How would you weigh gr ss of pseudoephedrine on a prescription balance with a sensitivity requirement of 6 mg and potential error of 2% or less?

(30) ℞

V-Cillin K®

800,000 units tid, 5 days

If the available tablets have a strength of 500 mg, how many tablets should be dispensed? It is known that one mg of penicillin K = 1600 units.

(31)

```
            Patrick Mills, M.D.
            61–40 Flushing Avenue
            New York, NY 12345
            Phone No. 555-1234

    Name : Magic Jordan          Age: 32
    Address: 96 Main St., NY 12345  Date: 3/9/96

    ℞
        Methyldopa 150 mg
        HCTZ          20 mg
        Lactose  qs

        Ft. caps.  # xiv

        Sig: i 8 A.M., and 4 P.M.

    REFILL  None

    DAW

                        PMills
                    Lic # 333444
```

Available tablets: Methyldopa 250 mg tablets weighing 500 mg each and HCTZ 50 mg tablets weighing 125 mg each. How would you dispense?

(32) Explain how you will make the following preparation.

Precipitated calcium carbonate USP   2 g
Sodium bicarbonate USP   2 g
Lactose qs   5.0 g
M. Ft. chart DTD #10

(33) The plasma concentration of a drug immediately following a 50-mg intravenous bolus dose of the drug was found to be 0.48 mcg/mL. What is the apparent volume of distribution of the drug?

(34) What is the average plasma concentration when a drug in a dose of 0.4 g is administered with an interval of 8 hours and has a volume of distribution of 50 L? It is known that the fraction of dose absorbed is 0.8 and the plasma elimination rate constant is 0.35 hour^{-1}.

(35) What would be the average plasma concentration of drug at steady-state if it is known that the plasma concentration at zero time point is 26 ng/mL when 0.25 g of the dose is given every 12 hours, and the elimination rate constant of the drug is 0.173 hour^{-1}?

(36) A clinical pharmacist has recommended that the dose of a cardiac drug be reduced from 0.25 mg to 0.22 mg in a renally impaired patient. In both the normal and renally impaired patients, the dosing interval was six hours. If the elimination rate constant of the drug in normal individual was 0.16 hour^{-1}, what would be the elimination rate constant value in the renally impaired patient?

(37) What should be the size of a dose of Nalfon® for an arthritic patient with a body surface area of 0.87 square meters? The usual dose of Nalfon® is 600 mg tid for arthritis.

(38) When a single 25 mg bolus dose of an antibiotic is given, the C_0 was found to be 2 mcg/mL and the elimination half-life was 1.5 hours. What would be the dose required to achieve a new minimum steady-state concentration of 0.45 mcg/mL with a dosing interval of 6 hours? Also what would be the new maximum steady-state concentration? Assume that the antibiotic follows linear kinetics.

(39) An infusion of 50 mg of nitroprusside in 100 mL of D5W is to be provided to a patient weighing 146 lb. What is the titration factor of this infusion between 0.5 to 1.5 mcg/kg/min to maintain mean blood pressure at 100 mmHg?

(40) For a five-week-old infant weighing 3 kg and suffering from shock, a physician prescribed 1 mcg/kg/min of dobutamine. The instruction was to add 6 mg of dobutamine in 25 mL of D5W and administer at a rate of 1 mL per hour. The available drug is dobutamine 150 mg/10 mL. Check if the dilution factor is accurate.

REVIEW SET 5

(1) A medication order for a 55-lb child calls for Sandoglobulin 0.2 g/kg IV. The supply on hand contained 6 g of Sandoglobulin in 100 mL. How many milliliters of this solution should be given?

(2) If a physician orders: "Lanoxin 0.25 mg p.o. q.d.," how many milliliters of Lanoxin® (digoxin) elixir containing 50 µg of digoxin per milliliter should be used?

(3) How many milliliters of water should be added to a liter of 1:1000 w/v solution to make a 1:6000 w/v solution?

(4) A medication order calls for prostigmin 0.25 mg IM. The only supply of prostigmin is 1:200 solution. How many milliliters of this solution would contain 0.25 mg?

(5) A patient has been instructed to take 10 mL of Vistaril® (hydroxyzine pamoate) oral suspension every four hours for four doses daily. How many days will a 6-fluidounce bottle of the suspension last?

(6) The dose of digoxin for rapid digitalization is a total of 1 mg in two divided doses at intervals of 6 to 8 hours. How many milliliters of digoxin elixir containing 20 µg/mL would provide this dose?

(7) If 50 mL of a Choldeyl® elixir containing 100 mg/5 mL active ingredient (oxtriphylline) is diluted to 500 mL, what will be the final strength of oxtriphylline?

(8) A medication orders 5.5 mEq Ca^{++}. What is the amount of calcium dihydrate (equivalent weight of $CaCl_2 \cdot 2H_2O = 73.5$) needed?

(9) What is the percentage of zinc oxide in an ointment prepared by mixing 140 g of a 8% zinc oxide ointment, 200 g of a 12% zinc oxide paste, and 160 g of white petrolatum (diluent)?

(10) Four lots of ichthammol ointment, containing 5%, 8%, 15% and 20% of ichthammol, are available. How many grams of each may he use to prepare 5 lb (avoir.) of a 10% ichthammol ointment?

(11) How much sodium chloride should be used in compounding the prescription?

B̧

Tetracaine Hydrochloride	1.0
Sodium Chloride	q.s.
Purified Water ad	30.0
Make isoton. sol.	

Sig. Eye drops.

(12) Freezing point depression of 1% atropine sulfate is 0.074°. Calculate the volume of iso-osmotic solution produced by 1 g of atropine sulfate.

(13) What molar ratio of salt/acid (sodium borate to boric acid) is required to prepare a buffer solution having a pH of 8.9? The pK_a of boric acid is 9.32 at 25°C.

(14) The drug Nitropress IV is administered by infusion at the rate of 3 μshkg/min. If a total of 20 mg of the drug is to be administered to a 150-lb patient, how long should be the duration of the infusion?

(15) A physician orders 2.5 g of an antibiotic to be placed in 1000 mL of normal saline solution (NSS). Using a reconstituted injection which contains 250 mg of the antibiotic per 1 mL, how many mL should be added to the NSS in filling the medication order?

(16) A medication order for an intravenous infusion for a patient weighing 140 lb calls for a 0.3 mEq of ammonium chloride per kg of body weight to be added to a liter of 5% dextrose injection. How many milliliters of a sterile solution containing 100 mEq of ammonium chloride per 20 mL should be used in preparing the infusion?

(17) 120 mL D5W IV was administered to a patient at flow rate of 20 gtt/min. The drop factor was 60 gtt/mL. What was the total infusion time?

(18) A patient has the following profile:

Sex: Female
Age: 43 years
Height: 165 cm
Weight: 85 kg

Calculate
a. REE in calories/day
b. Anabolic goal based on his body weight

(19) A medication orders: "D5 1/4NS 1000 mL." Calculate the amount of dextrose and sodium chloride in 1000 mL.

(20) A 280 MBq dose is ordered and the radiopharmaceutical activity concentration is 310 MBq/mL. What is the quantity to be dispensed to provide the necessary radioactivity?

(21) The following amounts of alcohol have been removed from a stock bottle containing 2.5 L; 0.00005 kL, 50 mL, 0.05 dkL, and 5 dL. How much alcohol will be left in the original stock bottle?

(22) How many ounces are present in gr XC?

(23) If a prescription is required for Phenergan VC with Codeine, 1 tbsp at bedtime for 15 days, how many fluidounces of the syrup would you dispense?

(24) Mr. John Doe has been suffering from diarrhea and Dr. Brown wants him to take 15 mL of Kaopectate®. How many teaspoonfuls of Kaopectate® should Mr. Doe take?

(25) ℞

Atropine Sulfate 0.2 mg

Sig: Administer intramuscularly.

If the available atropine vial reads gr 1/150 per mL, how many milliliters of the injection should be administered?

(26) Identify the errors and omissions in the prescription.

Henry Huxtable, M.D.
61-40 Flushing Avenue
Monroe, LA 71208
Phone No. 555-1234

Name : Fatima Khan   **Age**: 16
Address: 96 Havana Blvd., FL 31207   **Date**: 2/28/96

℞

Septra
                    #30

Sig: i bid, 7 days

REFILL _____

DAW ___✓_____

HHuxtable
DEA # AD 7973142

```
NORTHEAST PHARMACY
169 Hillside Avenue
Monroe, LA 71206    555-0342

℞ # 123456          Date: 2/28/96
Khan, Fatima
96 Havana Blvd.
Take one tablet twice daily for seven
days
Sulfameth/TMP 400/80 mg # 20
              H. Huxtable, M.D.
```

(27) A pharmacist measured 50 mL of syrup USP in a measuring cylinder, and transferred that amount to a beaker. To his surprise, he later observed that 10 mL of syrup USP was still left in the cylinder. What is the percent error in his syrup USP measurement?

(28) How would you weigh 25 mg g of aspirin on a Class A prescription balance with a sensitivity requirement of 6.5 mg?

(29) Explain how to weigh 0.025 grams of acetaminophen on a prescription balance having a sensitivity requirement of 1/4 grain.

(30) ℞

    Phenergan® tablets   12.5 mg
    Dispense 14 tablets

    Sig: qhs

If the pharmacist dispensed 25 mg tablets of Phenergan®, how many tablets should the patient take at bedtime?

(31) How would you dispense the following prescription? Show all the calculations, procedures, and the label for the product.

```
┌─────────────────────────────────────────────────┐
│              Patrick Mills, M.D.                  │
│              61-40 Flushing Avenue                │
│              New York, NY 12345                   │
│              Phone No. 555-1234                   │
├─────────────────────────────────────────────────┤
│  Name : Maliha Khan              Age: 3           │
│  Address: 96 Main St., NY 12345  Date: 3/9/96     │
│                                  Weight = 44 lbs  │
│                                                   │
│  R                                                │
│                                                   │
│    Sulfasalazine  30 mg/kg/24 hours               │
│    Prednisone  2 mg/cap                           │
│    Lactose  qs                                    │
│                                                   │
│    Ft. caps. DTD # xiv                            │
│                                                   │
│    Sig: Contents of i capsule in applesauce q6h   │
│                                                   │
│  DAW _____                                  │
│                                   PMills          │
│                               Lic # 333444        │
└─────────────────────────────────────────────────┘
```

Bulk powders for all the ingredients are available.

(32) Show how you will prepare the following prescription.

R

Iodine 2%
Boric acid 20%
Lactose qs 30 g
Ft.ℨ -iv

Sig: AAbid, UD

(33) The average blood concentration of a macrolide antibiotic observed in a panel of twelve adult males following oral administration of 250 mg of the antibiotic in a tablet dosage form are given below:

Time (hr)	0	0.75	1.5	3	4.5	6	8	10	12	14
C_p (mcg/mL)	0	0.33	1.3	1.44	1.44	0.61	0.27	0.13	0.06	0.03

Calculate the AUC, C_{max}, T_{max}, K_{el}, and $t_{1/2}$.

(34) To obtain an average plasma concentration of 15 ng/mL with a dosing interval of 8 hours, what should be the dose of the drug when the fraction of drug absorbed is 0.6? It is known that the drug has a volume of distribution of 75 L and has an elimination rate constant of 0.173 hour^{-1}.

(35) What would be the loading dose of an antibiotic drug with a 25 mg of maintenance dose, and half-life and dosing interval of 8 hours each?

(36) A clinical pharmacist has recommended that the dose of a diuretic be reduced from 50 mg to 25 mg in a renally impaired patient. In both the normal and renally impaired patients, the dosing interval was six hours. If the elimination half-life of the drug in normal individual was 4 hours, what would be the elimination rate constant value in the renally impaired patient?

(37) What is the average intravenous dose of Adriamycin® (doxorubicin) for a child whose weight is 50 kg and height is 142 cm? The average intravenous dose of doxorubicin for a child is 30 mg/m^2.

(38) Upon the administration of 0.5 gram of an aminoglycoside every 12 hours, the $C_{min\ ss}$ was found to be 8 mcg/mL, the plasma concentration at time zero was 40 mcg/mL, and elimination half-life was 6 hour^{-1}. If it is desired to increase the $C_{min\ ss}$ to 10 mcg/mL, what should be the dose of the drug, and the new $C_{max\ ss}$? Assume that the drug follows linear kinetics.

(39) An infusion of 80 mg of nitroprusside in 200 mL of D5W is to be provided to a patient weighing 186 lb. What is the titration factor of this infusion between 0.5 to 1.5 mcg/kg/min to maintain mean blood pressure at 100 mmHg?

(40) For a 5-month-old child weighing 14 lb and suffering from a serious asthma problem, a physician prescribed 0.85 mg/kg/min of aminophylline. The instruction was to add 50 mg of aminophylline in 500 mL of D5W and administer at a rate of 40 mL per hour. The available drug is aminophylline 2.5% w/v. Check if the dilution factor is accurate.

CHAPTER 1: PREREQUISITE MATHEMATICS REVIEW

Page 11

1. a. XXVIII
   b. XV
   c. XVII
   d. XXIII
2. a. 46
   b. 74
   c. 47
   d. 39
3. a. 19
   b. 14
   c. 4
   d. 171
4. a. XXXI
   b. VIII
   c. XXV
   d. XLIX
5. a. 64
   b. 47
   c. 45
   d. 16
6. 60 doses

7. 100/60 or 5/3 gr
8. 10½ tablets of medication A and 31 1/2 tablets of medication B.
9. 9.595 g
10. 1177/60 gr or $19^{37}/_{60}$ gr

Page 17

1. 27
2. 0.05 mL
3. 0.25 million units
4. 120 mg
5. 28.6% w/w
6. 3 g
7. 500 mg
8. 5.4 L
9. 36,111 mL or 36.1 L
10. 1 mL

Page 19

1. 125 mL
2. 0.16% w/v
3. 1% w/v
4. 3000 mL
5. 3900 mL
6. 24% w/v
7. 18 L
8. 250 mL
9. 1500 mL
10. 750 mL

Page 22

1. 1.285
2. 2.7
3. 1.22
4. 0.82
5. 18.6 g
6. 320 g
7. 38.46 mL
8. 4.73 kg

9. 85% w/v
10. 2160 mL

CHAPTER 2: SYSTEMS OF MEASUREMENT

Page 28

1. 20 mg
2. 0.032 g
3. 5 µL
4. 11.25 g
5. 10,000 tablets
6. 666.7 mcg
7. 400 mcg
8. 3420 mg
9. 0.74 mL
10. 0.4 L

Page 31

1. 16 prescriptions
2. 8.44 gallons
3. 240 minims
4. 3.6 scruples
5. 42 ounces
6. 119 fluidrams
7. 1/4 fl oz
8. 1/2 tablet
9. $4608
10. 320 capsules

Page 34

1. One day
2. 0.6 g
3. 7 drops
4. 6 ounces
5. 5 fl oz
6. 140 mL
7. 2.625 g
8. 36 tsp

9. No
10. 5 fl oz

Page 37

1. 0.386 gr
2. 123.1 gr
3. 0.33 oz
4. 6000 tabs
5. 32.5 mg
6. 59 g
7. 1 oz
8. 0.09 g
9. 2 tbsp
10. 5 glassfuls

CHAPTER 3: PRESCRIPTION AND MEDICATION ORDERS

Page 57

1. 50 days
2. 2 drops
3. 6.5 g
4. 10:00 P.M.
5. 2 capsules to be taken initially
6. 1/2 tsp at bedtime
7. 73 mL
8. 0.69 mL
9. 400 mL
10. 3 g

Page 63

1. a. Generic is dispensed instead of brand
   b. 30 tablets should be given and not 40
   c. Wrong DEA number
   d. Wrong instructions
   e. The drug is wrong
2. a. Wrong dosage form for an eight-month-old baby
   b. Wrong instructions: Until finished and not until Friday
   c. Wrong DEA number

3. a. Wrong instructions on the label
   b. Wrong medication strength
   c. Wrong DEA number
4. a. Wrong drug
   b. Wrong strength because Zantac® is unavailable in that strength, and it is the wrong drug
   c. Wrong DEA number
5. a. Wrong medication
   b. Wrong directions
   c. Wrong DEA number
6. a. Wrong medication strength
   b. Generic not allowed
   c. Wrong quantity of medication
   d. Wrong DEA number
7. a. Wrong medication (APAP and not ASA)
   b. Wrong directions: Every four hours and not four times
8. a. Brand should be given and not generic
   b. Single strength medication and not double strength
   c. Patient is allergic to sulfa: Bactrim® contains sulfa
   d. Wrong date
   e. Wrong DEA number
   f. One refill
9. a. Otic solution and not suspension
   b. Wrong directions
      4 drops and not 6 drops
      Right ear and not right eye
      Four times and not every four hours
   c. Wrong quantity: 10 cc and not 100 cc
   d. Wrong DEA number
10. a. Wrong strength: 50 mg and not 100 mg
    b. Wrong quantity: 100 and not 50
    c. Directions are missing
    d. Wrong DEA number

CHAPTER 4: PRINCIPLES OF WEIGHING AND MEASURING

Page 76

1. SR × 12.5
2. 0.1%
3. 80 mg
4. 15 mg

5. 16 mg
6. 4.63%
7. 40
8. 8.13 mg
9. 10%
10. 20

Page 85

1. $$\frac{120 \text{ mg of propranolol HCl}}{60 \text{ mL of stock solution}} = \frac{2 \text{ mg of propranolol HCl}}{X \text{ mL of stock solution}}$$

$$X = 1 \text{ mL}$$

Pipet 1 mL of the stock solution aliquot and transfer into the calibrated container. Add sufficient quantity of D5W to fill to the required volume of 120 cc.

2. $$\frac{65 \text{ mg of codeine}}{422.5 \text{ mg of stock mixture}} = \frac{10 \text{ mg of codeine}}{X \text{ mg of stock mixture}}$$

$X = 65$ mg aliquot of the stock mixture contains 10 mg of codeine.

3. $$\frac{1 \text{ mL of the L.C.D.}}{200 \text{ mL of the stock solution}} = \frac{0.005 \text{ mL of the L.C.D.}}{X \text{ mL of stock solution}}$$

$$X = 1 \text{ mL}$$

Take 1 mL of aliquot of the stock solution in the final container and add sufficient quantity of purified water to make 50 mL of the solution.

4. $$\frac{300 \text{ mg of pseudoephedrine}}{930 \text{ mg of the stock mixture}} = \frac{97.5 \text{ mg of pseudoephedrine}}{X \text{ mg of stock mixture}}$$

$X = 302$ mg aliquot of the stock mixture contains 97.5 mg of pseudoephedrine.

5. $$\frac{2000 \text{ mg of pseudoephedrine}}{5000 \text{ mg of stock mixture}} = \frac{97.5 \text{ mg of pseudoephedrine}}{X \text{ mg of stock mixture}}$$

$X = 244$ mg aliquot of the stock mixture contains 97.5 mg of pseudoephedrine. Since the LWQ is 300 mg, dilute the stock mixture to twice its amount with lactose and weigh out 488 of the diluted stock mixture.

6.

$$\frac{2 \text{ mL of the drug}}{10 \text{ mL of solution}} = \frac{0.6 \text{ mL of the drug}}{X \text{ mL of solution}}$$

X = 3 mL of the aliquot from stock solution should be measured to obtain 0.6 mL of the drug.

7.

$$\frac{3 \text{ mL of the drug}}{8 \text{ mL of solution}} = \frac{0.75 \text{ mL of the drug}}{X \text{ mL of solution}}$$

X = 2 mL of the stock solution

8.

$$\frac{325 \text{ mg of acetaminophen}}{1625 \text{ mg of the stock mixture}} = \frac{65 \text{ mg of acetaminophen}}{X \text{ mg of stock mixture}}$$

X = 325 mg aliquot of the stock mixture contains 65 mg of acetaminophen.

9.

$$\frac{1 \text{ mL of the drug}}{67 \text{ mL of solution}} = \frac{0.015 \text{ mL of the drug}}{X \text{ mL of solution}}$$

X = 1 mL of the stock solution which can be measured by the pipet.

10.

$$\frac{1 \text{ mL of the drug}}{25 \text{ mL of solution}} = \frac{0.12 \text{ mL of the drug}}{X \text{ mL of solution}}$$

X = 3 mL of the stock solution which can be measured by the pipet.

CHAPTER 5: CALCULATIONS INVOLVING ORAL LIQUIDS

Page 89

1. 300 minims
2. 66.7 times
3. 1.67 mL
4. 6 g
5. 2.25 mL of paregoric
   0.075 g of pectin
6. 3 gr
7. 200 mL
8. 95 mL
9. 250 mg
10. 6 days

Page 92

1. 100 mg
2. Noscapine 30 mg
   Guaifenesin 240 mg
3. 108.3 mg
4. 44 mg
5. 4.17 mL
6. 720 mg
7. 10 mg
8. 11.25 mL
9. 20 mL
10. 0.5 mL

Page 100

1. 48.33%
2. 18.92%
3. 7.69%
4. 35.71 mg per 10 mL or 0.36%
5. 2500 mL
6. 0.4% or 20 mg/5 mL
7. 600 mL of 20 mg/5 mL solution, and 400 mL of 30 mg/5 mL solution
8. 200 mL of 500 mg/5 mL solution, and 800 mL of 250 mg/5 mL solution
9. 20 mL of 100 mg/mL solution, and 80 mL of 125 mg/mL solution
10. Add 3 mL of water to 2 mL of 5% suspension

Page 105

1. 1.49 g
2. 9.13 g
3. 250 mg
4. 205 mg
5. 26.43 mEq/L
6. 2.1 g
7. 4.36 mEq/L
8. 73.13 g
9. 296 mg
10. 183.8 mg

CHAPTER 6: CALCULATIONS INVOLVING CAPSULES, TABLETS, AND POWDER DOSAGE FORMS

Page 108

1. 3 tablets
2. 2 capsules 3 times a day for 10 days
3. 60 caps
4. 6 tablets
5. None (extended release tablets cannot be split)
6. 2 days
7. 4 tablets
8. 30 tablets
9. 91 tablets
10. 1/4 tablet

Page 119

1. Crush 3 methyldopa tablets and weigh out 2.4 g. Crush 2 tablets of hydralazine and weigh out 0.4 g. Add 0.45 g of lactose, and mix geometrically. Fill 10 capsules appropriately. Capsule size 1 is needed.
2. 560 mg from three hydralazine tablets and 2240 mg of powder from 14 HCTZ tablets are needed. 14 capsules should be filled in capsule size 2 after adding 840 mg of lactose in the above mixture.
3. The following quantities of powders are weighed accurately.
   CPM* = 5 × 12 = 60 mg
   Pseudoephedrine HCl = 40 × 12 = 480 mg
   ASA = 300 × 12 = 3600 mg
   Lactose* = 60 mg
   Capsule size 0 is needed.

   *Since 60 mg of the drug is not weighable on a Class A prescription balance, aliquot method has to be followed. Lactose is used as a diluent. The drug and lactose together weigh 120 mg and are therefore weighable.
4. Amount of the ingredients needed for 12 capsules are as follows:
   Dimenhydrinate   30 × 12 = 360 mg
   Pantothenic acid   30 × 12 = 360 mg
   Thiamine HCl   10 × 12 = 120 mg
   Calcium carbonate   100 × 12 = 1200 mg

   Amounts of the first two ingredients are obtained directly by weighing the bulk chemicals. For thiamine HCl, 5 tablets of 25 mg are needed, and for calcium carbonate, three tablets of 500 mg are needed. The exact amounts of thiamine HCl and the calcium carbonate are obtained after crushing the needed tablets and obtaining the powders by using the following proportions:

$$\frac{125 \text{ mg of thiamine HCl}}{1000 \text{ mg of tablet powder}} = \frac{120 \text{ mg of thiamine HCl}}{X \text{ mg of tablet powder}}$$

$$X = 960 \text{ mg of thiamine HCl powder}$$

$$\frac{1500 \text{ mg of calcium carbonate}}{3000 \text{ mg of tablet powder}} = \frac{1200 \text{ mg of calcium carbonate}}{X \text{ mg of tablet powder}}$$

$$X = 2400 \text{ mg of calcium carbonate powder}$$

Capsule size 0 is needed.

5. 4523 mg of ASA powder from 7 tablets, 800 mg of ephedrine sulfate powder, and 900 mg of CPM powder from 6 tablets are needed. Final capsule size is 00.

6. 1200 mg of Benadryl® powder from 6 capsules, 1687.5 mg of prednisone powder from 10 tablets and 1612.5 mg of lactose are needed. Capsule size is #1.

7. After consulting the physician, phenobarbital dose is reduced to 0.025 g. 1800 mg powder of simethicone from 12 tablets, 300 mg of phenobarbital powder, 1200 mg of magnesium carbonate powder from two tablets and 600 mg of lactose are needed for the 12 capsules. Size of the capsules is #1.

8. 540 mg of warfarin sodium powder from 4 tablets and 3360 mg of lactose is needed to fill 12 capsules. 325 mg of the powder is filled in each of the size 1 capsules.

9. 15 mg of the prednisone is weighed by the aliquot method and 3000 mg of sulfalazine is added. After adding sufficient lactose, fill 260 mg each in 15 capsules of size #2.

10. CPM needed is $2 \times 15 = 30$ mg, APAP needed is $350 \times 15 = 5250$ mg, and pseudoephed sulfate is $30 \times 15 = 450$ mg. CPM cannot be weighed directly because of its small amount. Therefore use aliquot method. 120 mg of the stock mixture (120 mg CPM + 360 mg lactose), 5250 mg of acetaminophen, and 450 mg of pseudoephed sulfate are needed. Each capsule will weigh 388 mg. Capsule size 0 is needed.

CHAPTER 7: CALCULATIONS INVOLVING OINTMENTS, CREAMS, AND OTHER SEMISOLIDS

Page 137

1. 15.13 g, 75.67 g, 2179.20 g
2. 68.1 g, 4.54 g, 45.4 g, 9.08 g, 326.88 g

3. 0.1%, 0.01% w/w
4. a. 0.1% w/w
   b. 0.25% w/w
   c. 0.5% w/w
   d. 1% w/w
5. 8.06% w/w
6. 5.71% w/w
7. 1.48% w/w
8. 3.71% w/w
9. 5.23% w/w
10. 3.13% w/w

Page 146

1. 11:5:5
2. 8 g
3. 59 g
4. 5 g of 2% ointment and 15 g of diluent
5. 1.30 g
6. 22.11 g
7. 166.67 g
8. 4:1
9. a. 8.22%
   b. 414.66 g
10. 810.7 g of 5% ichthammol
    405.4 g of 12% ichthammol
    243.2 g of 20% ichthammol
    810.7 g of 25% ichthammol
    (or 405.4 g (5%); 810.7 g (12%); 810.7 g (20%); 243.2 g (25%))

CHAPTER 8: CALCULATIONS INVOLVING TOPICAL OPHTHALMIC, NASAL, AND OTIC PREPARATIONS

Page 161

1. 1.8
2. a. 0.18
   b. 0.19
   c. 0.20
3. 0.69 g
4. 0.048 g

5. 0.50 g
6. 54.44 mL of 0.9% NaCl and qs water to 100 mL
7. 5.8 g
8. 2.88 mL of 5% boric acid and qs water to 15 mL
9. 49.06 g
10. 0.173 g

Page 170

1. 1.79%
2. 2.74%
3. 1.68 g
4. a. hypotonic
   b. hypertonic
   c. hypotonic
   d. hypertonic
5. Dissolve 0.4 g of epinephrine sulfate in purified water to make 10.2 mL of an isotonic solution, and adjust the preparation to a volume of 40 mL with isotonic NaCl (0.9%) solution.
6. Dissolve 0.25 g of phenylephrine hydrochloride in water to make 8.9 mL of an isotonic solution, and adjust the preparation to 50 mL with isotonic boric acid solution.
7. 0.37 g
8. 0.519 g by cryoscopic method; 0.54 g by E method
9. 26.9 mL
10. 34.6 mL

Page 179

1. a. 4.56
   b. 1.04
   c. 7.47
   d. 3.24
2. 1.995×10^{-5}
   6.31×10^{-10}
   3.98×10^{-4}
   3.16×10^{-12}
3. 3.76
4. 8.36
5. 5.91
6. 5.01:1
7. 2.29:1

8. 4.76
9. 5.51
10. 0.46:1

CHAPTER 9: CALCULATIONS INVOLVING SUPPOSITORIES

Page 185

1. 1.5
2. 1.29
3. 3
4. 1
5. 3
6. 4.89
7. 2.82
8. 1.1
9. 1.29
10. 3

Page 188

1. Cocoa butter needed = 29.775 g and prochlorperazine needed = 0.45 g
2. Cocoa butter needed = 23.99 g and promethazine HCl needed = 0.24 g
3. Cocoa butter needed = 29.25 g and zinc oxide needed = 3.75 g
4. Prepare a 40% zinc oxide and cocoa butter mixture and fill in 12 suppositories
5. Cocoa butter needed = 19.75 g and phenobarbital sodium needed = 0.3 g
6. Cocoa butter needed = 16.92 g and dimenhydrinate needed = 4 g
7. Cocoa butter needed = 29.75 g and morphine HCl needed = 0.375 g
8. Cocoa butter needed = 22.8 g and bismuth subgallate needed = 3.6 g
9. Cocoa butter = 17.53, hamamelis extract = 2.5 g, and zinc oxide = 4 g
10. Cocoa butter needed = 23.86 g and promethazine HCl needed = 0.36 g

CHAPTER 10: CALCULATIONS INVOLVING INJECTABLE MEDICATIONS

Page 195

1. 63 drops/min
2. 33 drops/min
3. 42 drops/min

4. 50 drops/min
5. 21 gtt/min
6. 1.08 million units
7. 21 gtt/min
8. a. 8.4 mg
   b. 42 drops/min
9. 3.14 minutes
10. 63 drops/min

Page 205

1. 0.6 mL
2. 50 days
3. 39.8 units/mL
4. 28,800 units
5. 200 mL
6. a. 465.1 mg/mL
   b. 238.1 mg/mL
   c. 100 mg/mL
7. 0.6 mL
8. 4.0 mL
9. Reconstitute the powder to a final volume of 7.5 mL and withdraw 6.6 mL
10. 7 mL

Page 211

1. 1788 mg or 1.788 g
2. 6.25 mL
3. 6.15 mEq/mL
4. 4.1 mL
5. 17.26 mEq
6. 67.11 mEq
7. 3.0 mL
8. 555.55 mOsm/L
9. 431.63 mOsm/L
10. 455.1 mOsm/L

CHAPTER 11: CALCULATIONS INVOLVING NUTRITION

Page 221

1. 425 kcal

2. 1640 kcal
3. 150:1
4. 62.5:1
5. 50.6%
6. 47.5%
7. a. 630 kcal
   b. 8 g
   c. 53.13:1
   d. 32.54%
8. a. 2550 kcal
   b. 50 mEq
   c. 150 g of protein; 24 g of nitrogen
   d. 106.25:1
9. a. 2550 kcal
   b. 127.5 g
   c. 20.4 g
   d. 125:1
10. Potassium chloride 11.9 mL
    Calcium chloride 2.9 mL
    Sodium chloride 8.8 mL
    Insulin 0.12 mL

Page 226

1. 1455 kcal/day
2. 1042 kcal
3. 60 kcal
4. 1411 kcal
5. a. 1414 kcal
   b. 2475 kcal
   c. 2700 kcal
   d. 832 mL
6. a. 1268 kcal/day
   b. 2219 kcal/day
   c. 2250 kcal/day
   d. 7.46 L
7. a. 1459 kcal/day
   b. 2553 kcal/day
   c. 3375 kcal/day
8. 26 yrs
9. 111.4 lb

10. a. 1806 kcal/day
    b. 3825 kcal/day

Page 230

1. 1296
2. 1173
3. 1210
4. 1147
5. 1380
6. 1180
7. 492
8. 501
9. 837
10. 920

CHAPTER 12: CALCULATION OF DOSES AND DOSE ADJUSTMENTS

Page 240

1. 33.33%
2. 53.45 ng·hr/mL
3. 47.15 ng/mL
4. K_{el} 0.269/hr; $t_{1/2}$ 2.58 hr; C_{max} 422 ng/mL; T_{max} 2 hr
5. 97.25/94.75 = 1.03
6. Onset 1.4 hrs; intensity 0.6 mg/mL; duration 4.27 hr
7. 59.5 L
8. 4.5 mg
9. 79.65 mg·hr/mL; K_{el} 0.126/hr; $t_{1/2}$ 5.5 hr
10. 8.05 mcg·hr/mL; C_{max} 1.44 mcg/mL; T_{max} 3 h; K_{el} 0.387/hr; $t_{1/2}$ 1.79 hr

Page 244

1. 14.4 mcg·hr/mL
2. 43.29 hr
3. 19.2 mcg·hr/mL
4. 43.29 hrs
5. 3.24 mg
6. 3.848 mcg/mL
7. 92.4 hr

8. 4.3 mg
9. 9.47 hr
10. 4.3 hr

Page 249

1. 1.7325 L/hr
2. 22.53 L/hr
3. 11.3 L/hr
4. 4.53 L/hr
5. 9.87 L/hr
6. 127.4 mL/min
7. 80 mL/min
8. 81.9 mL/min
9. 126.02 mL/min
10. 101.9 mL/min

Page 253

1. $C_{max\ ss}$ = 28.57 ng/mL, $C_{min\ ss}$ = 3.58 ng/mL, $C_{ave\ ss}$ = 12.03 ng/mL
2. $C_{ave\ ss}$ = 23.12 µg/mL
3. $C_{max\ ss}$ = 13.67 µg/mL, $C_{min\ ss}$ = 9.77 µg/mL, $C_{ave\ ss}$ = 11.61 µg/mL
4. $C_{max\ ss}$ = 9.85 µg/mL, $C_{min\ ss}$ = 5.95 µg/mL, $C_{ave\ ss}$ = 7.74 µg/mL
5. 600 mg
6. 500 mg
7. 875 mg
8. 308.46 mg
9. 200 mg
10. 40 mg

Page 259

1. 205 mg
2. 9.72 hrs
3. 154 mg
4. 120 mg
5. 60 hr
6. 30 hr
7. 0.144 hr^{-1}
8. 0.162 hr^{-1}
9. 7.5 hr
10. 8 hr

CHAPTER 13: PEDIATRIC AND GERIATRIC DOSING

Page 267

1. 0.33
2. 1.25 mL
3. 0.2 mL
4. 0.7 mL tid
5. 0.625 mg
6. 2.23 mL every eight hours
7. 75 mL
8. 0.1 mL
9. 0.08 mL
10. 58.35 mL

Page 273

1. 5.7 or 6 fl oz
2. 30 tabs
3. 20%
4. 6 fl oz (or 182 mL)
5. 301.7 mg
6. 158 mg
7. 41.34 mg
8. 44.16 mg
9. 400.58 mg
10. 41.07 mg q3h

Page 278

1. Based on Table 13.1, dose can either be decreased or unchanged but the dosing interval should be increased.
2. 27.3 mg
3. 125.5 to 156.8 mg
4. 18 tablets
5. 2 tablets q4h 3 days = 36 tablets
6. New dose is 19.2 mg, and $C_{max\ ssn}$ is 2.37 mcg/mL
7. New dose is 625 mg, and $C_{max\ ssn}$ is 55.5 mcg/mL
8. Based on Table 13.1, increase the dose while keeping the same dosing interval.
9. New dose is 800 mg
10. New dose is 45.2 mg, and $C_{max\ ssn}$ is 4.26 mg/mL

Page 283

1. 246.66 mcg/min and 9.25 mL/hr
2. 380 mcg/min and 14.25 mL/hr
3. 26.7 mcg/drop, one would increase or decrease the infusion rate
4. 212.2 mcg/min or 7.96 mL/hr
5. 158.8 mcg/min or 5.96 mL/hr
6. 265.6 mcg/min or 9.96 mL/hr
7. 105.4 mcg/min or 3.96 mL/hr
8. 4.17 mcg/drop
9. 42.51 to 102.51 mcg/min or 10.2 to 24 mL/hr
10. 17.49 to 77.49 mcg/min or 4.2 to 18 mL/hr

Page 287

1. Concentration of solution required is 360 mcg/mL and the strength of dilution is 240 mcg/mL. Inaccurate dilution.
2. Concentration of solution required is 360 mcg/mL and the strength of dilution is 361 mcg/mL. Accurate dilution.
3. Concentration of solution required is 960 mcg/mL and the strength of dilution is 950 mcg/mL. Fairly accurate dilution.
4. Concentration of solution required is 1440 mcg/mL and the strength of dilution is 980 mcg/mL. Inaccurate dilution.
5. Concentration of solution required is 984 mcg/mL and the strength of dilution is 980 mcg/mL. Fairly accurate dilution.
6. Concentration of solution required is 1200 mcg/mL and the strength of dilution is 1210 mcg/mL. Fairly accurate dilution.
7. Concentration of solution required is 720 mcg/mL and the strength of dilution is 1210 mcg/mL. Inaccurate dilution.
8. Concentration of solution required is 7.01 mg/mL and the strength of dilution is 0.1 mg/mL. Inaccurate dilution.
9. Concentration of solution required is 28.05 mg/mL and the strength of dilution is 0.1 mg/mL. Inaccurate dilution.
10. Concentration of solution is 2.06 mg/mL and the strength of dilution is 0.1 mg/mL. Inaccurate dilution.

CHAPTER 14: CALCULATIONS INVOLVING IMMUNIZING AGENTS AND VACCINES

Page 292

1. 12.5 mcg

2. 850,000

3. 400,000,000

4. 80,000

5. 4

6. 500,000

7. 50 individuals

8. 90

9. 800,000 < usual recommended dose < 2,600,000

10. 0.5 mL

Page 295

1. 25

2. 100,000

3. 100,000

4. 50,000

5. 250,000

6. 13.5

7. 300 mg

8. 800

9. 125594321.6

10. 640

Page 297

1. 3 complete courses. 0.5 mL will be left.

2. 45

3. 60

4. 10

5. 15

6. 15

7. 100

8. 150

9. 100.5

10. 60

CHAPTER 15: CALCULATIONS INVOLVING RADIOPHARMACEUTICALS

Page 304

1. 0.74 MBq
2. 148 MBq
3. 0.99 or 1 mCi
4. 496.8 mCi
5. 9.25×10^6 Bq
6. 15 years
7. 12.8 hours
8. 0.0154 days^{-1}
9. 173.4 days
10. 78 hours

Page 313

1. 15.46 mCi
2. 27.35 mCi
3. 10.7 mCi
4. a. 1.3 mCi or 48.1 MBq
   b. 0.17 mCi or 6.3 MBq
5. 16.65%
6. 11.53%
7. 12.04%
8. 6.80%
9. 0.67 ml
10. 1.91×10^6 mCi/mg

REVIEW SET 1

1. 40
2. 0.038
3. 167
4. 1.25
5. 2
6. 18 mg
7. 21%
8. 9.93% w/v
9. 1 mg/g, 2.5 mg/g, 5 mg/g, and 10 mg/g
10. 8 parts of 2%, 5 parts of 10%, and 12% each
11. 0.384
12. 25.5 mL by White-Vincent Method, 26.9 mL by USP Method
13. a. 3.16×10^{-5}
    b. 6.0×10^{-9}
    c. 3.98×10^{-6}
    d. 1.6×10^{-8}
14. 21 drops/min
15. 250
16. 1211 mg

17. 408 kcal

18. 60.27

19. 55.5 MBq

20. 23.65

21. 800

22. 3.55

23. 1

24. 6.65

25. 7

26. Physician and the patient switched, wrong date, wrong address, wrong DEA#, no refills, and wrong amount of medication

27. 75 mg

28. Add 168 mg of lactose to 120 mg of salicylic acid and mix geometrically. Weigh 120 mg of the stock mixture, and it provides 50 mg of salicylic acid.

29. Measure 3 mL of the concentrate and qs with water to 200 mL. Measure 2 mL of this stock solution (gives 0.03 mL concentrate) and qs with water to 60 mL.

30. 42

31. Weigh out 4 HCTZ tabs and 8 triamterene tabs. Crush and add 60 mg of lactose per capsule in the crushed mixture. Punch 10 capsules containing 260 mg of powder in capsule size #2.

32. Need 0.6 g of iodine, 20 g of boric acid, and 99.4 g of lactose. Place iodine in mortar, add a few drops of alcohol and reduce to a fine powder. Then add boric acid and talc. Mix thoroughly until alcohol evaporates. Dry and sieve to break the lumps. Fill in a wide mouth 4-oz bottle and label appropriately.

33. AUC = 2.06 mg·hr/mL, C_{max} = 0.4 mg/mL, T_{max} = 4 hrs, $t_{1/2}$ = 2 hrs, and K_{el} = 0.346hr^{-1}

34. 7:30 A.M.

35. 6.1 L/hr

36. 0.19 mg

37. 36.8

38. Yes, the table shows that there is a need to increase the dosing interval to lower the $C_{min\ ss}$

39. 875 mg

40. Dose required = 400 mcg/mL and the doctor's order is providing 340 mcg/mL. Accuracy is off by 60 mcg/mL.

REVIEW SET 2

1. 10,000
2. 600
3. 4950
4. 1.176
5. 4
6. 216.67
7. 0.31%
8. 2.98
9. 9.5
10. 52.6
11. 0.435
12. 16.8
13. 10.36
14. 1536
15. 1600
16. 13.4
17. 25:1
18. 67.7
19. 615.6
20. 13.52 millicuries
21. 0.024
22. 8
23. 7
24. 0.19
25. 28
26. No prescription authority, wrong DEA#, wrong dosage form for infant, wrong refill information
27. 5 mg
28. LWQ = 120 mg; 120 mg of atropine sulfate + 323 mg of lactose to make a stock mixture. 120 mg of the stock mixture provides 32.5 mg of atropine sulfate
29. Weigh out 120 mg of gentian violet and dissolve in water to make 20 mL stock solution. Transfer 5 mL of the stock solution to calibrated container and qs with water to 120 mL.
30. 1.5
31. Correct the signa to DTD # 15. Crush 10 tablets each of ASA and phenobarb. Weigh 3 g of ASA powder and 0.3 g of phenobarbital powder.

Weight of each capsule = 3300 mg/15 = 220 mg. Therefore, add 40 mg/ capsule of lactose and fill 15 capsules of 260 mg each in capsule size #2.

32. Amounts needed are 1.5 g of iodine, 25 g of boric acid, and 123.5 g of lactose. Follow the procedure in the book for compounding.
33. 33 ng·hr/mL
34. 32.7 hours
35. $C_{max\ ss}$ is 8 mcg/mL, $C_{min\ ss}$ is 4 mcg/mL, $C_{ave\ ss}$ is 5.77 mcg/mL
36. New dose should be 411.8 mg
37. 17.5 mg/day
38. New dose is 163 mg, and the $C_{max\ ss}$ is 23 ng/mL
39. 4 mcg/drop
40. Dose required is 1296 mcg/mL and the concentration in the dilution is 980 mcg/mL

REVIEW SET 3

1. 9.75
2. 3.61%w/w
3. 180
4. 124 g
5. 70
6. 48
7. 0.28%
8. 6.67
9. 3.88
10. 31.58
11. 37.78
12. 176
13. 2:1
14. 83.3
15. 1200 units/hr
16. 20.13
17. 45.8% w/w
18. 1311.6 kcal/day
19. 15
20. 20,000
21. 7.5
22. 7.03

23. 3.5

24. 10.8

25. Wrong patient, wrong drug for an aspirin-allergic patient, and codeine abuse because the patient is also on Tylenol #3

26. 2

27. 5 × SR

28. Weigh 120 mg of aspirin, add 1320 mg of lactose to make 1440 mg of the stock mixture, and mix geometrically. Weigh 120 mg of the stock mixture.

29. Measure 1 mL of KI and qs with water to one liter. From the stock solution, measure 3 mL and qs to 50 mL in a calibrated bottle.

30. 1 day

31. Crush 5 methyldopa tablets and weigh out 2880 mg of the powder. Similarly crush two hydralazine tablets and weigh out 400 mg of the powder. Add the two powders to obtain 3280 mg of the total powder. Use capsule size #1 and fill 328 mg in each of the ten capsules. If the powder doesn't fill properly, add additional lactose and fill in capsule size #0.

32. All the powders are directly weighable. Weigh the ingredients as follows and mix geometrically:
Precipitated calcium carbonate 1 × 12 = 12 g
Sodium bicarbonate USP 0.5 × 12 = 6 g
Lactose 3 × 12 = 36 g
Fill in powder papers

33. Since the drug concentration doesn't reach MEC, there is no onset, intensity, or duration of action.

34. 14.4 mcg·hr/L

35. 200 mg

36. 10 mg

37. 16%

38. 68.2 mg

39. 13.33 mcg/drop

40. The concentration of solution calculated is 1296 mcg/mL, and the concentration of dilution is 980 mcg/mL. The accuracy is off by 316 mcg/mL.

REVIEW SET 4

1. 19.475

2. 3.9

3. 4000

4. 42.97 mL
5. 360
6. 125
7. 7500
8. 29.8
9. 3%
10. 2
11. 22.2
12. 7.7 mL of boric acid solution
13. 5.46
14. 6:20 A.M.
15. Add sufficient quantity of water in the Vancomycin 500 mg vial to make 7.5 mL. From this solution, withdraw 4.3 mL to obtain 286.4 mg of the drug.
16. 12.56
17. a. 3400 kcal of glucose
    b. grams of protein = 200 and nitrogen = 32
    c. 106.25:1
18. a. 1426.16 kcal/day for men
    b. 2496 kcal/day
    c. 3510 kcal/day
19. 120 mg/day
20. 8.05
21. 3333
22. 30
23. 5250
24. 0.73
25. 4.875
26. Wrong DEA#, wrong signa because the drug is a nasal adrenergic/decongestant
27. 0.2%
28. LWQ is 120 mg. Weigh 120 mg of APAP and 360 mg of lactose. Mix geometrically, and weigh 120 of the mixture.
29. LWQ = 300 mg. Weigh 300 mg pseudoephedrine. Add lactose to make 2769 or 2770 mg of the stock mixture. Weigh 300 mg of the stock mixture.
30. 15
31. Crush 9 methyldopa tablets and weigh out 4200 mg of the powder. Similarly crush 6 HCTZ tablets and weigh out 700 mg of the powder. Add lactose and fill in size 0 capsules.

32. Mix all the ingredients. Make 10 powder papers, each containing 500 mg of the powder.
33. 104.2 L
34. 2.3 mcg/hr
35. 12.5 ng/mL
36. 0.14 hr^{-1}
37. 302 mg
38. D_{o_o} = 83.95 mg, and C_{maxss_n} 7.17 μg/mL
39. 8.34 mcg/dop and 8.3 mcg/drop are accurate
40. Dose of the child = 180 mcg/mL, and the dilution concentration is 236 mcg/mL. The dilution is not accurate.

REVIEW SET 5

1. 83.3
2. 5
3. 4988
4. 0.05
5. 4.5
6. 50
7. 0.2%
8. 404.25
9. 7.04%
10. 1031.8 g of 5%, 515.9 g of 8%, 206.4 g of 15%, and 515.9 g of 20%
11. 0.09 g
12. 14.23 mL
13. 0.38:1
14. 97.8 min
15. 10
16. 3.8
17. 6 hours
18. a. REE = 1571.6 kcal/day
    b. Anabolic goal = 3825 kcal/day
19. 5 g of dextrose and 2.25 g of sodium chloride
20. 0.9 mL
21. 1.4 L
22. 0.195
23. 7.5

24. 3

25. 0.465

26. Septra DS is given as ibid, 14 such tablets are needed for seven days, brand drug should be dispensed, tablet strength for DS should be 800/160, and the DEA# is wrong

27. 20%

28. LWQ is 130 mg. Therefore, weigh 130 mg of aspirin and qs with lactose to 676 mg to obtain the stock mixture. From the stock mixture, weigh out 130 mg.

29. LWQ is 325 mg. Add lactose to make 1950 mg of the total stock mixture. Weigh out 325 mg of the stock mixture.

30. 1/2

31. Weigh out 2100 mg of sulfasalazine powder, 28 mg of prednisone (use aliquot method for weighing this quantity), and add sufficient lactose to obtain a total of 2730 mg of the powder. Fill 195 mg in each of the 14 capsules that are required to be dispensed.

32. Quantities needed are 2.4 g of iodine, 24 g of boric acid, and 93.6 g of lactose for four ounces of the powder.

33. $AUC = 8.21$ mcg/mL, $C_{max} = 1.44$ mcg/mL, $K_{el} = 0.387$ hr^{-1}, and $t_{1/2} = 1.79$ hr

34. 2.6 mg

35. 50 mg

36. 0.0867 hr^{-1}

37. 42 mg

38. 66.67 µg/mL

39. 6.6 mcg/drop

40. Concentration of solution is 8.11 mg/mL, and the dilution order is 0.01 mg/mL. It is not an accurate order.

Exponents

Many scientific measurements involve either very large or very small numbers, which may be conveniently expressed as *exponents*. An exponent may be defined as the power to which a number is raised. For example, 1500 may be expressed as 1.5×10^3, 25,000 as 2.5×10^4, 0.05 as 5.0×10^{-2} and 0.0015 as 1.5×10^{-3}. When numbers are expressed as exponents, two parts may be identified as follows:

$$\underbrace{1.5}_{a} \times \underbrace{10^3}_{b}$$

where

a = coefficient
b = exponential factor

In the above example, where 1500 is expressed as 1.5×10^3, the exponent "3" represents the number of places that the decimal point has been moved to the left, i.e.,

$$1\underbrace{5\ 0\ 0}.\ 0 = 1.5 \times 10^3$$

Likewise, when the decimal point is moved to right, the exponent takes the negative sign. As an example, the number 0.008 may be expressed as,

$$0\ .\ \underbrace{0\ 0\ 8} = 8.0 \times 1.0^{-3}$$

When multiplying the exponents, multiply the coefficients and add the exponents.

Example 1:

$$(2.0 \times 10^2) \times (1.5 \times 10^2)$$

answer: 3.0×10^4

Example 2:

$$(2.0 \times 10^4) \times (1.5 \times 10^{-6})$$

answer: 3.0×10^{-2}

Example 3:

$$(3.5 \times 10^3) \times (1.2 \times 10^{-7})$$

answer: 4.2×10^{-4}

When dividing the exponents, divide the coefficients and subtract the exponents.

Example 1:

$$\frac{(5.4 \times 10^4)}{(2.16 \times 10^2)}$$

answer: 2.5×10^2

Example 2:

$$\frac{(3.0 \times 10^{-3})}{(1.5 \times 10^2)}$$

answer: 2.0×10^{-5}

Example 3:

$$\frac{(2.5 \times 10^{-2})}{(6.25 \times 10^{-6})}$$

answer: 0.4×10^4 or 4×10^3

When adding the exponents, bring the exponents to the same base by moving the decimal points and then add the coefficients.

Example 1:

$$(1.5 \times 10^3) + (45.2 \times 10^2)$$
$$= 1.5 \times 10^3$$
$$+ 4.52 \times 10^3$$

answer: 6.02×10^3

Example 2:

$$(1.3 \times 10^4) + (4.8 \times 10^3)$$
$$= 1.3 \times 10^4$$
$$+ 0.48 \times 10^4$$

answer: 1.78×10^4

Example 3:

$$(2.6 \times 10^7) + (1.27 \times 10^8)$$
$$= 0.26 \times 10^8$$
$$+ 1.27 \times 10^8$$

answer: 1.53×10^8

Similarly, the subtraction of the exponential notation may be performed by changing the expressions to forms having the same common power of 10 and then subtracting the coefficients.

Example 1:

$$(1.8 \times 10^4) - (2.62 \times 10^3)$$
$$= 18.0 \times 10^3$$
$$- 2.62 \times 10^3$$

answer: 15.38×10^3

Example 2:

$$(7.5 \times 10^5) - (1.55 \times 10^3)$$
$$= 0.075 \times 10^3$$
$$- 1.55 \times 10^3$$

answer: -1.475×10^3

TABLE A.1.   The Rules of Exponential Notations.

$$a \times a = a^2$$
$$a \times a \times a = a^3$$
$$a^2 \times a^2 = a^4$$
$$a^4/a^2 = a^{4-2} = a^2$$
$$a^4/a^{-2} = a^{4-(-2)} = a^{4+2} = a^6$$
$$a^2/a^4 = a^{2-4} = a^{-2} = 1/a^2$$

Example 3:

$$(8.2 \times 10^{-3}) - (1.6 \times 10^{-3})$$
$$= 8.2 \times 10^{-3}$$
$$- 1.6 \times 10^{-3}$$

$$\text{answer: } 6.6 \times 10^{-3}$$

Rules of exponents are summarized in Table A.1.

Logarithmic Expressions

The word *logarithm* means exponent. The exponent that indicates to what power 10 must be raised to equal a given number is known as the common logarithm of that number. When we consider an expression such as,

$$3^x = 9$$

where x is the exponent on 3 which gives the number 9. In logarithmic expressions, the solution may be written as,

x is the logarithm on 3 which gives the number 9

i.e., $3^x = 9$

or $x = \log_3 9$

Similarly, $10^3 = 1000$ may be expressed as $3 = \log_{10} 1000$, i.e., exponent 3 to which the base 10 must be raised to give 1000 is called the logarithm of 1000. The number 1000 is referred to as antilogarithm of the number 3.

Example 1:

$$2^x = 32$$

$$x = \log_2 32$$

Example 2:

$$3^x = 8$$

$$x = \log_3 8$$

TABLE B.1.   Rules of Logarithm.

$\log ab = \log a + \log b$
$\log a/b = \log a - \log b = -\log b/a$
$\log aa = \log a^2 = \log a + \log a = 2 \log a$
$\log 1/a = \log 1 - \log a = -\log a$

Example 3:

$$5^x = 125$$

$$x = \log_5 125$$

The logarithm of 10 or any integral power of 10 is always a positive or negative integer. This is illustrated in the following examples:

Example 1:

$$\log 100 = 1 \times 10^2 = 2$$

Example 2:

$$\log 10,000 = 1 \times 10^4 = 4$$

Example 3:

$$\log 0.001 = 1 \times 10^{-3} = -3$$

The rules of logarithmic notations are summarized in Table B.1.

NATURAL LOGARITHM

In the previous discussion, when 10 is used as the base, the logarithm is referred to as the common logarithm. When the number 2.71828, designated as e, is used as the base, the logarithm is known as the natural logarithm.

$$\ln 1000 = 6.908$$

$$\log 1000 = 3$$

$$\ln/\log = 6.908/3$$

$$= 2.303$$

Therefore, 2.303 is the logarithm of 10 to the base 2.71828. The above expression may be rearranged as,

$$\log \times 2.303 = \ln$$

Thus, when converting to a common logarithm from natural logarithm, the above expression may be used as,

$$\log_{10} a \times 2.303 = \log_e a$$

Significant Figures

A significant figure is any digit that represents a quantity in the place in which it stands. The number zero is considered as a significant figure when it is placed between digits. However, if a zero is used only to locate the decimal point, it is not considered significant. For example, in the number 0.00050, the three zeros immediately following the decimal point merely used to show the location of the decimal point, and thus, are not significant. However the zero following the number 5 is significant. Thus, in the value 1.500, both zeros are significant. When the number 1500 is expressed as 1.5×10^3, it contains two significant figures. The rules of expressing significant figures are as follows:

(1) A zero, when placed between digits, is considered to be significant. For example, 4.005 has 4 significant figures.

(2) One or more final zeros placed to the right of the decimal point may be considered to be significant. For example, 2.0050 has 5 significant figures.

(3) A zero, when used only to locate the decimal point, is not considered significant. For example, 0.00025 has only 2 significant figures.

Some examples of significant figures are listed in Table C.1.

TABLE C.1. *Significant Figures.*

Number	Number of Significant Figures
15.	2
15.5	3
1.555	4
15.555	5
155.0	4
0.0015	2
15.0005	6
1.5×10^2	2
1.55×10^{-3}	3
150,005	indeterminate

Temperature Conversions

The intensity of heat, or temperature, is measured in Celsius (centigrade) or Fahrenheit scales, and expressed in degrees (°). The instrument that measures the temperature is called *thermometer*. Most thermometers in the United States use the Fahrenheit scale.

The Fahrenheit (F) scale establishes the freezing point of pure water at 32°F and the boiling point at 212°F. The Celsius scale establishes freezing at 0°C and boiling at 100°C. The difference between boiling and freezing points in the Fahrenheit scale is 180 and in Celsius scale is 100. Therefore, each degree Celsius is equal to 180/100 or 1.8 degrees Fahrenheit. By rounding the numbers one can express the same as "every 5 degrees measured in the Celsius scale is equal to 9 degrees as measured by the Fahrenheit scale."

A comparison of Celsius and Fahrenheit scales is shown in Figure D.1.

CONVERSION FROM °F TO °C

To convert the temperature from Fahrenheit scale to Celsius scale, the following expression may be used:

$$C° = \frac{F° - 32}{1.8}$$

Example 1:

Convert the normal body temperature 98.6°F to C°:

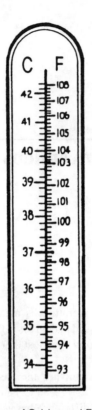

FIGURE D.1. Comparison of Celsius and Fahrenheit temperatures.

$$C° = \frac{98.6 - 32}{1.8}$$

$$= 66.8/1.8$$

answer: 37°

Example 2:

Convert 162°F to centrigrade:

$$C° = \frac{162 - 32}{1.8}$$

answer: 72.2

Example 3:

Convert −58°F to centigrade:

$$C° = \frac{-58 - 32}{1.8}$$

$$= -90/1.8$$

answer: −50

CONVERSION FROM °C TO °F

To convert the temperature from Celsius scale to Fahrenheit scale, the following equation may be used:

$$F° = 1.8°C + 32$$

Example 1:

Convert 26°C to Fahrenheit:

$$F° = 1.8 \times 2.6 + 32$$

answer: 78.8

Example 2:

Convert −35°C to Fahrenheit:

$$F° = 1.8 \times (-35) + 32$$

$$= - 63 + 32$$

answer: −31

Example 3:

$$F° = (1.8 \times 20) + 32$$

answer: 68

Useful Clinical Formulae

ANION BALANCE

The number of positively charged ions (cations) in the body must always be equal to the number of those negatively charged (anions). However, some negatively charged substances are not "measured" by the clinical laboratory tests, resulting in a net deficiency of anions between 8 to 16 milliequivalents/liter. This value is commonly referred to as the "anion gap," and it may be estimated as follows:

$$\text{"Anion Gap"} = \text{Sodium} - (\text{Chloride} + \text{Bicarbonate})$$

SODIUM OR WATER DEFICIT

The usual concentration of sodium in the serum is 135–145 milliequivalents/liter. If the values are higher than 145 mEq/liter, the amount of free water required to return these values to the normal range is calculated by the use of the following formula:

$$\text{Water deficit (L)} = [1 - 140/\text{measured serum Na (mEq)}] \times \text{body wt (kg)} \times 0.6$$

If the values are lower than 135 mEq/L, the amount of sodium needed to replace the deficit is calculated by using the following equation:

$$\text{Sodium deficit (mEq)} = [140/\text{measured serum Na (mEq)}] \times \text{body wt (kg)} \times 0.6$$

CALCIUM AND MAGNESIUM CORRECTION

The normal levels of calcium and magnesium are in the ranges of 9–11 mg% and 1.5–2.0 mEq/L, respectively. The levels of these cations in the body fluids may be corrected by using the following formulae:

$$\text{Calcium correction} = Ca^{2+} + (4.0 - \text{serum albumin}) \times 0.8$$

$$\text{Magnesium correction} = \frac{\text{total bilirubin} - 10}{3} \times 0.1 + Mg^{2+}$$

METABOLIC ALKALOSIS

The normal levels of carbon dioxide tension (pCO_2) are between 36–44 mm Hg and the normal bicarbonate levels, in adults, are between 21–30 milliequivalents/liter. Metabolic alkalosis may result when pCO_2 goes below 36 mm Hg or bicarbonate level goes over 30 mEq/L, causing a pH greater than 7.45.

Calculation of milliequivalents of HCl needed for the treatment of metabolic alkalosis is as follows:

$$\text{HCl (mEq)} = [103 - \text{measured serum Cl (mEq)}] \times \text{body wt (kg)} \times 0.2$$

METABOLIC ACIDOSIS

Metabolic acidosis may result when pCO_2 reads higher than 44 mm Hg or bicarbonate levels fall below 20 mEq/L, resulting in a pH lower than 7.35. A rise of 5 mEq/L of bicarbonate for every 10 mm Hg maybe necessary to normalize the pH.

Calculation of the amount of bicarbonate in terms of milliequivalents needed in the treatment of metabolic acidosis is as follows:

$$HCO_3 \text{ deficit (mEq)} = [24 - \text{measured } HCO_3 \text{ (mEq)}] \times \text{body wt (kg)} \times 0.5$$

SERUM OSMOLARITY

Volumes of the intracellular and extracellular body fluid compartments are kept constant by the osmotic pressure, which is created by the concentration of dissolved ions (electrolytes) in each compartment. The normal osmotic concentration is in the range of 280–310 mOsm/L.

Serum osmolarity may be determined as follows:

$$mOsmol/L = (2 \times serum\ Na^+) + \frac{serum\ glucose\ (mg\%)}{18} + \frac{BUN\ (mg\%)}{2.8}$$

where BUN = blood urea nitrogen

IDEAL BODY WEIGHT

The ideal body weight for a given height (IBW) serves as a reference standard against which the actual body weight can be compared. Ideal body weight can be computed as follows:

For males = 50 kg + (2.3 × inches > 5 feet)

For females = 45.5 kg + (2.3 × inches > 5 feet)

IRON DOSES

The average adult body contains approximately 4 g of iron, of which roughly two-thirds exists in the form of hemoglobin. Treatment of certain types of anemias usually consists of dietary supplementation or the administration of therapeutic iron preparations by oral and parenteral routes. Iron is often administered by i.m. as iron-dextran complex which is ferric hydroxide and dextran containing 50 mg of iron per milliliter.

Equations for calculating doses of elemental iron or as iron-dextran complex are as follows:

(a) mg of iron = W × (100 − %Hb) × 0.3

where
W = body weight in lbs
%Hb = measured hemoglobin expressed as a percentage of the normal hemoglobin concentration where 14.8% hemoglobin is considered as 100% concentration. If the patient weighs 30 lbs or less, the dose should be 80% of the calculated amount.

Dose in milligrams of iron may also be calculated using the following formula:

(b) Dose (mg Fe) = wt (kg) × 4.5 × (Hb_d − Hb_a)

where
Hb_d = desired hemoglobin value
Hb_a = actual hemoglobin value

Volume of iron dextran injection may be calculated as follows:

$$V = 0.66 \times \frac{(W) \times (D)}{50}$$

where

W = body weight in kg
D = % hemoglobin deficiency

Percent hemoglobin deficiency, D, may be calculated from the following equation:

$$D = 100 - \frac{Hb\ (g/dL) \times 100}{14.8}$$

Note: The maximum recommended daily dose of iron dextran is 25 mg for children weighing less than 5 kg, 50 mg for children weighing 5–10 kg, and 100 mg for children weighing more than 10 kg. In the IV therapy, the doses infused should be no faster than 50 mg/min.

REE CALCULATIONS BASED ON V_{O_2} AND V_{CO_2} VALUES

Sophisticated methods for assessing energy expenditures of hospitalized patients are now commercially available. One such method to calculate the REE involves the use of V_{CO_2} and V_{O_2} in expired air. An indirect calorimetric assay is employed to measure V_{CO_2} and V_{O_2} from the mechanically ventilated patient. REE can be calculated as follows:

$$REE\ (kcal/day) = [(V_{O_2} \times 3.9) + (V_{CO_2} \times 1.1)] \times 1.44$$

where

V_{O2}, mL/min = volume of oxygen consumption (or uptake)
V_{CO2}, mL/min = volume of carbon dioxide production (or output)

SUGGESTED READINGS

1. H. C. Ansel, N. G. Popovich, and L. V. Allen, "Pharmaceutical Dosage Forms and Drug Delivery Systems," 6th ed., Williams & Wilkins, Philadelphia, 1995.

2. G. S. Banker and C. T. Rhodes, "Modern Pharmaceutics," 2nd ed., Marcel Dekker, Inc., New York, 1990.

3. S. J. Carter, "Cooper and Gunn's Dispensing for Pharmaceutical Students," 12th ed., CBS Publishers, Delhi, 1987.

4. M. Gibaldi and D. Perrier, "Pharmacokinetics," 2nd ed., Marcel Dekker, New York, 1982.

5. H. A. Lieberman, L. Lachman, and J. L. Kanig, "The Theory and Practice of Industrial Pharmacy," 3rd ed., Lea and Febiger, Philadelphia, 1986.

6. A. Martin, "Physical Pharmacy," 4th ed., Lea and Febiger, Philadelphia, 1993.

7. I. K. Reddy and M. A. Khan, "Parenteral Therapy: Theory and Practice," Whittier Publications, New York, 1996.

8. "Remingtons: The Science and Practice of Pharmacy," 19th ed., (A. R. Gennaro et al., eds.), Mack Publishing Company, Pennsylvania, 1995.

9. S. Strauss, "Pharmacy Law Examination Review," 2nd ed., Technomic Publishing Company, Inc., Pennsylvania, 1990.

10. J. G. Wagner, "Biopharmaceutics and Relevant Pharmacokinetics," Drug Intelligence Publications, Illinois, 1971.

11. CDC Immunization of Adolescents: Recommendations of the ACIP, the AAP, AAFP, and the AMA. MMWR 45:RR-13, 1996.

12. "Pharmacotherapy: A Pathophysiologic Approach," 3rd ed., (J. T. Dipiro et al., eds.), Appleton & Lange Connecticut, 1997.